Writing for the Health Professions

Karl Terryberry

Daemen College

THOMSON ™

DELMAR LEARNING

Australia   Canada   Mexico   Singapore   Spain   United Kingdom   United States

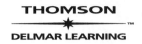

THOMSON
DELMAR LEARNING

Writing for the Health Professions
by Karl Terryberry

Executive Director:
William Brottmiller

Executive Editor:
Cathy L. Esperti

Acquisitions Editor:
Marah Bellegarde

Editorial Assistant:
Erin Adams

Production Coordinator:
Anne Sherman

Executive Marketing Manager:
Jennifer McAvey

Marketing Coordinator
Kimberly Duffy

Library of Congress Cataloging-in-Publication Data
Terryberry, Karl J.
  Writing for the health professions / Karl Terryberry.
     p. ; cm.
Includes index.
  ISBN 1-4018-4192-9
  1. Medical writing.
  [DNLM: 1. Writing. WZ 345 T329w 2005]
I. Title.
R119.T425 2005
808'.06661--dc22

                                    2004005275

International Divisions List

Asia (Including India):
Thomson Learning
60 Albert Street, #15-01
Albert Complex
Singapore 189969
Tel 65 336-6411
Fax 65 336-7411

Australia/New Zealand:
Nelson
102 Dodds Street
South Melbourne
Victoria 3205
Australia
Tel 61 (0)3 9685-4111
Fax 61 (0)3 9685-4199

Latin America:
Thomson Learning
Seneca 53
Colonia Polanco
11560 Mexico, D.F. Mexico
Tel (525) 281-2906
Fax (525) 281-2656

Canada:
Nelson
1120 Birchmount Road
Toronto, Ontario
Canada M1K 5G4
Tel (416) 752-9100
Fax (416) 752-8102

UK/Europe/Middle East/Africa:
Thomson Learning
Berkshire House
1680-173 High Holborn
London WC1V 7AA
United Kingdom
Tel 44 (0)20 497-1422
Fax 44 (0)20 497-1426

Spain (includes Portugal):
Paraninfo
Calle Magallanes 25
28015 Madrid
España
Tel 34 (0)91 446-3350
Fax 34 (0)91 445-6218

NOTICE TO THE READER

Dedication

This textbook is dedicated to my wife, Christine. Her efforts make my life easy.

Brief Table of Contents

Table of Contents

Preface

Writing for the Health Professions is designed to meet the needs of students in the allied health professions, in the preprofessional stages of their medical educations, and to be used as a reference for the practitioner. This reference teaches the principles of professional writing, writing for academic purposes, and writing in the health professions.

RATIONALE FOR A PROFESSIONS-SPECIFIC WRITING COURSE

The faculty and administration at various colleges with preprofessional health care programs recognize that writing has become an increasingly important element in the lives of allied health professionals, who may be called on to produce grant proposals, professional papers and presentations, and supporting documentation for legal purposes and for reimbursement from insurance companies or health maintenance organizations. The allied health field demands qualified professionals who can write well. Most students I have encountered in my teaching experiences, who are in their preprofessional or professional phases of their allied health coursework, have taken only required courses in writing, such as a first-year composition course. Many students are not challenged to write in their academic preparation, but they are required to write when they enter the workforce. Most never acquire the skills to write about research effectively, and many struggle to write their theses. However, as academic programs begin to recognize writing deficiencies in their graduates, they are taking steps to reinforce writing at an advanced level of study. Generic writing courses, however, are not focused properly on the issues that will allow these students to excel in the workplace. This book is designed to prepare these students to write for a variety of purposes. The objective of *Writing for the Health Professions* is to produce students who can write grammatically, mechanically, and structurally correct documents; who can write with professional style; who can research effectively and present the ideas of others in conjunction with their own primary research; and who will be able to write for any purpose in their jobs.

Most professionals who have returned to study in my classes claim that they wish someone had given them this information before they entered practice and made critical mistakes in their presentation of ideas. Reinforcing this need are several programs that have been created by large pharmaceutical companies. For example, some pharmaceutical companies hire writing consultants to provide seminars in writing to doctors, administrators, support personnel, and nursing staff. These programs offer simple and straightforward information about how to improve existing writing skills—and they are offered within the hospitals during the work day. The academic and medical fields are recognizing the importance of such training. This book will meet the needs of this advanced audience.

As the need for strong writing skills in this population increases, more writing courses are being developed. The courses are being taught primarily by English professors who have little or no experience writing for the medical profession and no text to guide them. Consequently, they use standard business, professional, or technical writing texts and supplement these with a text on research writing, writing in the sciences, or a narrowly designed text on documentation. Students in the health care professions desire a single text that speaks to their ability levels and their professional needs.

This book takes into account that its audience has a working knowledge of basic language skills, with the assumption that studying grammer for the sake of learning grammatical terms should *not* be the focus of a writing course. This has been the problem with writing textbooks aimed at specific professions in the past: None have presented a *functional* approach to grammar. In effect, they simply convert standard grammar texts, which are readily available to any writer, to manuals for the professions by adding professional writing samples or examples that use medical terminology. These offer grammar lessons in the same formats that have failed writers in the past. The authors of such textbooks simply try to offer examples with medical terminology and situations.

Organization of This Book

This book provides a clear formula for improving writing through the recursive writing process. Section 1 describes the phases of this writing process and follows these stages sequentially with chapters of instruction. The writing process described is a formula for success. The writer simply plugs in the values and addresses the topics sequentially.

In Chapter 1, "Phase One of the Writing Process," focuses on developing ideas through drafting. This is the essential message of the book: Any writing can be made better by rewriting. This phase emphasizes building a coherent and unified message.

In Chapter 2, "Phase Two of the Writing Process," the writer is asked to tackle grammar and mechanics, but these are functional lessons, not rules to be remembered. In other words, grammar lessons are supplied as part of the formula. The writer will examine the draft that was created in Phase One and applies these lessons for correctness. Furthermore, it is assumeed that the students can formulate sentences and can present ideas. It is not assumed, however, that they can identify the rules that govern sentence formation. Experience indicates that previous educational experiences have relaxed the rules that govern writing, focusing instead on ideas, not form or structure. However, most students crave knowledge about the rules because they know such rules exist, although they were never taught the rules or required to demonstrate competency. Consequently, many students are embarrassed by their inability to recognize grammatical parts of sentences or the characteristics of a sentence. However, few students have the time or interest to pick their way through a tangle of jargon and terms that are foreign to their field of study. As a result, I have developed a scheme to teach them the grammatical terms they need to know; this book does not teach grammar for the sake of teaching grammar.

Supporting the material on grammar and mechanics is a chapter on Phase Three of the process, devoted to developing a professional voice and style. Again, this information is presented as a logical stage in the writing process or part of the formula, not as an obtuse list of terms and functions that many books have used. More important, a section on verb-based writing, which is essentially ignored in most writing texts, is presented as a cornerstone of clear writing and for the development of clear and precise diction. The sections on sentence variation build on the processes of clear and precise sentence construction from the earlier sections of the text.

Chapters 4 and 5 cover, respectively, "Phase Four of the Writing Process: Creating Essays That Flow," and "Phases Five and Six of the Writing Process: Editing and Proofreading."

For each component of the writing process, specific writing assignments and a set of tasks have been included that can be used to reinforce these strategies.

Section 2 of the book addresses the academic side of writing. It presents the foundations of thinking needed to write well, such as rhetorical patterns and argumentation, and it offers instruction for research writing as well as for writing the thesis. Most important, this section of the book explains the significance of citing information accurately and avoiding plagiarism. These issues are of monumental concern for the student researcher.

Section 3 of the book offers writing instruction for documents that might be produced in the profession. Chapter 11 provides clearly defined guidelines for principles of documentation and the legal ramifications of poor writing, documentation, or presentation. Chapter 12 addresses professional communication in writing, writing for reimbursement, grant and proposal writing, and writing for review.

Throughout this book, the emphasis is on the importance of revising. The formula for success is to write a draft and rework it several times, with specific issues to address at each draft. To demonstrate this process, several different types of student writing samples are included.

Author Background

Karl Terryberry has been teaching writing at the university level since 1987 and, during a brief absence from academia, worked as a medical writer and a writer/editor in various business environments. Today, he is the Writing Coordinator for the English department at Daemen College, where a majority of the students plan to enter various allied health fields. He combines his expertise in the teaching of writing with his business and medical writing experiences to help students succeed. His success in the classroom has led to writing this book for students and practitioners alike.

Acknowledgments

I would like to offer special thanks to friends and colleagues who have made this book possible because of their willingness to guide me in my pursuits. Timothy McCooey, administrator for the Catholic Health System out of South Buffalo Mercy Hospital, shares my enthusiasm for writing well and guided me in the process of writing for administrative purposes. Additionally, I would not be in this profession if I was not guided and supported by Charles Bressler, my mentor at Houghton College. I am standing on his shoulders as I write this text.

Four former students, Lindsay Back, Janelle Hecker, Samantha Hoak, and Gabrielle Grubka, served as editors for the text and contributed some of the sample essays and examples. Without such students, my job would not be worthwhile. They represent the target audience for the intended learning experience of course work using this book. The following students also contributed sample essays or examples: Grace Golodolinski, Nicole Didas, Sarah Pilato, Melissa Galkowski, Jennifer Jordan, Mike Flanagan, Jeff Sommer, Ashley Lawton, Julie Schnepp, Jackie Mogel, Matt Paluch, and Sarah Wagner.

Most important, I would like to thank the faculty and staff at Daemen College for providing me with the necessary support to complete this project. Keith Taylor, Dean of the Division of Health Sciences, and Mike Brogan, Chair of the Physical Therapy Department, have been instrumental in giving me direction to develop this course. Peter Siedlecki, Dean of the Arts and Sciences Division, has been most reliable in providing administrative support, and my colleagues in the English department, Nancy Marck, Robert Morace, Gayle Nason, and Shirley Peterson, also have provided me with the emotional support to maintain these standards.

A very special thanks

to Timothy Quinlivan, deputy counsel for Independent Health, who provided the information about the legal ramifications of documentation.

I

The Writing Process

Key Terms

Audience   As a group, the intended or expected readers, which controls the type of language used

Coherence   Maintaining a consistent line of thinking throughout the essay to create a logical flow of ideas

Drafting   Reinventing the document-in-progress according to a plan or formula of the recursive writing process, as needed to restructure the thesis, reorganize the support paragraphs, and reinforce conclusions to build unity and coherence

Editing   Retooling sentences to address the formalities of language and grammar for precise communication

Functional grammar   Grammar learned for the sake of writing, not for the sake of knowing rules

Organizing   Planning the presentation of ideas through outlining

Proofreading   Scouring the final draft for problems in mechanics and formalities

Purpose   The thesis, which controls the information provided and the order of presentation

Recursive writing process   A writing process that depends on revision for a successful and effective product

Revising   Reading, rethinking, and making appropriate wholesale changes to the draft

Style   The attribute of writing that meets professional standards and accuracy while still maintaining the reader's interest by creating continuity and flow

Unity   Focusing all of the elements of the essay on a singular purpose, the thesis

section Objectives

On completion of this section, the reader should be able to

1. Understand the recursive writing process to develop a strategy for writing.

2. Demonstrate that writing should be approached in stages.

3. Reorganize and reinvent drafts while understanding that the smallest changes can and will affect the entire essay.

4. Recognize that writing is a skill made better with practice.

5. Differentiate between the linear approach to writing and the recursive process.

6. Write in stages, approaching the essay, the paragraphs, the sentences, and the words through a formula.

7. Approach writing in four stages: drafting, sentences and words, style, and editing and proofreading.

WHY WRITING IS IMPORTANT TO THE PROFESSION

I have worked outside of academics for a few years and have learned that writing well is important to success in any organization. In the many conversations I have had with chief executive officers (CEOs) and presidents of businesses and corporations, I learned that writing and communicating effectively often constitute an unwritten prerequisite to advancement. For example, I know good workers who stay on the bottom rungs of the corporate ladder because they have not taken the time to learn to write and, as a result, fail to represent themselves adequately or in a professional manner. In today's competitive market, this issue has never been as clear; a recent advertisement claims, "The number one reason for not hiring an applicant is the applicant's inability to communicate effectively." In fact, at one large company, I was instructed to sift through a pile of applications and cover letters from corporate executives to find the effective writers and to place their dossiers in the "A" pile, or the one to receive interviews. All other applicants would not receive consideration for employment. This alone should demonstrate that writing is important to success.

Additionally, many hiring executives are writing job descriptions that make effective oral and written communication the most important element of employment. They do this not only because writing is part of the everyday ritual of the job but because they consider that an employee's representation of himself or herself reflects directly on the company or organization of which he or she is a part. To an employer, good business results from the interaction of good people with the customer. Sometimes, the only mechanism a customer has for judging the merit of the company is through an employee's written or oral communication. The same is true in academic organizations and the health professions.

Many medical professionals, however, do not perceive their practice as a component of the business model and therefore do not think that writing, communicating, or representing themselves well matters. I once heard a medical student claim that "writing has nothing to do with science." Of course, this is not true. No one would advance the profession if the results of research were not written and published. Ultimately, effective medical writing requires the same principles of logic, organization, clarity, and precision that any science requires. Professionals of any kind must understand the importance of written communication and how it affects their status in the profession.

Furthermore, many successful physicians claim that 90% of their job is communicating with the public in some way or representing themselves professionally through communication mechanisms. Much of their work in the office requires verbal skills (conversing with patients); however, medical professionals also spend many hours writing explanatory or educational materials, writing responses for inquiries from organizations, writing to receive reimbursement, writing to the administration at hospitals to request equipment or to establish their position on a controversial issue, and writing research papers and conference proposals to better their standing in the field. They write these documents themselves because they cannot trust someone else to represent them and their ideas accurately. Their business is too important to leave the writing to a nonprofessional.

Think about communication from the patient's perspective and not the practitioner's. Every good doctor I know is considered "good" by patients because of his or her ability to communicate well. The successful health professionals I know are classic examples. Their practices are growing because they communicate with patients on the patients' level. They understand their audience's needs, and they tailor their communication to meet those needs. Furthermore, they understand that their audience is a group of consumers who usually can choose their physician or health professional freely. Most patients have few mechanisms or the technical expertise to judge the worth or expertise of the medical professional treating them, and the practitioner who makes the best impression does so through communication. Think about your experiences in the office of a medical professional. If the medical professional working with you explains complicated matters in terms that you can understand or is genuinely interested in conversing with you about your problems, you will feel confident in that professional's abilities, even though you may know nothing about the medical procedures performed. The same is true for communicating in written form. If you receive written instructions from a physician with clearly defined explanations, you will be more likely to complete the procedures asked of you. Patients are consumers, and if they are not satisfied with the experience or treatment, they will seek help elsewhere.

Writing for the health professions, however, involves much more than communicating with patients. Consider the other elements of writing that health professionals produce on a daily basis. For example, when I ask this question in writing seminars, many health professionals and students first choose charting and notes. Although these are important elements of your professional practice because you must be clear and precise in your assessments and documentation, they constitute a small fraction of the writing you must perform to be a successful practitioner. However, the type of writing for notes or charts often is informal and devised through a shorthand notation system. It is not the type of writing that requires critical thinking and analysis.

Think about how writing influences your profession in the following examples. You will enlist your colleagues' support if you can write to support your interests to administration or if you can write persuasively to garner support from others outside of your profession. You will raise your level of esteem if you can publish articles or books that take part in your field's scholarly dialogue. You will always be reimbursed for services rendered if you can adequately represent your work through writing to insurance companies or health maintenance organizations (HMOs). You will remain in business longer if you can defend your actions when reviewed or when legal issues arise. You can support your profession and your employing organization by writing grant proposals or by seeking the support of outside organizations. You become a logical thinker when you write and a clear articulator of ideas. If nothing else, consider this: Many qualified people are seeking employment in the health care job market or are competing for patients in the allied health professions. Writing well makes you more competitive.

This text, then, aims to demonstrate the importance of writing in the health professions, and it attempts to hone the skills of anyone who writes. To serve these goals, the text is divided into three sections: learning *how* to write, learning how to write for academic purposes, and learning how to write for the profession. This text will explain the need for effective communication in writing for the health professional, but more important, it will demonstrate how to represent yourself well and sell yourself and your ideas in a manner expected of you by the profession.

WRITING, THIS TEXTBOOK, AND THE PROFESSION

This text provides a clear formula for improving writing through the **recursive writing process**. According to this formula, writing well is accomplished through several phases of writing, **revising** (reworking on several levels), rewriting, and rewriting again. Each chapter describes the stages of the writing process and follows these stages sequentially. Using the recursive writing process as a formula for success, the writer simply plugs in the values and addresses the topics in a logical sequence.

The first section of the book describes the writing process and the most important elements of writing well. The chapters in this section reinforce the fact that developing ideas through drafting is essential. Any writing can be made better by rewriting. Follow the guidelines provided in this part of the text to accomplish this goal. This first section begins by outlining the formula for the writing process and its complexities. A successful writer will use most, if not all, of the strategies presented throughout this section because they are based on generally accepted principles of writing. If you learn one lesson from this text, learn that *good writing is the result of clear thinking made visible.* Clear writing is clear thinking, and acceptable writing requires time and a commitment to analyze, revise, and reinvent to produce a worthy product. Ultimately, these steps, the revision process, are grounded in the principles of critical thinking and critical reading. These chapters introduce the recursive writing process and direct the writer to focus on **audience** (intended readers) and **purpose** (thesis) to deliver a unified and coherent message in the first draft.

For the second draft, the text instructs the writer to tackle grammar and mechanics, but these are functional lessons, not rules to be remembered. In other words, grammar lessons are supplied as part of the formula. The writer will examine the draft that was created in Phase One and apply these lessons for correctness. Furthermore, I assume that students using this textbook can formulate sentences and can present ideas. I cannot assume that students using this textbook can identify the rules that govern sentence formation. My experience indicates that previous educational experiences have relaxed the rules that govern writing, focusing instead on ideas, not form or structure. However, most writers crave knowledge about the rules because they know they exist; perhaps they were never taught them or required to demonstrate competency. Consequently, many writers are embarrassed by their inability to recognize grammatical parts of sentences or the characteristics of a sentence. However, few writers or practitioners have the time or interest to pick their way through the tangle of jargon and terms that are foreign to their field of study. As a result, I have developed a scheme to teach them the grammatical terms they need to know; this text does not teach grammar for the sake of teaching grammar.

Supporting the material on grammar and mechanics is a chapter on the third phase of the process, devoted to developing a professional voice and style. Again, this information is presented as a stage in the process or part of the formula, not as an obtuse list of terms and functions, as used in many texts. More important, the concept of verb-based writing is essentially ignored in most writing texts, but I have emphasized it as a cornerstone of clear writing and for the development of clear and precise diction. The sections on sentence variation build on the processes of clear and precise sentence construction from the first sections of the text. With each stage of the process, I include specific writing assignments and a set of tasks that are designed to reinforce these strategies.

Revising is the key to successful writing. The formula for success is to write a draft and rework it several times with specific issues to address at each draft. To demonstrate this process, I have included several different types of student writing samples. Some are designated as model essays; others are examples of poor writing that can be made better.

The second section of the text then applies the writing process strategies to the documents and assignments that you will be required to produce as a student in the field. These assignments involve the principles of reasoning and logic that accompany argumentation and writing to inform your audience. Additionally, to argue well or to appropriately inform your audience, you will need to learn and practice the methods for research writing and the modes of explaining information. (This text follows the guidelines presented by the American Psychological Association [APA] for research writing formats.)

Finally, the third section of the text takes the student out of the classroom and into the profession. The types of writing assignments and discussions surrounding various writing forums are consistent with the practical world of writing for the medical practitioner and the student of the profession. The text provides instruction for a variety of informal and formal writing: daily office exchanges, writing for administrative purposes, patient education literature, and writing for publication.

Follow the guidelines presented and apply the principles of the recursive writing process to be a successful writer in the health professions and a successful practitioner. This text provides a formula for writing success. Plug in the values and approach writing as a process. Writing well, for the health professions, is not an art but a skill, and any skill can be improved with practice.

THE RECURSIVE WRITING PROCESS

"I don't see why we have to take a writing class. Writing has nothing to do with my job."

"I was never taught how to write, so don't expect much from me."

You have heard these statements before, or you are thinking them at this point in your academic career. Such common statements indicate the awkward feelings that most people have about writing. Many people enter writing classes armed with these excuses for several reasons. First, most people are embarrassed by the fact that rules for writing exist and they do not know them. Our elementary and secondary school education put terms in our vocabulary such as "adjective," "direct object," or "nominative absolute," but we received them with indifference because these terms are abstractions that were offered in examples of sentences we would never write. Most writers were never challenged to use this information in practical situations. These terms were learned but never put into practice, and over time, we forgot how to use them. In most cases, we were never required to demonstrate our knowledge of them, or we were never held responsible for them because we did not write often or for an audience who cared. Now, when asked to employ that knowledge we learned in elementary or secondary school, we are embarrassed by our inability. This is a normal reaction, and the excuses are a logical product of such weak preparation.

This text will reintroduce you to those grammatical terms or procedures not as abstractions but as part of a process or formula for putting ideas on paper in a professional manner. It will not ask you to memorize jargon from the grammar field, or to memorize rules. This text will serve as a guidebook to writing well.

"Writing is a skill, and any skill can be made better with practice."

You should not fear your inability to write well because your instructors do not expect you to know how to write professionally when you enter this stage of your academic preparation. You have, most likely, taken introductory writing courses, and you might have taken an upper-division course or two that demanded heavy writing. Completing such courses does not mean that you are prepared to write for the profession. Just like medical practitioners, academicians teach to various practices or theories. Your instruction, up to this point, may have stressed the less formal techniques of writing. This text will help you build an expertise in the formalities of writing and to correct any bad habits you may have developed over time.

You can become a better writer only if you practice what you learn and incorporate these lessons into your thinking. Writing is a skill, not some magic gift. You can establish yourself in your profession by honing this skill and developing it into an expertise.

Writing instructors often hear the following excuse for poor writing skills:

"I'm not a good writer. I don't have any talent. I'll never be a good writer."

This claim assumes that writing is a talent on loan from some higher power. Some people *are* gifted crafters of words and sentences; they are artists with their words, but these authors do not inherit these words from Divine Providence. They work at their craft by writing, revising, rewriting, and rewriting again. Their work is never done, because words, phrases, sentences, paragraphs, and essays take time to create and even more time to craft into powerful meaning. For example, I once spent an entire semester in graduate school learning how to write a ten-line poem. This text does not ask that you learn how to write poetry, nor does it ask you to express ideas in abstractions; it *does* ask that you understand the importance of words and the impact of their meaning. Every mark on the paper has meaning, and you will soon recognize that to garner support for your ideas, you will grapple with the language and struggle to find the exact words and combination of words to express your ideas clearly.

The Process

Begin your journey into the world of professional writing by understanding that the process of writing is endless, because a text can always be improved. The entirety of this textbook is based on the following premise: *When we write, we invent a product; when we rewrite, we make the product better.* Ultimately, what we put on paper becomes a puzzle of meaning to be reworked and re-solved. Consequently, to write well, you must be willing to create the puzzle and then rework it several times to find the exact meaning you need to present to your reader. Writing instructors have often told me that writing is a deliberate act of problem solving. Our scientists and medical practitioners, then, should be excellent writers because they solve problems for a living.

The first lesson any writer needs to learn is that good writing is not produced in a linear fashion over a short period of time. Look at Section Figure 1-1. In this diagram, consider that a writer receives an invitation or reason to write at point A and the product is finished at point B. If a writer follows this linear process, he or she would not revise or rework the document. The writer would sit at the keyboard, begin typing, and print the final copy in one, short process. Because of the demands on our time, we would like to think that this *is* the writing process. We would like to think that our ideas are clearly organized in our heads, our sentences already

A – B

| Section Figure 1-1 Linear Process of Writing

crafted, and our words already chosen, all in grammatically and mechanically correct form. The only part left is the process of taking the finished document out of our heads and putting it on paper. This is impossible to do. No one should put this type of pressure on himself or herself, but people do because they do not understand the complexities of writing. Successful writers must learn and understand that what they create in this linear process is nothing more than a preliminary or rough draft.

Analyzing the Linear Process of Writing

Beginning writers feel that the linear process is the most direct and thus the best method to use because it requires little time. An uneducated writer may look at the final draft and not feel satisfied with the end result. Consequently, he or she may add another phase to the linear process by proofreading the text and making both substantive and cosmetic corrections. This type of writer, although misguided and uninformed, has realized an important element of the writing process: Writing improves if approached in stages. This text will demonstrate that writing must be approached through a series of revisions that attack specific problems in each draft produced.

Consider the following checklist of all of the components of writing:

OVERALL ESSAY:
- [ ] audience
- [ ] clarity/coherence
- [ ] depth/details
- [ ] informal tone
- [ ] organization
- [ ] purpose
- [ ] redundancy
- [ ] thesis development

PARAGRAPH LEVEL:
- [ ] introduction
- [ ] cohesion
- [ ] conclusion
- [ ] paragraphing
- [ ] transitions
- [ ] verb tense shifts

SENTENCE LEVEL:
- ☐ object-based
- ☐ passive voice
- ☐ structure: parallelism, modifiers, mixed
- ☐ sharp transitions
- ☐ variation

DICTION:
- ☐ wordiness
- ☐ vagueness
- ☐ trite phrases and clichés
- ☐ idiomatic expressions
- ☐ slang
- ☐ word confusion
- ☐ words missing

GRAMMAR:
- ☐ comma splices
- ☐ run-on sentences
- ☐ sentence fragments
- ☐ subject-verb disagreement
- ☐ pronoun-antecedent disagreement

PUNCTUATION:
- ☐ comma
- ☐ semicolon
- ☐ colon
- ☐ dash
- ☐ quotation marks
- ☐ apostrophe
- ☐ hyphen

MECHANICS:
- ☐ capitalization
- ☐ numbers
- ☐ spelling
- ☐ proofreading and editing

No writer can consider all of these topics and address them all when writing in the linear process. Each category requires a commitment of time and editorial energy to ensure a readable and acceptable product of communication.

For example, no writer can begin writing about a subject without thinking about the topic or **organizing** ideas about the topic. Consider also that a document created in this linear process probably begins by discussing one subject but ends proving an entirely different idea. Consider also that sentences and paragraphs may not be adequately connected to carry the thought process, and the words and phrases used may not be the precise terms needed to effectively communicate the message. A document may contain all of these problems, and we haven't even addressed mechanical or grammatical correctness yet.

To write well, a successful student of the profession must learn to write in stages. We should approach any writing assignment with the expectation that the document will take several drafts to complete and that the process of **drafting** absorbs enormous amounts of time. This is often the most difficult concept for students of writing to comprehend. Students, more than most people, face unrealistic demands on their time. They are saddled with course work that requires hours of preparation and reading. Furthermore, instructors claim that *their* courses are the most important, and shortcuts to student preparation should be taken in "someone else's class." Realistically, students will not have enough time to complete the writing assignments in any class to the best of their abilities because writing well requires days, weeks, and sometimes months of preparation, revision, reassessment, and rewriting.

The demands on your time for these writing assignments will be great; expect the demands and prepare for them now. Many writers perform poorly because they have not allocated enough time to manage the complexities of writing. As a result, they attempt to write, revise, and rewrite the day before an assignment is due. This abbreviated process will earn you grades below your expectations and produce writing below professional standards. Learn now that the writing process requires time; successful writers will afford themselves the time to work consistently across the allotted time for the assignments through the stages that follow.

The Phases

Consider Section Figure 1-2 compared with the linear diagram presented in Section Figure 1-1. The phases of the recursive writing process diagrammed in the figure are represented in the chapters that follow in this text. However, a brief overview is needed here.

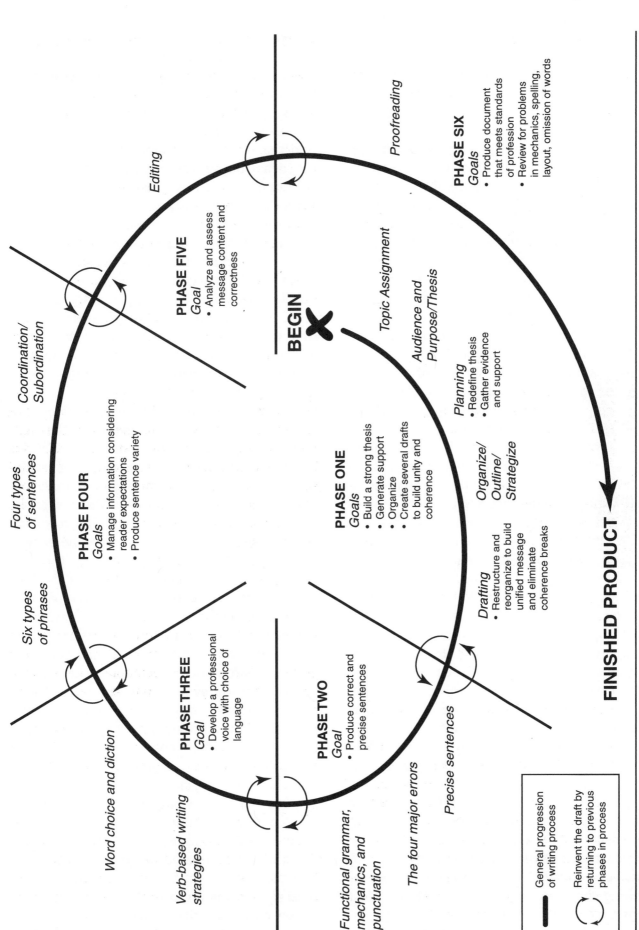

BEGIN ✗

Topic Assignment

Audience and Purpose/Thesis

Planning
• Redefine thesis
• Gather evidence and support

Organize/ Outline/ Strategize

Drafting
• Restructure and reorganize to build unified message and eliminate coherence breaks

PHASE ONE
Goals
• Build a strong thesis
• Generate support
• Organize
• Create several drafts to build unity and coherence

Proofreading

PHASE SIX
Goals
• Produce document that meets standards of profession
• Review for problems in mechanics, spelling, layout, omission of words

FINISHED PRODUCT

Editing

PHASE FIVE
Goal
• Analyze and assess message content and correctness

Coordination/ Subordination

Four types of sentences

PHASE FOUR
Goals
• Manage information considering reader expectations
• Produce sentence variety

Six types of phrases

Word choice and diction

PHASE THREE
Goal
• Develop a professional voice with choice of language

Verb-based writing strategies

Functional grammar, mechanics, and punctuation

PHASE TWO
Goal
• Produce correct and precise sentences

The four major errors

Precise sentences

	General progression of writing process
⟳	Reinvent the draft by returning to previous phases in process

Section Figure 1-2 The Writing Process

First, the diagram is spiral in nature to demonstrate that the stages of production require constant reassessment and reconsideration of your audience and purpose. The solid line represents the general progression of attacking writing, and the breaks indicate a new phase or the development of a new stage in the production process. Ultimately, the process spirals back to the beginning to send the message that no stage of writing can accomplish its purpose if it somehow detracts from the overall effectiveness of the paper or assignment. Furthermore, at every phase of production, the writer must develop ideas that support the intended purpose and use words that are appropriate to the audience. No writer should approach these phases of writing without reconsidering and reassessing the impact each phase has on the specific purpose of the paper, or thesis. Ideas and language that drift from the intended purpose need to be reshaped to fit the mold established by the thesis. To support the need for constant reinvention, the diagram includes "recycling" arrows after each phase to demonstrate the fact that no phase can be complete without considering the phases that have come before it. Follow the recycle symbols back in the process, and consider the changes that may be levied on the previous stages. Any change to one phase can damage the foundation that has been established by others.

The first phase of writing, then, is often the most important because it is the first layer of the foundation. In this phase, building **unity** and **coherence** in the document is the most significant goal. Unity, maintaining a consistent thought process throughout the document, is established by the thesis statement. The thesis statement provides the direction the paper will take. The remainder of the paragraphs, sentences, and words written will somehow support that thesis. Your goal in the first phase is to build a draft that coherently supports that thesis statement. Obviously, how you plan, gather ideas, and organize your ideas will support your efforts. However, the first phase of drafting that you engage in will be the most important.

Phase One: The Drafting Process

In the drafting process, you will constantly reassess how the body paragraphs you have written support your thesis. If you find that paragraphs do not support the thesis, you will reinvent the paragraphs until they do. If you find that your body paragraphs fully develop the ideas you want to present but they still fail to support the thesis, then you must reassess your thesis and reinvent it. Ultimately, while drafting, you want to build a message that can be traced lucidly throughout your text. If you present information that does not support your thesis directly, or is off track, your reader will not receive your intended message. If your reader struggles to sift through your ideas to find your message, you have not done your job as a writer. Easy reading comes from hard writing, and easy reading is coherently shaped and logical.

As you attempt to build a unified essay, you will begin to notice how other parts of the essay connect and build a consistent line of thought. When they deliver your message clearly, without interruption, your essay is considered coherent. If your sentences address separate topics in your paragraphs without any clear indication of how they connect, coherence is lost. As you build a coherent message throughout the essay, the same principles of thinking can be applied to the connections between paragraphs and the entirety of the message in the essay itself. Provide clear transitions between sentences and between paragraphs to send a coherent message to your reader. If your paragraphs and evidence do not support your purpose (thesis), unity is lost. If your ideas shift unnecessarily and sentences and paragraphs seem disconnected, coherence is lost. Unity and coherence take the guesswork out of reading. They provide a clear purpose and carry that singular purpose through the text without creating confusion. Your text, you should note, should not be a puzzle for the reader to solve.

Many underprepared writers make the claim that the reader is at fault for not "getting" the message. This is not true. The reader can only gather what the writer provides.

Your writing should be a clear representation of your thinking. If your thoughts are misguided or if you are not sure about your message, your work will reflect that uncertainty with a lack of unity and an incoherent message. Your profession demands a unified message written in a coherent fashion.

Unity and coherence are the main goals of the first phase of the writing process. The writer cannot attempt to fine-tune writing if the message is not clear and precise. For many beginning writers, this is the most demanding of the stages in the process. You will be required to critically analyze all that you have written and to challenge your own thinking or what you have written. Be prepared to create several drafts of your paper at this stage. When the focus of your paper changes, begin a new draft. Do not let uncertain ideas from a previous draft infiltrate your new, more precise draft. Once you have a draft that is unified and coherent, you finally have a rough draft. Now, employ other strategies to fine-tune your work. These are included in the other phases of the recursive writing process, which is the process depending on revision for a successful and effective product.

Phase Two: Developing a Professional Style with Words and Sentences

Once you as the writer have established a clear path to prove the thesis statement, creating a unified and coherent draft, begin considering ways to develop a professional writing **style** (writing that meets professional standards and accuracy while still maintaining the reader's interest by creating continuity and flow) and addressing grammatical correctness. Phase Two, the second stage of the writing process, should be devoted to these two pursuits, which refine sentences and words. These strategies will require the understanding of lessons in **functional grammar**: grammar that is needed to help the writer create precise sentences and to communicate on a professional level.

In Phase Two, the writer should be concerned with grammatical correctness. The paper has been clearly organized and its purpose defined; now the sentences should be scrutinized for accuracy and precision. The writer at this stage should understand the seriousness of grammatical errors such as sentence fragments, comma splices, fused sentences (run-on sentences), and subject-verb disagreements. Although most writers at this stage of their professional training can avoid these errors, some people cannot. Allowing any of these errors in your writing is damaging to your academic reputation. Anyone at the professional level will expect writers to be astute in basic grammar. To be grammatically precise, a writer also needs to understand some rules of punctuation. These rules should be learned with the rules of grammar in this stage of the writing process, but catching and correcting such errors require careful reading and scrutiny of the text. Expect to challenge every sentence in your work in terms of grammatical accuracy; every mark on the paper has meaning. Consequently, other problems related to sentence clarity should be considered: lack of parallel structure, dangling modifiers, and incorrect pronouns. These basic errors result in incoherent thought and language that is impossible to understand for concrete meaning.

Again, creating grammatically correct sentences will take much time, and addressing each of the potential problems may require a separate draft, or at least a separate reading.

Once the writer is sure of grammatical correctness, he or she can begin refining the sentences and words used to fit the demands of the audience. Because the audience is educated, the writer will choose language appropriate to support the cause or purpose. Consequently, writers should employ standard verb-based writing strategies. These will force the writer to unravel sentences and rebuild them using a clear *who-does-what* focus. In doing so, the writer will employ strong verbs, which essentially requires the close scrutiny of all words and their precise meanings in the sentences. Choosing the words that most accurately represent your meanings is the focus of verb-based writing and the development of professional diction.

Phase Three: Sentence Variety for Continuity and Flow

As the writer changes sentences into a clear formula (the *who-does-what* focus), the sentences will inevitably become formulaic and lose their spontaneity or flow. Often, meanings will change, and the writer must guard against this. Consequently, the writer must review the overall purpose of the essay again and relate the paragraphs and sentences back to the thesis at the appropriate places. Once this has occurred, the writer can be concerned with continuity and flow. The formulaic sentences resulting from verb-based writing strategies can be enhanced with the addition of phrases and clauses. In adding these grammatical constructions, the writer must be aware of the impact these changes make on the reader. The writer should ensure that information placed in a phrase or in a dependent clause is subordinate to the information contained in an independent clause. Likewise, information must be appropriately subordinated or coordinated, and this can be accomplished with the use of a few sentence variation techniques. Once the writer is secure in the fact that the essay flows, has appropriate diction and style, is grammatically correct, and is unified and coherent, he or she can consider the fourth and final phase of the writing process: editing and proofreading.

Phase Four: Editing and Proofreading

The final stages of the writing process, **editing** and **proofreading**, require the most time, because scrutinizing your work demands that you as the writer carefully dissect every sentence and word for exact and precise meaning. To do so, you need to become a critical reader and thinker. A successful writer will read through the text and search for problems in reasoning, ask questions about the relevance of information presented, consider how others might interpret the language and misconstrue the meaning intended, and find ways to communicate complex thoughts effectively to the audience. When the writer is assured that the document meets these demands, he or she edits one more time for grammar and mechanics and then proofreads the work with attention to paper format, glaring errors, or documentation style. A sense of objectivity is needed here. A polished writer always uses another person or persons as editor and proofreader to objectively and critically examine the text. Attempt to objectify your experience by distancing yourself from the text and returning to it with a fresh perspective. Many writers do not have the time to dedicate to this endeavor, but it works.

The key to understanding how to be a good writer is to understand the complexities of the diagram. Continually reinventing the document allows the writer to restart from various stages. Once the writer begins putting ideas on paper, the ideas can then be reshaped and crafted to better communicate the intended message. Again, writing well is actually a process of rewriting and revising, but a writer cannot revise without words on the paper. Put together a draft, no matter how horrible it is, and rework it. As you practice, your initial drafts will improve and the phases of rewriting will be less time consuming.

Follow the design of the diagram for the recursive writing process, and understand that the conclusion of each section offers new opportunities to restart or reinvent. Recognize also that the whole diagram is circular in nature, indicating that the writer's work is never done; it always reinvents itself. Any document can be made better with a commitment of time and editorial energy. This is the formula for success.

▌CONCLUSION

The writing process is indeed a formula for writing success, but it is not a rigid formula. Try the steps in the process first and adopt the strategies that work well for you. Then, recognize your weaknesses; address those strategies that do not work well for you, and omit those that do not.

Understanding that we all need editors and we all need help clarifying our ideas is a sign of a mature writer. No one who writes professionally sends anything to be published unless someone else who can give feedback and constructive criticism reads the document. We cannot realistically know everything about writing well, but we can know where to find answers to our questions, and we can know whom to ask for help.

The central concept of this text is that writing is a skill, and any skill can be improved and made more effective. The application of this concept will involve a variety of skills. Obviously, certain mechanical aspects of standard written English must be addressed: grammar, mechanics, and stylistic elements. However, effective communication goes far beyond these elements. It involves the ability to generate ideas, to clarify one's purpose, to analyze and address an audience, to arrange ideas in a rational format, to select words appropriate for the target readers and specified purpose, and to construct paragraphs that develop ideas clearly and thoroughly. Consideration and application of all of these elements equal the writing process, and the end product of using this process effectively is a document that expresses our ideas clearly and concisely to our intended audience.

The sections of this book take you through the writing process and explain each phase: building the essay through drafting, developing correct sentences and appropriate wording, developing a professional writing style, and editing and proofreading your final product. This formula, if followed and put into practice, will produce writing that will be acceptable at any professional level.

1

Phase One of the Writing Process: From Idea to Draft

Key Terms

Body paragraphs The paragraphs that provide support for the thesis

Conclusion The paragraph or paragraphs at the end of the essay that reinforce that you have proved your stated thesis

Informative writing States facts through synthesizing existing information; also called *expository writing*

Introduction The first paragraph or paragraphs of the essay that introduce the subject matter and that house the thesis statement

Persuasive writing Attempts to influence the reader to choose one position over another; also called *argumentative writing*

Tone The choice of words that dictates objectivity or subjectivity

Transitions Sentences, phrases, or words that connect two related sentences or paragraphs to continue a line of thought

chapter objectives

On completion of this chapter, the reader should be able to

1. Understand the preliminary stages in developing a first draft.
2. Identify audience and tailor language to meet audience needs.
3. Understand the purpose for writing and choose appropriate language.
4. Create a workable thesis and support it throughout the essay.
5. Create a draft that is both unified and coherent.
6. Understand the roles and purposes of the introduction, body paragraphs, and the conclusion.
7. Create workable thesis statements.
8. Create transitions to provide a continuous flow of ideas that will build unity and coherence in the essay.
9. Identify problems in unity and coherence.
10. Read and revise the first draft to build a unified and coherent message.

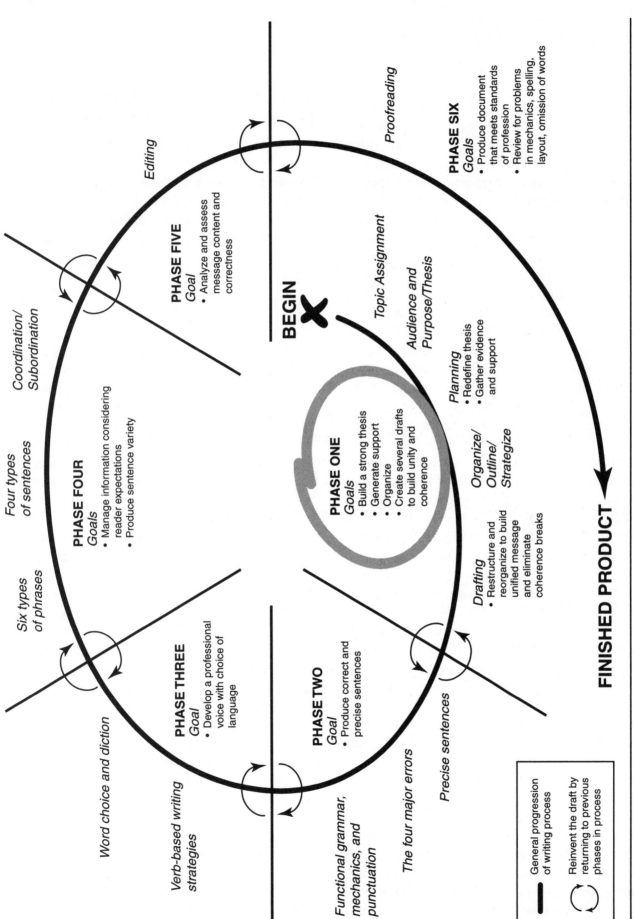

Figure 1-1 The Writing Process: Phase One

BUILDING THE ESSAY

Before any writing can be performed, the writer must identify the intended reader and write with a specific purpose. Without this information firmly in place, the document is adrift. You cannot reasonably expect to write anything unless you have a clear indication of what you want to communicate, and you cannot choose the appropriate language to communicate your points if you do not know to whom you want this message delivered. These are the first steps in the first phase of the writing process, as depicted in Figure 1-1.

Once you understand a direction that you will want to take, you can begin formulating a working thesis. No paper can successfully operate without one. It is the rudder that steers your ship of ideas. Consider also that the thesis is not provided for the writer's use. It is provided for the reader, to indicate the writer's message or to provide a controlling idea that guides the reader's reactions. Your reader can then hold the controlling idea in the forefront of his or her mind while reading the remainder of the text and challenge your ideas and evidence against the claim that you have made. The reader should not be charged with the task of piecing together bits of information to solve a puzzle. Your reader will want direct answers and information. Using the controlling idea, the reader can see the direction the writer intends to follow and can then make assessments about the support given in terms of the thesis. The remainder of the text and the messages that are delivered in it should clearly support the thesis in all facets of the document. Using the thesis well allows the writer to build a coherent document, and coherence makes for a pleasurable and informative reading experience. Consider the adage "Easy reading comes from hard writing."

With the thesis firmly in place, the writer can then begin planning and organizing the essay around it. To generate ideas, many writers gather ideas by using various techniques: mind mapping, zero drafting, brainstorming, freewriting. Find the mechanism that works best for you and use it regularly. To organize the text, many people use outlines; others simply like to begin drafting. Do what works best for you. These issues this text will not address.

The First Stage: Considering Audience, Purpose, Planning, and Organization

You cannot begin writing unless you have a purpose and know to whom you will be writing. Actually, you could begin writing, but you would not be clear in your focus because you need to understand your direction before you launch into supporting it. Consequently, you should answer the following questions as you begin any writing assignment:

Who is my audience?

What is my purpose?

The successful writer will keep the purpose at the forefront of any discussion in the paper. Constantly referring back to the thesis or logically proving the thesis allows the reader to revisit the purpose and to assess the writer's ideas in relation to that purpose. Furthermore, the successful writer will always consider the audience in the presentation of ideas. Doing so will help the writer make appropriate choices for words, sentences, and paragraphs that make the reading experience exact and informative.

Many writers fail to recognize these simple elements of good writing. Unskilled writers are egocentric in that they assume that anyone who reads their work should know their terminology and should be able to follow their process of thinking. This is the most damaging mistake to make as a writer. Your job as a writer is to communicate ideas to your audience, not exercise your intellect. Be considerate of your audience and guide your readers through the process. I often use the metaphor of pushing the reader down a line of train tracks for the central goal of good writing. An educated writer will put his or her readers on a set of tracks and push them down the line until they reach their destination. The readers have no means to veer off the path other than those that the author chooses. Weak writers present ideas in the form of a maze. Dead ends and false paths lead the readers away from the true purpose of the work. The work of these writers is confusing because the reader is not prepared to discover clues and deduce a meaning. The job of a reader is to be guided and directed. Strong writers understand these facts and are considerate of their readers' needs. They write to meet the demands of their audience, and this type of thinking makes them successful.

Purposes

In academic or professional writing, you will usually write in either of two arenas: to *inform* or to *persuade*.

Informative writing (sometimes called expository writing) provides the reader with information, or it helps to explain a set of circumstances. It is most often used in the medical profession to set forth the findings in a study. This type of writing requires the writer to back up or support his or her claims with hard facts or data. Informative writing assignments never take on a subjective slant; they are written with an objective eye for accuracy and clarity. Consider what you read in journals or textbooks as classic examples of expository writing; these forms of writing educate the reader. Educational material should not be slanted, and its results should be verifiable by anyone interested in contesting the information presented. Conversely, some people think that newspaper and news magazine articles are written in this mode. This is not always the case, as some authors carefully conceal their biases and ultimately seek to persuade the reader. This is not expository or informative writing. Expository writing uses conventions of organization to plan out the approach to explaining a set of circumstances. Usually, these include methods such as definition, cause and effect, and comparison and contrast, to name a few.

Persuasive writing (often called *argumentative writing*) attempts to reinforce an already existing opinion or to sway a reader to change opinions. Some writing instructors teach the persuasive essay as a mechanism of argument because in it the author presents one side of an argument and then is expected to reinforce it with evidence. Indeed, the persuasive essay is

an argument. However, the effective argument is well supported with convincing evidence. Most persuasive essays are written in the health professions through professional forums, such as newspapers or journals, or through administrative writing to convince administrators or others in the field to shift their stance or support a claim on a debatable issue.

Many beginning writers fail to comprehend the purpose of this form of writing—the persuasive essay or argument assignment—because they believe that their *opinion* on a subject constitutes an *argument*. This is not the case, because everyone's opinion is not truly valid for academic or professional purposes until it is supported with some verifiable evidence or experience. Using personal experience is often considered a weak form of evidence because it may not be reproduced easily. Consequently, you, the writer, are saddled with the responsibility of supporting your ideas with facts and hard evidence.

Use the following formula as a general guideline to building the persuasive or argumentative paper.

Formulating the Persuasive Essay:

Introduction: A. Establish that an argument exists by discussing background.
B. Take a position (thesis).

Body: A. Provide evidence paragraph(s) to defend your position.
B. Refute the opposition with evidence paragraphs.

Conclusion: Restate your position in terms of argument defended and/or refuted.

Notice that section B of the body paragraphs might be devoted to refuting the opposition's claim. If this is possible, it is a strong strategy. If it is not possible, then avoid the weak sides of your position as best you can. Your goal is to convince your reader to believe your claim and to understand how your support mechanisms warrant that claim. In other words, if you support your side well, you might not need to refute the opposition.

The important element to remember when writing a persuasive essay is that everyone has an opinion, and some or most of your readers might disagree with your stance on the issue that is being debated. Tact and understanding should be applied liberally. Your goal here is not to offend those who disagree but to present information in such a way that those who disagree might change their opinion. This requires understanding your audience and using the correct **tone** in the words you choose.

Audience

Although the main goal of an essay is to inform, persuade, or argue, knowing the audience is the key to success. Using appropriate language, or language written on the same intellectual and emotional level as that of the audience, helps align you with the audience, dissenters and all. Remember, you are writing neither to clear your head of ideas nor to verify that you can think. You are writing essays and argumentative documents to convince others to believe what you believe, or at least to believe that you have provided a rational argument with reasonable claims. If you fail to realize that you are writing for others, you will never be a successful writer.

Tone

Understanding your audience will allow you to make clear and conscious decisions about the words that you choose. (See "Word Choice and Diction" in Chapter 3.) When considering the formulation of your essay, you may feel passionate about the subject discussed and be tempted to use forceful words that drive your point into the heart of the dissenters. This is not wise. You should choose your words carefully to elicit the desired response. Although you may easily be able to make your point with some words, you may be able to reach more of your audience by using language that indicates that you understand both sides of the issue but prefer one side over the other. Politicians use an old saying from the public relations field to illustrate this point: "It's not what you say that's important; it's how you say it." You want to send the message to your reader that you understand both sides, but you have weighed the options and have taken this stand with diligence.

The uninformed are usually exposed in formal writing assignments because they may have an opinion, but they rarely know why. When they begin to write to communicate their stance, their words reveal their weak argument. A student once came to talk to me about writing an essay on removing a piece of modern art from a park because she thought it was offensive. I asked her to tell me why she thought it was offensive, and she could only tell me that she was raised to believe that exposing the human body in public was indecent. Looking at her issue in terms of a paper posed some problems. Her opinion was valid to her, but not to others. Her personal issues had not been universalized for use in an essay, and consequently, she moved on to another topic.

The purpose of writing to inform or writing the argumentative essay is to provide the reader with necessary evidence that is convincing. The writer is forced to assess his or her belief system or, often, to put personal preferences on hold. Often, writing is an academic exercise to build clarity of thought. Writing your ideas on paper and defending them forces you to analyze them from the perspective of an objective observer or to exchange ideas with others in a rational format or venue. As you write, you must consider others and understand how your words affect your audience. These types of assignments force you out of your comfort zones and into the world of thinking for and about others. To do so, you must engage in the processes of critical thinking and analysis.

Producing the First Draft

With these issues in mind, begin the essay and produce a draft. Your goal in this first phase of the writing process is to create a unified document by reworking your ideas in several drafts. Once you have ideas in place that are governed by logic and reason, you can begin to scrutinize your words and build a coherent argument. Nothing, however, can be accomplished if you do not have words, sentences, and ideas with which to work. Consequently, some writers begin typing and keep writing until they run out of ideas. Some turn their monitors off and write as much as they can. In both cases, the writers are not concerned about the formalities of writing. They are simply putting words on paper to help them clarify or visualize their thoughts. Others create detailed outlines of their ideas and write to follow the direction they have planned. This may save time, as the writer can perform the difficult thinking in the notes stage and organize thoughts in a logical fashion before typing.

The key to getting started is recognizing which strategy works best for you. Experiment with many strategies and gauge your success. In any case, the real writing process begins with the scrutinizing of these words *after* you produce a draft.

ATTACKING THE FIRST DRAFT: BUILDING STRUCTURE, UNITY, AND COHERENCE

Every essay you prepare should contain an **introduction** that contains your thesis statement, **body paragraphs** that serve as evidence to support your thesis, and a **conclusion** to reinforce your thesis and your supporting material. Of course, not every essay can be neatly packaged in this format, but this organizational structure should be applied to composing your work to build coherence and structure into your writing.

Examine Figure 1-2. The diagram suggests that all parts of the essay must support each other in some way. If all of the points made in a body paragraph support a single purpose for the paragraph and if all of the paragraphs support the thesis statement, the essay is unified. If they do not, you have built inconsistencies into your document that ultimately lead to incoherence and disrupt clear communication. Unity and coherence problems are

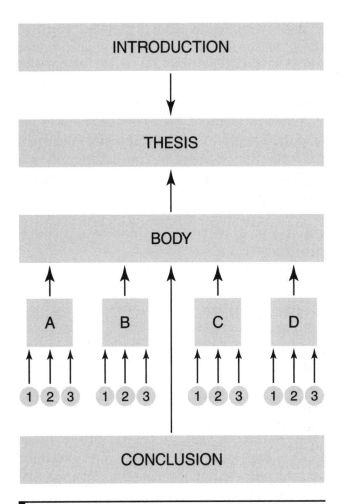

Figure 1-2   The Structure of a Unified Document

major concerns for any writer because they interfere with the transfer of the intended message.

To build coherence and unity into your documents, you must plan your approach to writing assignments and organize this information strategically with regard to your audience and purpose. Many writers begin the process of unity building when they begin planning the essay or gathering ideas. How you gather ideas and plan your approach is governed by your own needs and understanding of the subject. For some topics of which you know little, you will be required to spend time working through topic discovery and narrowing procedures: mind mapping, zero drafting, brainstorming, or free-writing. For other topics with which you are familiar, you may only need to piece together an outline.

You cannot adequately proceed through these phases if you do not know your intended purpose. Consequently, you must articulate a thesis statement and build your organizational structure around it, as dictated previously.

A thesis statement directs your readers to the singular point or message you wish to deliver. It governs every element of your writing, in that nothing should appear in the essay that does not in some way support the thesis. All sentences and words support the main point of the paragraph, and all paragraphs support the thesis in the essay. This is unification.

Even if you do not have a clearly written thesis, start by writing what you intend to prove at the top of the page. This assumes that you have performed the necessary thinking and studying to even write a direct statement that you can prove. If you have not thought through your subject, the process of writing your thesis and following it will be difficult. You may find that your ideas, once you write them in an essay, may not directly satisfy the needs of the thesis. In this case, you will change your thesis or rewrite your essay, whichever is more appropriate. This is part of the drafting process. If you are not sure what you are trying to prove, do not expect to write a clean draft your first time through. If you are organized in your thinking and have a clear direction, you should easily write your thesis statement and control your essay with it.

Save yourself some time by thinking through your topic and organizing your ideas before you begin to write. You would not leave for a vacation unless you had mapped a destination.

The Thesis Statement

Developing a thesis statement requires detailed thinking and strong organizing of ideas. The key to writing any thesis statement and embarking on the academic journey to prove that thesis is to narrow its focus. Many writers begin to write about a subject that interests them. For example, a student recently came to me with her research paper topic and claimed that she planned to prove that aquatherapy is an effective treatment modality for physical therapists. I immediately asked her to list all of the categories of ailments that therapists treat. As she listed them, I asked her if aquatherapy would benefit those ailments, and she could not demonstrate that this form of therapy would be beneficial for *all* ailments treated by physical therapists. Although aquatherapy would benefit osteoarthritis patients, it would not benefit patients with neuromuscular degenerative disorders. Consequently, she could not prove her thesis, and she could not do so because the topic was too broad. We concluded that she should focus on researching the benefits of aquatherapy for osteoarthritis patients, and her investigation revealed a topic even more specific.

The lesson here is to think and strategize about writing and proving the thesis before actually writing. As you think and strategize, you will inevitably gather information that will help you clarify your specific purpose.

Examine the changes that the following statement undergoes to become a strong thesis statement:

ORIGINAL: There are many kinds of buildings in Buffalo.

BETTER: Most people see the varied architecture in the city of Buffalo, but few realize the impact of famous architects such as Green and Wright.

FINAL: The buildings in Buffalo designed by E.B. Green and Frank Lloyd Wright derive from an architectural style that was fashionable at the turn of the nineteenth century, but the two architects have contrasting styles.

From this final statement, you can now provide a clear and focused essay in which all the parts relate back to the thesis. The charge to the writer is to compare styles of architecture of two prominent architects who worked in a specific place during a specific period. The thesis statement sets up the organization of the paper as well. A simple introduction could discuss turn-of-the-century architecture and identify Wright and Green as players. Other introductory or body paragraphs could describe the works of Wright and Green in the city of Buffalo, which will inevitably lead to the purpose of the paper: to compare their styles. Ultimately, the thesis statement controls the outcome of the paper's organization and provides the reader with a clear path to follow. This is your goal.

Examine the weaknesses in the other examples. In the original example, the writer could discuss any or all buildings that exist in Buffalo. They could be architecturally significant or not. Everything from houses to park bathrooms would have to be included. As a result, the writer would have to categorize the variety of buildings that exist and fit specific examples into those categories. This would be a monumental task that no writer has time to tackle.

In the second example (better), the purpose is clearer but not specific enough to direct the remainder of the paper. For example, the operative words in this example are "impact of famous architects." The term *impact* is too broad. It could mean that Green and Wright created some of their masterpieces in Buffalo that affected the universe of architecture and its study. It could mean that Green and Wright influenced others in this area of endeavor to create a unique style. Ultimately, the problem here is that the purpose is not evident, and uncertainty will mislead or confuse the reader. Professionals will not tolerate such weaknesses in writing.

The Introduction

An introductory paragraph leads the reader into the subject at hand with general statements or background information that is easily recognizable. Once the foundation for the subject is poured, the thesis statement sits on top. Consequently, the thesis statement usually follows any introductory element such as background information.

As a general rule, avoid using direct quotations or statistical evidence in your introductory paragraph. Your introduction should simply lead the reader into your thesis by providing general information. Quotations and statistics are usually used as evidence to support the writer's ideas; consequently, evidence and support belong in evidence or body paragraphs.

As many writers begin to formulate their thesis, they simply write out what they intend to accomplish. Because the thesis is not in its perfect form, the language used to construct it is in its developmental phase as well. The result is a statement that focuses not on the subject but on the writer. Again, as a general rule, avoid overly direct statements about your thesis or you as the writer of the thesis, such as "I am going to prove . . . " or "This essay will show . . . ." These types of lead-ins can easily be removed. Provide your thesis without telling your reader that you are providing your thesis.

Transitions

Transitions—either words, phrases, or sentences—help your reader move from one point to another without losing sight of the thesis. They are the language constructs that build coherence and unity. A good practice is to end a longer section or a paragraph by relating your subject matter back to your thesis statement. By doing so, you have common ground on which to make a transitional statement for the next paragraph. Your transitional sentence should demonstrate that it derives from your effort to prove your thesis and then allows the reader to move to a separate and different piece of evidence that supports the thesis.

A favorable method of providing transitions is through this general rule: *Always relate your paragraphs back to the thesis.* Your readers will never forget the purpose of the work if you can constantly remind them of it, and you will have a consistent point in your body paragraphs to connect ideas in other body paragraphs. Think of the train tracks metaphor as you develop your work. Your job is to place your reader on a set of rails or tracks and then push the reader down the line to your main purpose. Do not allow the reader to leave the rails—to be distracted by superfluous or unrelated information. If you feel that the reader may stray from the purpose of the essay after being misled by the information you provide, return the reader to the main focus by relating your points directly to the thesis statement or by eliminating the misdirecting information. If you feel that you are overstating your thesis, adjust accordingly by removing the redundant material. However, no reader will complain about your tendency to be direct and clear. Most readers will find disjointed, incoherent writing unacceptable and clear, direct writing pleasurable.

The Conclusion

The concluding paragraph pulls the essay together by summarizing the main points that have been discussed. Like the introduction, the conclusion should not offer new evidence, as evidence belongs in the body paragraphs, nor should additional direct quotes be used. Many people feel that a pithy phrase or the words of someone else will help them close their paper. This is a mistake. Put *your* signature on the paper by concluding with *your* words. Do not depend on the words of others to make your points for you. You are the writer, and you know the main thrust of your essay. Build a conclusion around the major thrusts that *you* have set forth.

Also, avoid rewording your introduction. Your introduction sets the stage and offers your thesis. The conclusion reinforces in your reader's mind that the evidence you have provided proves the thesis you have stated. Again, to use the metaphor of keeping your reader on track, the reader should successfully reach his or her destination in the conclusion. In fact, the reader should not have any means to doubt your thesis or your evidence, unless you misdirect him or her into other avenues of thinking.

ATTACKING THE FIRST DRAFT AGAIN: BUILDING COHERENCE AND UNITY

An important element of the writing process begins with the drafting stages and should focus on building coherence and unity. A draft requires that you put your ideas down on paper. Following the procedures already listed, you will have in place your purpose, audience, and general organization principles. You should recognize that you can and should change your purpose, audience, or organizational structure if you find that your paper requires such changes. Be aware, however, that even the slightest changes may alter the entire thrust of the document—which may then have to be revised accordingly.

To assess the effectiveness of the draft you have written, you must read your work as a reader would: objectively. Distance yourself from the work and approach it from a fresh perspective, with no assumptions. Put the paper aside for a few hours or even a day. Clear your mind of the topic and give your brain a rest. Then, return to the paper with an agenda. Ask questions and challenge the assumptions you have made. Find fault with your reasoning. Look for ways to be distracted from the thesis. This type of exercise is covered more fully under "Revising Your Argument: Critical Thinking and Reasoning" in Chapter 7. A good writer is always a demanding reader. However, reading for coherence and unity is your main priority when you attack your first draft.

Reading Your Writing: Revising for Coherence and Unity

If you have defined your audience and purpose and have assured yourself that you have connected ideas in a rational structure, you can now begin your first reworking of your first draft. A good practice to help you maintain your focus is to write your thesis statement and your targeted audience at the top of the page and begin reading with a singular purpose: to determine if you have supported that thesis.

Your task at this point is to write and read only for your thesis. Gather your ideas from your outline or your notes and scour your paragraphs looking for the supporting information for the thesis. Press on by asking yourself to answer questions about the thesis and to clarify your thinking. Do not concern yourself with spelling, sentence structure, grammar, mechanics, or style. These are all elements of the writing process that will be addressed in later drafts. Here, you want to create a foundation of your paper that stays on task. You can bulk up your argument later and fine-tune your sentences and words later. Your argument and your sentences are not worth the paper they are written on if the document is not coherent and unified. If you stall out while reading or feel distracted, reread what you have written to jump-start your thinking and to press on. If you find yourself distracted while reading, take note of this distraction. This is a sign of a problem. Stop reading and return to the previous paragraph to assess the effectiveness of the argument. If you are distracted at this point, imagine what your reader is feeling. You may be supplying your reader with opportunities to get off the metaphorical train tracks. Reread, looking for potential distractions causing the reader to lose interest or focus. These are the coherence breaks that will damage your authority as a writer. Supply the reader with the information that is applicable to the thesis, and connect these ideas with the information and evidence that surround them. Revise the paragraphs by considering what the reader needs to connect ideas together. Does the passage require re-organization so that ideas flow in a logical order? Does the passage require further development of ideas so that similar ideas in different concepts connect with each other? Can the disconnection between ideas be mended by providing transitional words and phrases to blend ideas in different sentences?

Overall, consider the following to be your charge in this phase of the writing process: *Simply read and produce paragraphs that are representative of your thinking and recognize that every part of the paper can be scrutinized and changed.* I italicize this sentence because it relates to the writing process in general: All text is and should be changeable.

When you are certain that you have a clear direction, reread your introduction and revise it by providing some background information and by proposing your thesis to your reader in a manner that is logical and supportive of the text you have created in your body paragraphs. The thesis, as you know by now, is the most important element of your paper, because it will guide your reader to your purpose and create a set of expectations. If your document fails to meet the reader's expectations, you have not done your job well. Examine your thesis in terms of the evidence you have provided.

Other Ideas to Help the Writer Scrutinize Words and Ideas

Once the initial draft is written, you can now scrutinize every word in your text. You should consider this task as an attempt to build clarity into the document. Clearly constructed thoughts are the mark of an organized mind and a well-trained writer.

Look first at your paragraphs (and consequently at the whole of the body and conclusion of your draft) and ask, "Does the message get through?" Secondarily, make sure that the body paragraphs support the thesis. If they do not, you have two choices: Change the direction of the paragraphs or change the thesis. You have the option. Many successful writers will assess the initial quality of their essay by reading the conclusion and comparing the ideas there with the thesis and the introduction. If your conclusion and your introduction offer differing approaches or directions, you have a unity problem. You must finish the document as you intended in your introduction. Also, eliminate coherence breaks; try connecting ideas with transitional words, phrases, sentences, or passages.

Your task in building the first draft is to put ideas onto paper in order to scrutinize them in terms of your thesis and for organizational strategy. Once the initial draft is on paper, you can then restructure your thesis, reorganize your ideas in your body paragraphs, add support to your paragraphs, reinforce your conclusion, and then rewrite the introduction to provide a powerful lead-in to your thesis. Put your ideas on paper and organize them into a rational, logical progression that proves a singular point or makes your case. When all of this has been accomplished, you have a *rough draft*.

REVIEW: FIRST PHASE OF DRAFTING

Once you have organized your thoughts and planned them to follow your thesis, you can begin crafting your words, sentences, and paragraphs into an essay. The first attempt at drafting the essay should have a singular goal: Prove your thesis. If you fail to stay focused on your thesis, your essay will "drift" (resulting in a unity problem), and you will lose your reader. Remember that you are writing not for your own purposes but to communicate to an audience. Keep the reader in mind as you work your words into sentences and your sentences into paragraphs.

To produce a flawless draft in your first attempt is impossible; consequently, you should set a reasonable goal for yourself. Your goal, as just stated, is to prove your thesis, but you may not be able to prove it fully to your liking and your readers' liking the first time through. Many writing instructors will ask you to jump in and put something down on paper. This is a good method to use because it allows you to at least have something on which to work your editorial pen. To take advantage of this method, you must always move ahead, even if you stall. Keep writing and proving your thesis, and once the message is through, you can then retreat to the beginning and begin cutting the excess and paring down your words to elicit an exact response.

In another approach, the writing of the first draft is done in stages. The writer divides the essay into its component parts and sets out to prove them one at a time. This is a useful approach if you are well organized before you begin to write. Not all of us are organized enough to attack the essay in this manner.

In either approach, your focus should be on the thesis. Do not worry about the details yet. If you refer back to the recursive writing diagram, you will see that the details—grammar, mechanics, spelling, and sentence variation—will be addressed in stages. Your goal is to prove the thesis in your first draft, and nothing more. The key words are unity, coherence, and order.

Your thesis is the tool that directs the essay's energy, but it is also the main tool for building unity in your work. Nothing can exist in the essay that does not support the thesis. Your essay must be unified if you plan to communicate clearly with your audience. For many people, this is a difficult task. It asks you to put yourself in the shoes of your audience and to be rational and precise. We are not often challenged to think this way when we communicate verbally. Consequently, you will not "write as you speak" or put together your words in a haphazard fashion. You will be required to be directly on target. A unified essay is one in which all parts of the essay support the thesis. Consequently, all topic sentences in your paragraphs support the thesis, and all the elements of support you use in your paragraphs support the topic sentences.

Your essay must also be coherent as well as unified. A coherent essay is one in which all of the elements of support blend into each other. Often, this is accomplished with transitional words and phrases that indicate relationships between ideas, sentences, paragraphs, or whole parts of essays. Some writers can achieve coherent connections by repeating words or phrases or by creating parallel constructions that provide rhythmic equality to equally weighted parts of the whole. Consider how your words can be crafted to push the reader down that metaphorical set of train tracks. You do not want to allow your reader to get off the tracks because you have set up diversions with your words. Build a straight and narrow line of tracks for the reader to follow.

FINAL SUGGESTIONS: REVISING WITH PERSPECTIVE AND OBJECTIVITY

Many people think that they have in their heads an essay that is to be written. They only need to tap into their brain and the words will flow out onto the page. Unless you are a genius, this probably does not happen for you. Most of us need to engage in the process of revision at this early stage to assure ourselves that the essay is on track. Others feel that if you must revise, you must not be a clear thinker or a good writer. The opposite is true. The best writers spend hours and days revising their work to make the exact impact they want on the reader.

Good writers are excellent readers who can evaluate their work with an objective eye. You should work to build this skill because it will help you develop critical thinking and critical reasoning skills. Your task, once the essay is put down on paper in rough draft form, is to assess your work as you read it. Your goal in the revision of your first draft is to make sense to your reader. You have followed your thesis in the first phase; now, you must bring all the elements together to create that unified and coherent whole.

To revise successfully, you need to understand that revision is the most time-consuming part of the writing process. If you do not plan to revise and rework the essay, you will not have adequate time to produce a document of high quality. To revise well, you need to distance yourself from your work in order to come back to it with objectivity. If you are too close to your draft, you will not see the critical mistakes that your reader will. Take a walk, go to the gym, do anything that does not require heavy reading or thinking. Distancing yourself from your work will rest your brain and allow you to face your work with a fresh perspective when you return to it. This fresh perspective is the most important element of the process of revision. You need to make clear and rational judgments that often call for you to cut large sections from your paper or to rewrite pages. You should understand and recognize that this type of cutting and reworking the essay is standard practice with excellent writers. You should plan for huge blocks of time to be absorbed by this activity.

Read through the essay looking for problems in reasoning or sections that do not relate to the thesis, faulty connections between sentences or paragraphs, or portions of the essay that create confusion. You should feel obligated to read as your audience will read. Do not simply let the words drift into your mind and out. Think about what you read and compare these thoughts to the thesis at every point of the essay. Read for continuity and read for purpose. As you read, make notes to yourself and then find ways to revamp the words to make sense. When you make your corrections, go back to the previous paragraph and reread looking for similar mistakes. When you have finished the entire essay, go back and reread the entire essay again and again for the types of problems associated with lack of unity, coherence, or failures to support your thesis. Once the essay is in a format that you feel is strong in unity, coherence, and supporting its thesis, try reading the essay aloud or giving it to someone else to read. Remember that you are not fixing the grammar or mechanics, or working on sentence correctness or style. You are simply trying to present an issue and stay focused on it in a way that any reader can follow.

Exercises

COHERENCE AND UNITY

■ Recognizing Coherence Breaks

Directions: Following are examples of incoherent paragraphs. Study each one and determine various means to solve incoherence: organization, development of ideas, or transitions. In all cases, the reader's expectations have not been met.

1. Tom and Jim crouched in the old shed, waiting for someone to discover them. He thought that the farmer had passed by. He felt safe in the silence, but he looked at Jim's foot and he knew he couldn't go on. He was happy to be there with Jim. They were a long way from home.

2. The Rocky Mountain summer was hot and dry. Steve wanted to go trail riding. His friend, Tom, wanted to go rock climbing. Tom was a great rock climber because he had a low center of gravity. The summer days were long, and the boys were free to roam the countryside.

3. When the doors of the stadium opened, thousands of fans rushed in. The seats were the last to fill up as the mass of people flooded the floor. The stage extended across the field, and the sound of sirens could be heard. This will be the best show of the year.

4. The Eastern coyote hunts mainly for mice and rabbits. Jones was deep in the Adirondack Mountains, and the noise of the village and the highways could not be heard. Many hunters had seen the coyotes, and a few had been shot. Their carcasses were hanged on the fence rows to warn others of their fate. Jones' mission was to rid the neighbors of these rascals that have been trading rabbits and mice for the neighbors' small dogs and cats.

5. Prince Edward Island is busy during the summer. The grasses have grown tall over the season, and weeds surrounded the old house. Some of the windows needed painting. Shutters were hanging loosely from their frames. Soon, the fields will be plowed under and the preparations for winter will begin.

■ Building Unity and Coherence

Directions: Find the breaks in the line of reasoning. Fix all coherence problems by considering a thesis, connecting ideas clearly, and offering mechanisms to help guide your reader to that singular purpose.

Mrs. Jones, a female born on November 1, 1970 has five primary complaints. She has pain when showering, brushing her hair, washing dishes, dressing and driving. The patient suffers extreme stiffness in her right shoulder and has low strength. She complains of pain when moving her shoulder and arm with limited coordination. Mrs. Jones stopped work. The problems of strength, reduced mobility, and pain need to be improved.

Mrs. Jones will be shown how to use an elastic band for her home exercises. The band will improve her mobility and stiffness. She will be doing weight lifting. The patient will have two short-term goals. She will return to her previous functioning and her discharge date is set for three months. The patient does not need long-term goals because the duration of treatment is short. Mrs. Jones completed physical therapy three times with the same complaint. When discharged, she improved her status, but her condition deteriorated over time. No home exercises were prescribed on the time of discharge.

■ Identifying Unity and Coherence Problems

The following sample is a student's essay before it was revised. This was the first attempt at putting words to paper.

Coherence breaks are identified with the following symbol: ^. Notice that the sentences before the indicator carry forward a particular subject. The sentence following the indicator starts a new idea but fails to carry the reader from the previous point to the present.

Problems in unity are identified using this symbol: ~. Notice that the sentences following the indicator suggest a topic or an idea that is not on task. The essay contains a thesis, and the information provided in the paper should support that thesis. If you provide information that is related to your thesis, explain that tangential connection to your reader. Do not ask your reader to make such connections.

Punishing a child teaches children what is right and what is wrong. Many parents punish their children by talking to them or by reward and punishment. ^ Child abuse consists of hurting a child physically, mentally, or emotionally.

(Notice that the first two sentences discuss the issue of punishment. The sentence after the indicator defines child abuse. These two ideas are not connected in any way. Any reader could make the connection, given the time to do so, but this task is not the reader's job. It is the job of the writer.)

~ There have been parents beating their children for hundreds of years.

(In this example, the borrowed information suggests that parents have been beating their children over time. How does this information support the thesis? It does not, and consequently, this error leads to a mistake in unity.)

Some punishments do consider spanking but do not hurt the children. Spanking a child is considered a soft slap to show the children that they did something wrong. Beating a child leaves bruises and psychological problems. ~ Unfortunately, there are parents all over the world who deliberately hurt their children. Child abuse causes many unresolved issues that usually do not get explored. Discipline can often be used in different ways. In case a child does not relate to a certain way, the parent can approach them in different ways to teach them morals.

As hard as it is to punish children, it needs to be done. ~ Our society focuses on parent-child relationships and specializes in natural parenting. Punishment gives children a sense of what proper behavior is. Children need to learn the difference between right and wrong. Punishing children can be done in many different ways. One example to discipline a child is isolation. When a child is left alone they get bored easily. When they are forced to pursue something they do not get motivated unless they want to do it. Then they realize what they did was wrong. Another way to discipline children is by reward and punishment. When children are young, they react well to this. They realize that when you take something that they want away, they did something wrong, but when they do well or if they do something that you ask them to do, they get a reward. People believe that reward and punishment works well with children. This creates problems because every time they do something right, they expect to get something in return. If they know that they are not going to get something in return, they may not do what you ask them to do. If this happens, you may have to approach the situation in a different way. ^ Lastly, talking to children begins a great relationship and tells them what is right and what is wrong. In this case, punishment may not be the answer, but explaining to them what is wrong can create an image of what is right. Speaking to your children can be a powerful tool for explaining morals. ^ ~A theme is created from experiments and it shows the relations between a parent who wants to raise their children properly and the society in which they live. If you talk to children, it teaches them to trust you and to respect you and the decisions you make. The examples you set for your children also teach them what is wrong and right by your actions.

Many parents do not understand the concept of talking to your children like they are human. This is when spanking gets too far. ^ Child abuse creates mental, physical, and emotional problems. Children who are hurt constantly deal with numerous problems and side affects. Some examples include becoming sensitive to pain, destructive, and depressed. The child becomes unlovable and is likely that they will not be loved by anyone because of their behavior. ^ Usually when there seems to be child abuse in a family, the parent is usually the one with the problem and they hit the child to blame someone else. ~ As a society we project problems of child abuse and try to concentrate on helping the parents. They are usually dealing with mental health issues or they have expectations of their children to do unrealistic things. In many cases, the child gets stressed out and needs to take his or her aggression out on someone who won't fight back. ~ Child abuse is used as a form of control but sometimes the child is left with destructive organs or even death.

Directions: Now read the remainder of this essay and use the given symbols to identify the problems in coherence (^) and unity (~).

Child abuse stems from stress or the parents' childhood. Changes have occurred by giving the parent therapy and treatments. The parent may think that beating a child is normal if they were hit as a child. The parents need to recognize what they are doing to their children and realize the relationship that they could have with them. It has been shown that the link between economic and social atmospheres affect families that are involved in child abuse. Physical abuse normally occurs with low-income families because they have too much stress keeping control in their life and to support their families. Evidence proves that there is a relationship between child abuse and low-income families. They get stressed easily because of poverty and become likely that they are unable to support their families. Emotion becomes very natural to a human being in how they respond to certain situations. In the past, it has been shown that people are embarrassed to deal with the poor. Emotional abuse usually takes place within a high income-tax family, because they don't seem to spend enough time with their children and they search for attention. Rich families create a life worth living but do not create time to spend with their children. Parents involved in this need to realize that they need to care for their children and give them guidance.

Children who are in an abused situation usually need psychological help. After a child is abused they suffer many side effects. These side effects include that they cannot trust, they have shame and doubt in anything they do, and they become destructive with people and property. It strains their brain and creates an image so they perceive themselves as not being good enough. Many abusive parents have low self-esteem and some do not even know who they are. Hitting a child is wrong and often enough parents who do this need mental and emotional help as well as the children. For some reason, the parents believe beating someone satisfies their urge to control something and forces them to believe that it is right. Child abusers form discipline into an extreme level. The parent's attention should be on the child and what they can do to help them, not what they can do to help themselves. Discipline creates morals and behavior, so telling them to do something right by doing something wrong and hurtful is not the right approach. Sadly, child abuse is done in many ways. They may not be hitting them, but child abuse can also be from not taking care of them.

Some examples are leaving a baby in a hot car for hours, not cleaning up after the children, or even not feeding them. If these parents can't take care of themselves then they should not be taking care of children.

Control is an issue that needs to be resolved before the children are born. Control helps life and releases some stress. Control leads to a natural relationship between parents and their children. They can learn how to discipline them by finding out what their children react to and how they can learn. If a parent is stressed, they should seek help if they cannot control it. Control seems to be one of the main problems because if they can't control something in their life, they need to control something else. Lack of self-control usually leads to child abuse. Punishment deals with a child's behavior and teaches them what they did wrong. It does not physically harm them. Child abuse is not discipline. It controls the way a parent reacts to certain situations. When trying to discipline children, hurting them is not the point, teaching them a lesson is. Parents need to understand that and if they don't, they need psychological help. This will help parents deal with their problems and create new relationships with their children.

■ Identifying and Correcting Coherence and Unity Problems

Directions: Examine the following sample student essay and find coherence breaks and problems with unity. Provide possible transitions to solve some of these problems.

A New York study found that most people would support a restriction on the use of cell phones (Holsendolph, 2002), then on November 1st, 2001, New York State introduced a "hands free" law for all automobile drivers to follow while driving. "Hands free" implies that all drivers must have both hands on the wheel at all times while driving. The driver must be clear of interference, ensuring that he has complete control of his car. When implemented, the law focused on the increasing number of drivers talking on cell phones while driving.

When asked about talking on cell phones while driving, Chuck Hurley, of the Illinois-based National Safety Council claimed "It's not where the hands are, but where the head is" (as quoted in Hands-free . . . , 2001, p. 19). When used in certain circumstances, hand-held cell phones can lead to reckless driving (Copquin, 2002).

Ernest Holsendolph (2002) tells of a situation that he encountered while driving on the Atlanta Interstate that has attracted attention from safety experts. He observed a white Ford Bronco that drifted toward the right lane, then back into the original lane. Then, the driver of the SUV spotted a car she was about to crash into, she then turned to the right lane, again. Gradually, the SUV then drifted back to the center lane. Ernest then pulled up next to the SUV to observe the driver holding a cell phone in her right hand, distorting her view of the righthand lane (Holsendolph, 2002).

Once implemented, "hands free" tried to decrease the number of automobile accidents caused by drivers being distracted while driving. The law specified the use of cell phones while driving and not other distractions that occur every day: applying makeup, eating fast food, shaving, changing the radio or station, and smoking cigarettes. Any of these distractions impairs the driver from having complete control of their car, yet, none are illegal except for the use of cell phones. The law does not state that eating a cheeseburger while driving is equivalent to talking on a cell phone. Still, one hand is needed to hold the cheeseburger, which would be the same hand that would be holding a cell phone while you were talking on it. The same argument could be presented for shaving, applying makeup, smoking, or adjusting the controls of your vehicle. Tom Wheeler, president and CEO of the Cellular Telecommunications and Internet Association concludes, "Any activity a driver engages in, besides the task of driving, has the potential to distract" (as quoted in Hands-free . . . , 2001, p. 19). Driver distractions lead to 20–30 percent of all crashes as estimated by the National Highway Traffic Safety Administration (Hands-free . . . , 2001, p. 19).

Since the introduction of the law, companies have introduced "hands free" kits for talking on cell phones while driving. Earpieces that connect to the phone, and then attach to your ear, are most common. These earpieces must connect to the phone once it rings, causing attention to drift from the road to the preparation of the device. Claudia Copquin of *The New York Times*, said "I don't know what to do first: insert the ear jack or press the talk button?" She also admits that she struggles to keep her eyes on the road when her phone rings, as her head drifts from the road to the phone itself (as quoted in Copquin, 2002). One study showed that hands-free devices do not actually reduce driver distraction (Hands-free . . . , 2001, p. 19). Even with the use of these "hands free" kits, distraction still exists while talking on the phone.

In one test, it was found that there was no significant difference between drivers using hands-free devices and those using hand-held phones (Hands-free . . . , 2001, p. 19). The law states that the driver is to have complete control of their car. The focus of the driver even while being "hands free" is still on the phone call. The drivers' hands may be on the wheel now, but their attention still drifts to the person on the other end of the conversation. David Stayer, a University of Utah psychologist, found that listening and talking on a phone while driving were both distractions (as quoted in Holsendolph, 2002). The person talking to the driver doesn't know what types of conditions the driver is occurring, (weather, road work, and hazards) and doesn't realize the distractions that the driver occurs. Stayer further concluded:

> There is a different quality of communication between two people in a car and people on phones. The people in a car share the awareness of how demanding the driving may be, and they tailor their conversation accordingly, getting quiet if the driver had to do certain maneuvers in busy traffic, and talking more relaxed if they are traveling on a quiet street. (Holsendolph, 2002, p. 1)

"Hands free" was originally implemented to allow a driver to have complete control of his car and to be free of distractions. Free of distractions would imply that nothing interferes with the driver. Stayer says that using cell phones can be dangerous, because talking makes drivers "sluggish" (as quoted in Holsendolph, 2002). University of Utah researchers concluded that the distraction with cell phones is caused by the concentration on the conversation, and not by dialing or holding the phone (Hands-free . . . , 2001, p. 19). If a driver's attention is focused on a phone call, their attention is diverted, endangering not only themselves but other drivers on the road as well. Also, Stayer

claims, "When you're talking, you're impaired" (as quoted in Holsendolph, 2002). The goal of the "hands free" law was to decrease the number of accidents caused by distractive driving: car crashes, pedestrians and animals being hit, and speeding. Yet, all of these accidents still occur due to the drivers' attention still not being focused on the road. A study involving nearly 6,000 Canadians proved that a driver using a cell phone "quadrupled the risk of a collision" (Holsendolph, 2002). The law has managed to ensure that both hands are on the steering wheel at all times, but it has done nothing to ensure that the attention of the driver is on the road at all times.

The mistake that was made when introducing the "hands free" law was the extent to what was considered a distraction while driving. Anything that distracts a driver while driving should be included under the law, not just the banning of talking on a cell phone while driving. The number of car accidents caused due to cell phone use while driving increase daily. Studies have also proven that the use of hands-free phones has made no difference in crash risk compared to the use of hand-held phones. Now, the law must state clearer what is considered distractive, and what should take a "hands free" approach.

References

Copquin, C. G. (2002, September 1). I can't talk now. Call me back! *The New York Times*, p. 17.

Hands-free cell phones distracting: Study finds device no boon to safety. (2001, August 17). *Houston Chronicle*, p. 19.

Holsendolph, E. (2002, January 13). Hand-held? Hands-free? Critics say it doesn't matter—cell phones are not safe to use while driving. *The Atlanta Journal*, p. 1.

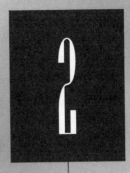

CHAPTER

2

Phase Two of the

Writing Process:

Developing Precise

Sentences

Key Terms

Comma splice   Two independent clauses incorrectly joined by punctuation

Dangling modifier   An introductory phrase that fails to modify its intended antecedent

Mechanics   Marks on the text that standardize text according to manuals or rules of usage (capitalization, italics, apostrophe, hyphen)

Parallelism   Like elements in similar grammatical constructions are coordinated in form

Pronoun agreement   The pronoun and its antecedent reflect each other grammatically

Punctuation   Marks on the text that dictate separation of elements or help clarify meaning (comma, colon, semicolon, dash)

Run-on sentence   Two independent clauses incorrectly joined without punctuation

Sentence fragment   An incomplete thought posing as a complete thought

Subject-verb disagreement   Verbs do not match nouns in number or form

Verb tense shift   Unnecessarily changing verb tense within a sentence or paragraph

Chapter Objectives

On completion of this chapter, the reader should be able to

1. Identify and correct pronoun disagreement.
2. Identify and correct dangling modifiers.
3. Identify nonparallel constructions and create parallel ones that coordinate ideas.
4. Identify verb tense shifts within sentences, paragraphs, or essays and create a unified approach to verb use.
5. Recognize the importance of creating grammatically correct sentences and the formalities of writing such as punctuation and mechanics.
6. Identify and correct basic grammar problems: subject-verb disagreement, comma splice, run-on sentence, and sentence fragment.
7. Demonstrate an ability to use punctuation that promotes clear communication.
8. Recognize that standards exist for mechanics and abide by standards set in style manual.

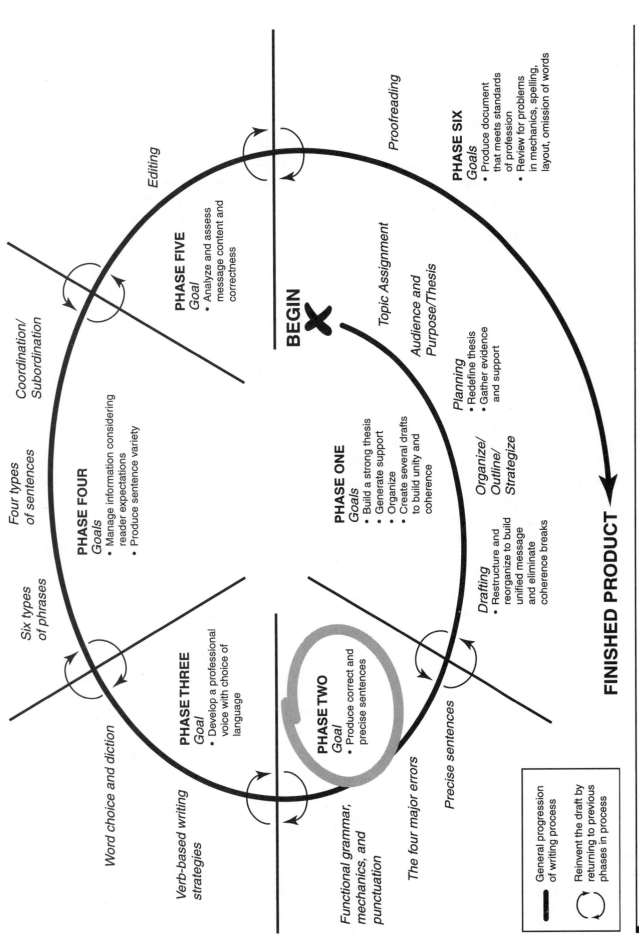

Figure 2–1 The Writing Process: Phase Two

BUILDING AND REFINING SENTENCES

Just as you scrutinized your thoughts in paragraph form in the rough drafts, you will scrutinize your thoughts at the sentence level in this stage of the writing process (see Figure 2-1). Understand that you will spend at least a draft or two on this process, which will take more of your valuable time.

Your first task is to build precise sentences. This process requires that you weed out unnecessary words and phrases, develop parallel structures, coordinate and subordinate appropriate parts of the sentences, and make your sentences concise to create powerful ideas that make an impact on your reader.

After you have developed precise sentences, you will now read through the document to determine whether the sentences you have created are indeed sentences. Here, you will begin to employ some knowledge of grammar and mechanics, but these are functional lessons that will serve you well and that every reader will expect. You cannot afford to embarrass yourself in your profession by not writing in complete sentences or following the standard rules of grammar and usage.

As the essay begins to take shape through the initial drafting process, you can now begin to focus on crafting the paper into a professional document with precise use of sentences and words.

Agreement of Pronouns and Their Antecedents

Pronouns, as you know, take the place of nouns for readability. For example, no one would find the following sentence readable: "The girl pulled the thorn from the girl's foot." Obviously, a better sentence would read: "The girl pulled the thorn from her foot."

As writers create pronouns and their antecedents, they must be conscious of **pronoun agreement** problems that can arise. Most people will recognize that the following has an agreement problem: "The girl pulled the thorn from their foot."

Not every agreement problem is evident, however. Consider the following example:

Each of the girls has (her/their) own desk.

In this case, the subject of the sentence is *Each* and is singular. Therefore, the correct pronoun is *her*. Many people will think that *their* is correct because *girls* is plural. This is not the case. *Girls* is the object of the preposition and not the word to receive a pronoun antecedent.

The following words are singular and take singular antecedents:

each	everybody (one)
every	somebody (one)
none	no one
either	nobody
neither	anybody (one)

Consider the following examples:

Everyone is required to bring *his* or *her* coat.
Neither of the men has *his* book with him.

Take into consideration also the collective nouns that can sometimes confuse.

The team won (its/their) first game.

Either could be correct, depending on whether the team is acting as a unit or as individuals.

Pronoun References

Just as writers need to be cognizant of agreement issues, writers also need to recognize that antecedents may not always clearly reflect the pronoun intended. Sometimes, more than one word could serve as the antecedent.

The student told the nurse that her chart has been misplaced.

In this case, *her* could refer to either the nurse or the student. The meaning is not clear, but it should be to the savvy reader and writer. Here, as in many cases, the pronoun *her* should represent the subject of the sentence (*The student*) instead of the noun that happens to be closest to it (*the nurse*). Rework such sentences for clarity and accuracy.

Other beginning writers use pronouns to represent particular ideas when the particular idea is not clear. For example, many writers will create a lengthy paragraph with various ideas. To make their point, they will wrap up the paragraph with a sentence that begins with "This proves that . . . ." If the paragraph contains several ideas, the reader will not know which concept to attribute to *This*. As a general rule, pronouns should reflect precise terms or words, not refer to a broad idea or concept.

Consider the following example:

She talked endlessly about the operation, and *this* was boring.

This refers to a broad and unclear concept that is not clearly mentioned in the sentence. Try reworking the sentence:

She talked endlessly about the operation, and this blathering was boring.

Consider the problems created in the following by unclear pronoun usage:

When she stuck the needle into his arm, it began to bleed.

Does *it* refer to *needle* or *arm*?

When a woman marries, *you* take on new responsibilities.

If the *woman* takes on the responsibilities, the correct pronoun is *she*.

All those planning to enter the contest should submit *your ballot*.

Probably the writer means *their ballots*.

Exercises

PRONOUNS

■ Choosing the Appropriate Pronoun

Directions: From the options in parentheses, choose the appropriate pronoun in each sentence.

1. All of the employees on the unit believed that (their, his or her) actions were medically necessary.

2. Both the charge nurse and the nurse manager found (their, his or her) schedule too busy to attend to all of the needs of their patients.

3. In the event of an emergency, the therapists understand the procedures to care for (their, his or her) patients.

4. The patient insisted that the technician make copies of the CT scan films and send (it, them) to his doctor.

5. The results of the study provoked debate because of (its, their) controversial nature.

6. Although ovaries produce estrogen, the anterior pituitary gland regulates (its, their) activity.

7. The anterior pituitary produces hormones, and (it, they) effect various biological processes.

8. After discovering that they both had the same disease, the patients discussed (their, his or her) treatment methods, and neither patient could determine the appropriate course of action for (their, his or her) disease.

9. Neither of the doctors decided on (their, his or her) position on the embryonic stem cell issue.

10. Both the doctor and the nurse documented (their, his or her) actions during the surgical procedure.

■ Correcting Pronoun Inconsistencies

Directions: Find and correct any pronoun inconsistencies in the following sentences.

1. The doctor informed his patient that his test results were negative and that he could be discharged from the hospital immediately.

2. The surgical resident was pleased with its outcome and had a positive ending to his day.

3. I injected the patient with a 2-m bolus of lidocaine, and this relaxed the patient.

4. If the results returned insufficient, it would be necessary to repeat the procedure.

5. The doctor, a successful cardiologist, discussed it openly with his neighbors.

6. I informed the patient's daughter of her grave condition and inquired into her wishes for end-of-life care.

7. The chest x-ray films provided by the radiology department demonstrated their role in the diagnosis.

8. The paper reported the results of the new drug, and it discussed many positives to its use.

Identifying and Correcting Dangling Modifiers

A modifier, in the form of a word or group of words, connects to another word or group of words to explain it or them further or to describe. A **dangling modifier** is a group of words that is intended to modify an element of the sentence (usually the subject) but fails to modify the correct word. Consider the following example:

Walking down the street, my ticket appeared in the gutter.

This is a classic example of a dangling modifier because the sentence claims that a ticket was "walking down the street." The phrase *walking down the street* should modify the subject of the sentence, but the subject is *my ticket*. In no way was that ticket walking; consequently, the writer has created a dangling modifier. The sentence should read in the following manner:

Walking down the street, I found my ticket in the gutter.

In this corrected example, *I* is the subject of the sentence that takes on the modification of *walking down the street*.

Consider the meanings indicated by these sentences:

At the age of two, my uncle took me for a plane ride.

Your uncle was talented at age two.

Hearing the alarm, the hospital's hallways were cleared.

The hospital hears the alarm.

Using an antidepressant, Dr. Jones was able to treat the patient.

Dr. Jones used an antidepressant.

After 6 hours of labor, Dr. Jones delivered the baby.

Dr. Jones labored for 6 hours.

Exercises

DANGLING MODIFIERS

■ Exercise Set 1

Directions: Use the example provided to revise the following sentences.

EXAMPLE: Believing what the labels and advertisements say, their minds believe it to be true and trick their body into thinking the same.

The writer should ask himself or herself the following: Whose mind believes?

For correct revision of the sentence, the implicit and explicit subjects must be identical.

REVISION: As people believe what the labels and advertisement say, they believe the information on the label or in the advertisements to be true and trick their bodies into thinking the same.

1. The results of the test underwent extensive reviews, thus finding some cause of the flaw.
2. Having finished the chores, the television was turned on.
3. Realizing the need for more time, the agency delayed its decision.
4. Further comparative studies were conducted, hoping to find the most efficient method.
5. On the achievement of higher degrees in physical therapy, direct access is being considered.
6. Realizing the need for more practice, weekend schedules were implemented.
7. After reading the study, the article remains unconvincing.
8. By receiving intercessory prayer, their minds believe they will achieve healthiness.

■ Exercise Set 2

Directions: Correct all sentences containing dangling modifiers.

1. The patient's left leg measured 2 inches larger than the right, caused by the accident.
2. Having declared an emergency situation, the charge nurse ordered the removal of the patients from the unit.
3. To easily remove the dressing, sterile water was poured onto the wound.
4. Discovered in the closet, the nurse used the Kelly clamps to secure the drainage tube and stabilize the patient.

5. On the IV pole that I had found on the floor upstairs, I hung the saline solution.

6. During manual muscle tests, the patient's right shoulder demonstrated less strength than the left, resulting from the trauma.

7. After reading the chart, the patient was put on strict "npo" status by the physician.

8. Due to his progress in therapy, the therapist recommended Mr. Smythe's discharge.

9. Following an insulin injection, the nurse recorded a low blood glucose reading on the patient.

10. Resulting from prolonged exposure to second-hand smoke, the doctor diagnosed the patient with lung cancer.

11. Due to an increased dosage of anesthesia, the nurse believed the patient felt better.

12. During the surgery, the anesthesiologist nearly administered 3 units of O positive blood.

13. I instructed the patient to do only 10 repetitions of each exercise prescribed by the therapist.

14. After running multiple tests, the laboratory reported the patient's blood pH at 7.5 almost.

15. While preparing the settings on the ventilator, the respiratory therapist only set the VIO$_2$ at 80%.

16. The heart monitor nearly registered the patient in bradycardia for 5 minutes.

17. Following examination by the doctor on call, the patient was admitted almost with a 3-inch-diameter wound.

18. The patient swiftly attempted to rehabilitate from the surgery and, as a result, aggravated the injury.

19. Admitted to the emergency room for dehydration, the patient received an IV saline solution that the nurse hung for over 3 hours.

20. The patient bravely and willingly accepted the diagnosis and treatment options.

21. The wound indicated the extent of the accident, obviously beyond repair.

Developing Parallel Structure (Coordination of Ideas)

Writing for your profession often requires establishing equality between ideas for clarity.

To create such equality, or coordination, use parallel grammatical constructions.

In any sentence where similar ideas are expressed, be sure to employ **parallelism**, or parallel structure, for that grammatical sequence. That is, match nouns with nouns, verbs with verbs, prepositions with prepositions, and so on.

EXAMPLE: At camp, our students like *to bike* and *to fish*.

Notice that the italicized words are parallel because they are both infinitives. The following example is incorrect because the elements are not parallel:

At camp, our students like fishing and to bike.

To correct this problem in parallel structure, change *to bike* to *biking*.

To make sentences parallel, writers often repeat words as needed to reinforce parallelism. This usually occurs in longer sentences in which the item modified is obscured.

EXAMPLES

Acceptable: The instructor wants to meet those students who play rugby and organize a team.

Better: The instructor wants to meet those students who play rugby and *to* organize a team.

Acceptable: He thought that the economic conditions were improving and the company was planning to increase dividends.

Better: He thought that the economic conditions were improving and *that* the company was planning to increase dividends.

Exercise

PARALLEL STRUCTURE

Directions: Examine the following sentences and correct the problems in parallel structure.

1. I have an apple and pear.

2. In the group were a carpenter, locksmith, a painter, and plumber.

3. I am hot, tired, and I wish I had something cool to drink.

4. She hoped to fly to Buffalo and that she could rent a car there.

5. My friend can tutor students who need help in English and lead orientation sessions.

6. Some examples include becoming sensitive to pain, destructive, and depressed.

7. Towards females, the media portray Barbie doll-like women as successful in life and can achieve anything.

8. The methods help you achieve a state of mind, not cure illnesses.

9. Treatment will include the use of a hot pack, various stretching techniques, aerobic activity on a stationary bike, and conclude with ice on the back of his neck.

10. The exercises will help him keep the muscles loose, flexible, and eventually recover full range of motion.

Eliminating Unnecessary Verb Tense Shifts

Verb tense shifts are created by failure of the writer to maintain a consistent time frame with his or her choice of words. In other words, a writer may report some information in a paper in the present tense, and then, for no reason, begin discussing other information by using the past tense. Such a shift will confuse the audience by asking the reader to manage time changes that are not significant to the meaning of the text.

Most often, writers fail to recognize the appropriate verb tense to use when they write about the works of others or when they discuss research. As a general rule, when writing about literature or any other publication, use the present tense. Literature exists in a continual present. This means that a reader can pick up the document today and read it to gather information; a reader can pick up the same document ten years from now, read it, and gain the same message or information. For example, if discussing the impact of *The Adventures of Huckleberry Finn* on modern American literature, a writer might use the following:

> Twain presents Huck as a noble savage, and this archetypal character resurfaces in most American novels that followed as authors champion the underdog.

For managing issues in the historical past, a writer may be tempted to use the past tense. Past tense is not appropriate in discussing the written word. Indeed, Twain wrote the novel over the course of time, and it was published in 1884. If we were discussing an act that Twain performed, then we might consider using the word *presented*. However, the impact of Twain's writing extends far beyond 1884 or the days leading up to the publication date. We study Twain today as others would have in the late nineteenth century. Consequently, his words and ideas have the same impact now as they did then and require a present-tense verb.

Furthermore, the discussion of the works of other authors in the twentieth and twenty-first centuries maintains the present-tense verbs for the same reasons. It would be awkward to attempt to shift verb tenses in the middle of this sentence because Twain's act preceded the other authors' acts. Furthermore, the impact of Twain's writing is still being felt. Consequently, the present tense should be applied:

> Twain presents Huck as a noble savage, and this archetypal character resurfaced in most American novels that followed as authors championed the underdog.

This example, however, could be acceptable if the discussion focused on the changes in American literature over time. In other words, Twain's effects have stopped being felt. To show a shift from the past to the present, the writer might consider using a past-tense verb to dictate the end of the era.

Science writers experience a different set of problems. They often discuss the works of others to establish a research foundation, and consequently, they should hold to the rule: Use present tense when discussing the writing of someone else. However, in most articles written for the medical profession, the authors discuss the experiments that they performed in the past and relate this information to their findings. These experiments were organized and applied at a time in the past and will require a past-tense verb. Consequently, when discussing the actions of someone that occurred in the past, use past tense; when discussing the writing of someone else, use present tense.

Such a verb tense shift in the following example is acceptable and expected. Words in *italics* indicate present forms; underlined words indicate past:

> Although experts have proved electrical stimulation (ES) effective for use on muscles, many therapists *do not perform* ES therapy. Studies *show* that ES in combination with traditional therapy *increases* muscle mass in unutilized limbs, allowing the patient to regain control over gait patterns earlier than with conventional therapy alone. Weiler and Stein measured the effects of ES on the walking ability of patients with spinal cord injuries and demonstrated that different injuries responded to ES therapy in varying degrees. Their experiment *indicates* that ES is effective for various injuries.

Exercise

VERB TENSE SHIFTS

Directions: In the following sample essay, mark the unnecessary shifts in verb tense.

> Throughout the course of reading the short story "The Story of an Hour," the reader begins to wonder what traits make up the character of Mrs. Mallard. Her character is mysterious and peculiar. She experienced several emotions that can be interpreted differently by different people. The author wrote in such a manner that leaves the reader asking questions about Mrs. Mallard's character.
>
> The story begins with an element of foreshadowing. The reader is told that Mrs. Mallard has heart trouble. This statement leads the reader to believe that, later in the story, Mrs. Mallard's physical ailment will be a factor. When Mrs. Mallard hears the news of her husband's death, she cries uncontrollably in the arms of her sister and retreated to her bedroom. Then, a look of intelligent thought came over her face. She reflected on life without her husband and thought about the possibilities of her new freedoms. Such ambiguity in this situation forces the reader to interpret the relationship between her husband and she. Later, a force came and "takes over" Mrs. Mallard. She could have been feeling guilt for feeling freedom.

FUNCTIONAL GRAMMAR, PUNCTUATION, AND MECHANICS

After you have cleared unnecessary and awkward errors from your work in the first part of this stage of the writing process, you will now read through the document to determine if the sentences you have created are indeed sentences. Here, you will begin to employ some knowledge of grammar, punctuation, and mechanics, but these are functional lessons that will serve to meet the standards expected by your audience. You cannot afford to embarrass yourself in your profession by not writing in complete sentences.

The Four Major Errors: Subject-Verb Disagreement, Comma Splices, Run-On (Fused) Sentences, and Sentence Fragments

Nothing is more damaging to a document or paper than simple grammatical incorrectness. Often, readers will become frustrated with a writer's inconsistencies and inaccuracies and lose concentration on the message. In some cases, the errors cannot be ignored because the grammatical incorrectness creates drastic problems in the basic elements of written communication. Not only do these major errors distract your reader, but they also send messages about your education, training, or commitment to details. Incomplete sentences often tell an educated audience that you, as a writer, were not trained to understand the simple construction mechanisms of sentences. This may not be true, but the reader can judge your credibility only by the document you present.

Everyone who reads this text was trained to recognize complete sentences and to create agreement between subjects and verbs but, over time, may have failed to put that knowledge into practice. Without practice, the ability to recognize such problems may be lost. Creating major errors in building sentences tells your reader that you did not receive such an education (which is not true), that you have lost that knowledge, or that you do not care to demonstrate your knowledge in this area. In any case, you are sending the wrong message to your reader. Your reader may now decide that you lack practical education or that you are not detail oriented. Anyone in today's competitive market would not want to be labeled in such a manner.

Ultimately, people judge you by your presentation of ideas. Consequently, successful professionals formulate relationships with people who operate on equal intellectual planes. If coworkers or patients believe you are not professional in your actions, you will have a short career or an unfulfilling one. Learn these simple grammatical rules and avoid the four major errors.

Subject-Verb Disagreement

Subjects and verbs must match in number (singular or plural) and person (first, second, and third), and they must match in any independent or dependent clause in which they exist. If they do not, these constructions create an unforgivable error termed **subject-verb disagreement**. Usually, most writers will not have difficulty making subjects and verbs agree. Most if not all of us recognize that the following sentences are incorrect:

The people runs down the street.
The book were not convincing.

We know that *people run* and that *the book was*.

In some cases, however, the subject and the verb are separated or hidden from each other, but the mistake is the same: subject-verb disagreement. Follow the set of instructions to learn the troublesome constructions and how to fix or avoid them.

- Recognizing Plural and Singular Nouns

  The *data are* accurate. The *datum is* accurate.
  Rickets *is* [not *are*, because it is one disease] not contagious.

- Collective Nouns

  The class *wants* a vacation. The class members *want* a vacation.
  The crew (sails/sail) the ship. [They *sail* or it *sails*, depending on your intent.]

- Separating Subjects from Verbs with Phrases or Clauses

  To avoid embarrassing subject-verb disagreements, find the subject of the sentence and the verb connected to it for every sentence you write. Make them agree without allowing any intervening words to confuse you or your reader. In the following examples, the subjects of the sentences are italicized. Notice how phrases intervening between the subject and the verb can create uncertainty with subject-verb agreement.

  A panel of experts (agree/agrees) that this procedure is best.
  The charts containing the problems of the patient (was/were) placed on the nurse's desk.
  The patient as well as her family members (consents/consent) to the treatment.
  Cancer of the lung, along with cancer of the skin and breast, (is/are) treatable.
  Sometimes, *the contributions* of a person to human progress (remain/remains) unknown.

- Subject Placed after Verb

  There (is/are) several reasons for this mistake.
  In the group (was/were) a carpenter, a painter, a locksmith, and a plumber.

- Compound Subjects

  Compound subjects usually require a plural verb. Consider substituting the word "they" for the compound subject and then connect subject and verb:

  Correctness and precision (is/are) requirements of good writing.
  (They) are requirements of good writing.

  In other cases, the "compound" subject may not actually be compound. Often, the word *the* will unify the compound subject into a singular subject. Consider the following example:

  The correctness and precision of the document (make/makes) it easy to read.

  In this case, *The correctness and precision* refers to a singular attribute of the document. Read the subject as "It," and use "makes." This, however, is an unusual case. When in doubt, throw it out and start the sentence over.

- Indefinite Pronouns and Adjectives as Subjects

Each, every, none, either, and *neither,* as well as *everybody* (*everyone*) and *anybody* (*anyone*), all are singular. To solve this dilemma, as in the previous examples, read each sentence with the word "one" after the subject, and eliminate words between the subject and the verb.

> *Every* nurse, doctor, and hospital employee (need/needs) to sign the document.
>
> Every (one) needs . . .
>
> *Each* of the administrators (has/have) an agenda.
>
> Each (one) has . . .
>
> *Either* of you (is/are) fit for the job.
>
> Either (one) is . . .

"None" may be singular or plural. Consider the object of the preposition:

> None of the candidates (is/are) competent.

- Either . . . Or and Neither . . . Nor

Singular subjects require a singular verb, but a sentence containing both a singular subject and a plural subject creates a problem, solved by applying the following rule: The verb agrees with the closer subject.

> Either the nurse or the doctors were at fault.
>
> Neither the administrators nor the board of trustees has seen the document.
>
> Neither my colleagues nor I am going to the luncheon.

Comma Splices, Run-On Sentences, and Sentence Fragments

Before launching into a discussion about comma splices, run-on sentences, and sentence fragments, we need to incorporate some terminology that will help clarify parts of sentences. Such clarification will establish the strategy to avoid major errors.

Independent clause: A complete thought containing a subject and a verb

> I never had the ambition to work in the field.

Independent clauses are sentences. They can stand alone because they contain a subject and a verb and they create a complete thought.

Dependent clause: A group of words that may contain a subject and a verb but does not express a complete thought

> Although I wanted to work in the field, I never had the ambition to do it.

Dependent clauses are not sentences and therefore cannot stand alone. They must be connected to an independent clause in order to exist.

Comma Splices

A **comma splice** is composed of two or more independent clauses joined only by comma.

> Health professionals must now collect payment for services rendered, they must also provide clear documentation to do so.

In this example, *Health professionals must now collect payment for services rendered* is an independent clause. It can stand alone because it creates a complete thought through its subject and verb. The second part of this example, *they must also provide clear documentation to do so,* is also an independent clause. It too can stand alone, because it creates a complete thought with its subject and verb.

This construction becomes grammatically "illegal" when two independent clauses are connected by a comma. Basic grammatical instruction will tell you to separate these independent clauses with a period. A document that failed to separate sentences with a terminal mark of punctuation would lead to communication chaos.

Although the period is the logical means to connect these independent clauses, other means exist. Consider the following:

Three Ways to Join Independent Clauses — and to Correct the Comma Splice

- Period + capital letter on next sentence opener

> Health professionals must now collect payment for services rendered. They must also provide clear documentation to do so.

- Comma + coordinating conjunction (*and, but, or*) [Sometimes *for, so,* and *yet* are used as conjunctions, but these are used in informal constructions. Professional writers should be concerned with formal constructions and use *and, but,* and *or* as the standard coordinating conjunctions.]

> Health professionals must now collect payment for services rendered, and they must also provide clear documentation to do so.

- Semicolon

If two independent clauses express two closely related thoughts, use a semicolon to connect the independent clauses. Stylistically, this move will tell your reader that you recognize that the constructions are independent clauses, but you want to convey the message that these independent clauses should be considered together or closely connected. Likewise, the independent clauses might be closely connected in their presentation of ideas, but the writer needs to employ a transitional word or phrase to clearly connect the ideas. In this case, connect the independent clauses with a semicolon before using a conjunctive or transitional adverb, such as *however*, *therefore*, or *consequently* (see list later on). These transitional elements are not conjunctions but are used in a similar fashion. Coordinating conjunctions require a comma; conjunctive adverbs require a semicolon. Some examples follow:

> Health professionals must now collect payment for services rendered; they must also provide clear documentation to do so.
>
> Health professionals must now collect payment for services rendered; however, they must also provide clear documentation to do so.

Note: Some writers may want to begin a standard independent clause with a transitional adverb. Although this has generally been accepted, it is stylistically weak for a formal paper. If you know the rules, employ them.

The following is a list of other transitional or conjunctive adverbs. Use a semicolon before these for effective connections between independent clauses.

however	consequently
then	hence
therefore	moreover
thus	accordingly

Be careful not to confuse independent clauses with compound elements of a sentence. Doing so may cause you to insert unnecessary commas. Notice the lack of punctuation after the coordinating conjunctions in the following examples. These are compound elements, not two independent clauses, joined by coordinating conjunctions:

> The room was blue and yellow.
> The maniac blocked the elevator and pulled the fire alarm.
> He drove up the coast and into Maine.

When two independent clauses are joined, you must use a comma:

> He drove up the coast, and he drove into Maine.

Notice that the insertion of *he* makes the latter part of the original sentence an independent clause, because it now contains a subject and a verb, which together create a complete thought.

As a general rule, when revising for grammatical correctness, look for coordinating conjunctions and perform this test. Cover the coordinating conjunction and all the words following it. If it creates a sentence, you have an independent clause. Perform the same test by covering the coordinating conjunction and the words before it. If you have another independent clause, you are required to insert a comma.

EXAMPLE 1:

The maniac blocked the elevator ~~and pulled the fire alarm~~.

This is an independent clause.

~~The maniac blocked the elevator and~~ pulled the fire alarm.

This is not an independent clause. No comma is required.

EXAMPLE 2:

Health professionals must now collect payment for services rendered and they must also provide clear documentation to do so.

Is a comma required after "rendered"?

Health professionals must now collect payment for services rendered ~~and they must also provide clear documentation to do so~~.

This is an independent clause.

~~Health professionals must now collect payment for services rendered and~~ they must also provide clear documentation to do so.

This too is an independent clause. You now have two independent clauses joined by a coordinating conjunction. You are required to include the comma before the conjunction.

Note: This rule can be relaxed if the independent clauses are both short and closely connected. Eliminating the comma in such constructions may be desirable if the reader aims for continuity.

CORRECTED VERSION: Health professionals must now collect payment for services rendered, and they must also provide clear documentation to do so.

Run-On Sentences

A **run-on sentence** is formed by joining together two or more independent clauses without using punctuation or a conjunction. To an objective and intelligent reader, this mistake leads to confusion.

Use the same rules for joining independent clauses as discussed in the preceding section on comma splices to fix the following sentences:

Health professionals must provide documentation to receive payment for services insurance companies require it.

Sharks contain cartilage they do not have a bone in their bodies.

These two examples demonstrate a lack of understanding of sentence structure and are representative of communication chaos.

Sentence Fragments

A **sentence fragment** is an incomplete sentence punctuated as a complete sentence. It is often the result of a missing subject or verb, or of combining words that do not create a complete thought.

Following are examples of missing subjects and verbs. These errors should be caught easily by careful proofreading.

A broken, leaning schoolhouse standing in a field.

This example is missing a verb. The schoolhouse has to *do* something.

Was standing in a field with broken shutters and doors.

This example is missing a subject. *What* was standing in a field?

Other types of fragments are created when we borrow from our conversational voices and take mental shortcuts to communicate. These examples you will find in informal passages:

She wanted to go back to college. *Although she did not complete her schooling.*

We left the auditorium early to beat the traffic. *Because he had seen the demonstration before and did not need to see it again.*

The receiver caught the pass and ran 80 yards to the end zone. *And I thought the game was over.*

In each of these cases, the italicized groups of words are sentence fragments, not because they do not contain subjects and verbs; instead, they are fragments because the initial words indicate that the following words are connected to another complete thought. In fact, most sentence fragments are dependent clauses masquerading as sentences, but we know, as a grammatical rule, that a dependent clause cannot stand on its own. It is *dependent*, meaning that it depends on something else in order for it to exist. It depends on an independent clause.

To solve this problem, look for trigger words that indicate dependency. We also know that *and* is a coordinating conjunction, and it must "coordinate" two like elements. Consequently, *and* and the other coordinating conjunctions (*but, or*) cannot start sentences. When they do, they are the culprits that create sentence fragments.

Consider ways to correct the following fragments:

EXAMPLE: I liked working in the office as an assistant. Although I didn't like getting paid less money to do the same work.

REVISION: Although I didn't like getting paid less money to do the same work, I liked working in the office as an assistant.

EXAMPLE: No need to explain.

REVISION: You have no need to explain.

Many people will read these examples and claim that they see this type of mistake often—

in newspapers, magazines, or other print forms or on television, They do indeed exist, and they appear too often. That is the problem: Because they appear frequently, many people begin to accept them as the standard. Just because they are used (misused) often does not make them right.

Ultimately, comma splices, run-on sentences, and subject-verb disagreements are not used regularly or used in convention because they create huge gaps in reasoning and disrupt the communication process. Sentence fragments, however, have been used for stylistic purposes because they represent the way most people talk. When you write, you are not talking. Writing requires precision and accuracy, because when you put words on paper, your reader can analyze and scrutinize them for exact meaning. If you fail to communicate, you have not accomplished your purpose. Speaking, on the other hand, is the form of communication that is less permanent. Words you hear are more difficult to scrutinize, and as a result, speakers can "get away" with inaccuracies and vague language because they will expect the listeners to piece together the puzzle. As a writer, you do not have that luxury. You will want to create exact and precise language that cannot be confused or misinterpreted.

Consider the work of the television journalist and the print journalist. Television journalists may make outrageous statements, sometimes with little repercussion. A print journalist, however, is often heavily scrutinized by his or her readership. Letters to the editor appear frequently in newspapers, magazines, and journals because the readers have taken the time to closely analyze the language and have made clear judgments about what was communicated. The message and the language used to communicate that message become the target. This is the result of the more permanent nature of writing, allowing close scrutiny for errors. Writers must be clear and precise; otherwise, their message will not reach its audience, or their message will be misinterpreted.

The reader is not at fault if he or she misinterprets the message; the writer is.

Exercise

THE FOUR MAJOR ERRORS

Directions: For each of the following sentences or groups of words, make sure each is grammatically correct.

1. Every one of the professional golfers donate their time to charity.
2. When I watch television, desires to look like the actresses fills my mind.
3. The young viewers never see behind the scenes, they only witness the final product.
4. Although he had been well recommended by his former employer.
5. The mission is dedicated to serving the following countries; China and Guatemala.
6. The driver spotted the car, therefore, she avoided the crash.
7. Some of the collection was not sold.
8. Acquiring alcohol as a teen is easy they have someone buy it for them.
9. The officer, climbing out of his check-station and taking out his pencil and book.
10. The more things change; inevitably, the more they stay the same.
11. In the group was science, English, foreign language, and the health professions professors.

Punctuation Rules and Correct Sentences

This section provides information in list form for easy reference. Learn these **punctuation** rules and apply them to your work. If you are ever unsure of your practices, refer to these pages and make the correct decisions.

Rules of Grammar and Punctuation for Connecting Independent and Dependent Clauses

- Commas are required to separate independent clauses. Commas are not used to separate coordinate elements of a sentence such as modifiers or phrases.

EXAMPLES

We must provide clear documentation to receive payment for services, and we must do so because insurance companies require it.

I have always wanted to work in the field but never had the motivation to do it.

* Commas are used to separate introductory dependent clauses from the independent clause.

EXAMPLE: Although I wanted to work in the field, I never had the ambition to do it.

* Commas are used to separate items in a series, and the comma before the coordinating conjunction MUST be present.

EXAMPLE: I make coffee, toast, and cereal for breakfast.

* Commas SHOULD be used to separate introductory prepositional phrases from the independent clause. Some grammar texts will allow you to omit the comma as an option. You will never be wrong if you include it. Play it safe and include it.

EXAMPLE: In the morning, I make coffee for breakfast.

Restrictive and Nonrestrictive Phrases and Clauses: That *versus* Which

Successful writers can recognize the correct usage of *that* versus *which* to introduce phrases and clauses. The general rule is as follows:

* *That* indicates that the phrase or clause following it is restrictive and therefore requires no comma.
* *Which* indicates that the phrase or clause is nonrestrictive and requires either a set of commas or a single comma if at the end of the sentence.

Examine the following sentences and observe how meaning changes with the use of *that* and *which*.

EXAMPLE Using *that*

The computer that is broken is in the equipment closet.

In this example, the writer wants the reader to understand that more than one computer is in the equipment closet, and the one that is broken is under consideration.

EXAMPLE Using *which*

The computer, which is broken, is in the equipment closet.

In this case, the message the writer intends to send is that the computer is in the equipment closet, and, incidentally, it is broken. Only one computer exists in the frame of reference of the reader and the writer. The fact that it is broken is incidental to the intended meaning of the sentence. As a result, this information (being broken) is set off, appropriately, by commas and introduced with *which*.

To apply the general rule stated earlier, cover the information if you think you should use *which*, and then read the sentence. If the sentence maintains its meaning, use *which* and a comma. If the sentence cannot be completed because you have covered the information that helps the sentence communicate its meaning, use *that*.

Exercise

THAT VERSUS *WHICH*; ESSENTIAL VERSUS NONESSENTIAL

Directions: Insert the appropriate word, *that* or *which*, into the following examples using the information provided earlier.

1. Please help me with my duffle bag _____ is third in line.

2. The stewardess helped me stow my duffle bag _____ I had brought with me on the trip.

3. After much searching, we found a store _____ sells authentic Scottish kilts.

4. After much searching, we found the liquor store _____ was selling gin at a discount.

5. I am walking because I own only one car _____ is now being repaired.

Rules of Semicolon Usage

- Semicolons are used to connect two independent clauses that are not connected by a coordinating conjunction. These sentences should be closely related.

    EXAMPLE: I finished my exam early; it was easy.

- Semicolons connect independent clauses that are joined together by a conjunctive or transitional adverb.

    EXAMPLES

    I finished my exam early; however, no one else in the class did.

    I finished my exam early; consequently, I think I failed it.

- Semicolons can also be used to separate elements of a sentence that have heavy internal punctuation. These are usually items in a series that are internally punctuated.

    EXAMPLE: We went to Niagara Falls, New York; Niagara Falls, Ontario; and then to Niagara-on-the-Lake, Ontario.

- Use a semicolon to separate an independent clause joined by a coordinating conjunction if the sentence is heavy with internal punctuation.

    EXAMPLE: Although we traveled around the Niagara peninsula, becoming tired, which caused me to doze off, we finally arrived at the aquarium with Jim, Donna, and Fred's two sisters, Jane and Jean; but we regained our energy at the winery.

Rules of Colon Usage

Do not confuse the roles of colons (:) and semicolons (;). A semicolon divides two complete sentences; a colon separates a complete sentence from an explanatory element, usually a list. The colon, however, should never be used in formal writing unless a complete sentence precedes it.

- Use a colon to introduce a list after a complete sentence.

    EXAMPLE: The gift basket was filled with the following: oranges, chocolates, and crackers.

    INCORRECT: The gift basket was filled with: oranges, chocolates, and crackers.

- Use a colon to clarify a previous statement.

    EXAMPLE: We could perform only one procedure: radical surgery.

If you use a colon to introduce a list or explanatory phrase that is a complete sentence, be sure the first word in the sentence is capitalized. Incomplete sentences or lists, as noted previously, will not take capitalization.

    EXAMPLE: We could perform only one procedure: We would remove the limb.

- Use a colon to introduce a direct quote after a complete sentence.

    EXAMPLE: Jones recommends that we use three procedures: "To treat a cold, give the patient fluids, rest, and antihistamines."

- Use a colon in the following specific cases:
    - Salutation of a business letter   Dear Dr. Jones:
    - Time   7:15 A.M.
    - Biblical verses   Genesis 2:1
    - To separate titles and subtitles   "The Nagging Cough: A Disturbing Trend in Sleep Disorders"

Rules of Comma Usage

Use a comma . . .

- Between independent clauses linked by a coordinating conjunction:

    I built the deck next to the house, and the wind toppled a tree onto it.

- To set off introductory phrases and clauses:

    A. Long, introductory prepositional phrases:

    Before making any assessments of the patient's condition, try performing this test.

    Exception: You have the option to set off short, introductory prepositional phrases:

    In the closet, I left my coat. *OR* In the closet I left my coat.

    B. Introductory dependent clauses:

    When I learned the price of the prescription, I realized that I could not afford it.

    C. Introductory participial phrases:

    Suffering from lung disease, the people in the emergency room coughed and wheezed.

Note: Do NOT use a comma to set off intro-ductory gerund phrases:

> Seeing the starving people encouraged many to move their families out of Ireland.

D. Introductory infinitive phrases:

> To appreciate the size of freighters, you should visit Port Dalhousie.

E. Absolute phrases:

> The rain having stopped, the people began to exit their shelters.

F. Introductory words:

> Initially, the group protested, and eventually, they revisited the issue.
>
> However, the plane arrived on time.
>
> Consequently, we finished the report and went home.

- To separate elements in a series:

> I went to the store and bought milk, bread, and eggs.

- To separate coordinate modifiers:

> The clear, smooth finish of the table reflects my image.

- To set off nonrestrictive phrases and clauses:

A. Dependent clauses:

> The registrar, who had to give me the schedule, is not in her office.

B. Nonrestrictive participial phrases:

> Michael's car, parked on the street, will receive a ticket soon.

C. Nonrestrictive appositive phrases:

> Janelle, coauthor of this chapter, provided me with several examples.

- To set off parenthetical elements:

> Terraforming Mars, I am convinced, is necessary.

- In comparative/contrastive constructions:

> We are naive, not stupid.

- With interjections:

> Oh, I can't believe she said that!

- With direct address:

> The new contract proposal, ladies and gentle-men, is not legally binding.

- With direct quotations:

> Jones claims, "The real evidence of indigenous groups can never be discovered."

- With tag questions:

> You can't defend him in court, can you?

- With dates, addresses, and numbers:

> About 110,000 people have lived at 15 Center Street, Tempe, Arizona 97401, since Monday, April 4, 1960.

- To prevent misreading:

> Inside, the cave was filled with bats.

Exercises

COMMAS

■ Commas with Nonessential Elements

Directions: Consider the use of commas with nonessential words, phrases, or clauses to make any necessary corrections in the following sentences.

1. Slee Hall the recently completed fine arts building is acoustically perfect.
2. The toy that I wanted to buy is no longer available.
3. Dr. Jones decided however that this proce-dure was best.
4. The Genesee River which flows north into Lake Ontario flows through the city of Rochester and is used to make beer.
5. Watching the mouse intently the cat crouched in the grass.
6. Mark Twain, one of America's greatest story-tellers, worked as editor of the *Courier Express.*

■ Commas with Introductory Elements

Directions: Identify the introductory element in each sentence and apply the appropriate mark of punctuation.

1. As my fishing line tightened the reel began to scream.
2. Having changed her major Kara had to enroll in biochemistry.
3. Consequently she now has time to meet me for lunch.

4. Changing her major has been a positive experience for her.

5. When she was in high school she did not know what career path she should choose.

6. To gain a full understanding of the program Kara met with faculty members.

7. To make a lot of money has been his goal.

■ Commas in a Sample Student Essay

Directions: Read the following student essay. Then identify the problems in punctuation and offer suggestions for revision.

One of the most common neurological disorders, Parkinson's disease affects both men and women and the disease most often develops after the age of 50. A cause of Parkinson's disease includes the progressive deterioration of the nerve cells of the portion of the brain that controls muscle movement. The brain normally produces dopamine a substance used by cells to transmit impulses. The degeneration of the brain reduces the amount of dopamine available to the body. An insufficient amount of dopamine disturbs the balance between this substance and other transmitters such as acetylcholine. Resulting from the insufficient amount of dopamine a loss of muscle function creates an inability of the nerve cells to properly transmit messages. The reason for deterioration of these cells remains unknown. The disorder may affect one or both sides of the body, with varying degrees of loss of function. To help minimize the degree of functional loss for a patient without Parkinson's the stretching and manipulating of muscles can be helpful; consequently this research aims to determine whether physical therapy can assist Parkinson's patients in maintaining their current muscle strength. A physical therapist can aid the patient in maintaining the muscle that she possesses.

Physical therapy undertakes a significant role in the muscle maintenance of a Parkinson's patient and it uses active and passive exercise, gait training, practice in normal activities, hot or cold treatments, water therapy and electrical stimulation. To stretch and manipulate the patient's muscles the therapist uses passive exercises and the range of motion [ROM], coordination, and speed of the patient improve by active exercises. In order to maintain ROM and lessen abnormal posture physical therapists should teach Parkinson's patients useful relaxation techniques. Preliminary research regarding Parkinson's patients indicates that physical therapy intervention is unlikely to permanently reverse the rigidity which is directly affected by the nervous system.

Physical therapy plays a significant role in patient education. During physical therapy the therapist must emphasize the importance of self-relaxation to reduce rigidity and to apply the patient's remaining postural response methods by encouraging them to subconsciously practice correct posture voluntarily. Physical therapy would be a practical way to teach patients methods in which they can compensate for the physical weaknesses associated with the disease and the therapists demonstrate methods that reduce the potential for the impairments to return. When relaxation techniques and strengthening exercises are assigned by the physical therapist the patient reduces rigidity and maintains a stable ROM and he decreases atypical posture and encourages musculoskeletal change. Using relaxation methods first allows the therapist to develop the intervention to active mobility and stretching once the patient becomes facile with self-relaxation.

To achieve mobility throughout each segment of the spine the therapist encourages exercises. The following experiment presents an explanation for physical therapy in identifying the provisions that eventually result in disability and immobility. Our team of researchers, Jones, Davies and Scott conducted an experiment with 20 out-patients, affected with the Parkinson's disease to determine the importance of strengthening exercises and to conclude the degree of ease that the exercises provided the patients to help change their body position. The test group consisted of 12 males and 8 females ranging from the age of 64 to 83 years of age. Motor training for the patient various exercises repeated 5–10 times, twice a week for 5 consecutive weeks included mobilization exercises for the trunk, upper and lower limbs, and the individual divisions of the spine. To rectify movement and rid the patient of atypical posture the therapist practiced the previously listed exercises. The results of the study showed a general improvement in all exercises performed in all but four patients the reason 4 of the original 20, patients failed to improve has not been determined.

New research addressing musculoskeletal detriments, by the therapist, allows the patient to gain sufficient ROM for automatic movements which permits the therapist to focus on balance impairments. A Parkinson's patient's ability to successfully survive everyday activities of reaching, dressing and being jostled in a crowd centers on the patient's capability to weight shift and to balance. Patients with gait impediments demonstrated significant improvement when performing exercises of standing balance and weight shifting. Implicated in essential activities gait patterns require the ability to move in a continuous and slow motion, composed weight shifts and changes in the direction of movement.

A recent article presented two case studies which were conducted according to the intervention described above depicting the early treatment of patient's with Parkinson's disease. One of the two cases involved one man not taking medication for Parkinson's disease and a second man receiving medication for the disease. In case one a man age 67, experienced impaired balance and difficulty with functional movements. He was referred to physical therapy for the necessary exercises to delay the intervention of pharmacology. Treating the individual for 1 month three sessions each week for approximately 1 hour each time, made it possible for the ROM of his limb to nearly return to its original measurement. The second case involved a man age 68 and he initially experienced a tremor in his right hand and gait complications. He chose to receive a medication that reduces rigidity and assists him in contending with the disease. His symptoms at the time of physical therapy intervention, included balance complications and poor functional difficulties. Case two patient attended physical therapy for 6 weeks three sessions per week and 1 hour per session these treatments concentrated on gait and functional activities. When 6 weeks of physical therapy were completed his everyday functional activities and his gait improved.

In light of the literature that was previously reviewed we can assume that this disease needs to continue to be studied and researchers must determine the necessity of physical therapy for Parkinson's patients. The experiments conducted by researchers demonstrated the importance of physical therapy in maintaining the muscle that she possesses and they prove that strengthening and manipulating muscles can help to minimize the degree of loss of function for the patient.

■ Punctuation Reading for Rules of Comma Usage

Directions: The following passage abides by the rules of comma usage listed in this chapter. Read the writing sample and identify the rules governing each comma insertion.

In light of the research, physical therapy helps Parkinson's patients maintain the muscle that he possesses, and this can be proved in the following discussion.

Parkinson's disease (PD) affects movements; therefore, exercising may assist patients to improve their mobility. Some doctors prescribe physical therapy or muscle-strengthening exercises to tone muscles and to develop underused and rigid muscles through a full range of motion. Exercises will not prevent disease progression, but they may improve body strength. Schenkman's conclusion supports the previously stated ideas: Exercise does not have the ability to end disease progression, but it can develop the patient's body strength:

> "Physical therapy may not be very effective in remediating the direct effects of pathology of Parkinson's [disease] on the integrative mechanisms for balance. Physical therapy, however, could be effective in reducing contributions of other impairments, such as loss of trunk and pelvic mobility, in remediating balance impairments" (Schenkman et al., 1989, pp. 544–545).

Also, exercises improve balance, helping people overcome gait problems, and they strengthen certain muscles that allow people to speak, swallow, walk, and function better.

Physical therapy, extremely important for the Parkinson's patient, usually follows an approach that uses active and passive exercise, gait-training, practice in normal activities, and if needed, hot or cold treatments, water therapy, and electrical stimulation. Giving particular emphasis to upright posture, gait training, and extension exercises for the neck, trunk, and legs stabilizes the patient. Passive exercise, mainly stretching and manipulating muscles by a physical therapist, aim at preventing muscles from shortening. An active exercise program, used to help ROM, coordination, and speed, that begins with slow and gentle exercises and becomes progressively more intense, may improve mobility in patients with early and mid-stage Parkinson's disease (WebMDHealth). Relaxation techniques that the patient is capable of using should be taught to the patient in order to reduce rigidity, and these will maintain ROM and lessen abnormal posture. Essentially, physical therapy encourages the well-being of patients; it acts as a common denominator in patients who are able to maintain productive years.

Responsibility for teaching the Parkinson's patient a formal home exercise program that will guarantee continued effective intervention and will provide the patient with some control over the disease depends on the physical therapist. According to Schenkman in *Physical Therapy* (1989), on the intervention that consists of teaching the patient self-relaxation of rigidity, assisting the patient in maintaining flexibility and ROM, and restoring the patient's automated movement patterns through repetition, the patient should continue in a home exercise program that continues to maintain flexibility, ROM, and movement; once the patient has achieved maximum therapeutic gains, the patient must continue to maintain those gains through self-exercise. Postural reeducation, an important aspect of the home exercise program, incorporates the flexibility acquired in therapy into appropriate postural alignment throughout the day.

Physical therapy intervention reduces disabilities by improving the patient's ability to function. Schenkman and Butler state that ". . . functional activities should be incorporated into mobility exercises" (1989, p. 948). Any form of exercise is beneficial, although task-specific exercises are the most effective; this concept supports the notion that physical therapists are necessary to assist the patient in performing the exercise effectively. Once the physical therapist establishes exercises, the patient's role revolves around efforts to practice movements, even simple ones, such as marching in place, making circular arm movements, and raising the legs up and down while sitting. Therefore, the template exercises established by the physical therapist enable the patient's physical activity.

Muscular and articular restrictions, which are ultimately caused by Parkinson's disease, contribute to reducing muscle content. Exercise, when coupled with sensory reinforcements, proves efficacious for Parkinson's patients. An experiment reported in *Disability and Rehabilitation* (1999) presents an explanation for the physical therapist to encourage exercise to achieve mobility. The results in this study supported "the rationale that physical therapy intervention is to identify the underlying and composite mechanisms which gradually lead to disability and immobility." This case study supports the demand for continuing study on the effect of physical therapy on patients suffering from Parkinson's disease; the results confirm that "the degree of disability in PD can be reduced by adding a simple physical therapy programme to the [patient's] pharmacological treatment" (Viliani et al., 1999, p. 73).

The studies suggest that the disability of Parkinson's disease can be reduced with early physical therapy intercession as gains are made in musculoskeletal flexibility, alignment, and overall functional movement. Schenkman and colleagues (1989) demonstrate the necessity of physical therapy, and the two case studies exemplified the changes that occurred in two Parkinson's individuals who received physical therapy early in disease. The study concluded that " . . . physical

therapy intervention contributed to [the] changes, although further study will be necessary to establish [a] relationship" between the changes in the patients and physical therapy treatment (p. 925).

Physical therapy successfully combats the rigidity and the ROM losses in Parkinson's patients. Preliminary assessment of physical therapy reveals beneficial results for Parkinson's disease patients, but continued research regarding these effects on patients remains necessary. Gait training, posture, mobility, and functional activities will improve with the assistance of physical therapy.

References

Parkinson's disease. Retrieved from http://my.web-med.com/content/dmk/dmk_article_40066

Schenkman, M., & Butler, R. A. (1989). A model for multisystem evaluation treatment of individuals with Parkinson's disease. *Physical Therapy, 69,* 932–940.

(July 1989). A model for multisystem evaluation, interpretation, and treatment of individuals with neurologic dysfunction. *Physical Therapy, 69,* 538–547.

Schenkman, M., Donovan, J., Tsubota, J., Kluss, M., Stebbins, P., & Butler, R. B. (1989). Management of individuals with Parkinson's disease: Rationale and case studies. *Physical Therapy, 69,* 944–955.

Viliani, T., Pasquetti, P., Magnolfi, S., Lundardelli, M. L., Giorgi, C., Serra, P., & Taiti, P. G. (February 1999). Effects of physical training on straightening-up processes in patients with Parkinson's disease. *Disability and Rehabilitation, 21,* 68–73.

Young, R. (1999). Update on Parkinson's disease. *American Family Physician.* Retrieved from http://www.aafp.org/afp/990415ap/2155.htm

Mechanics

Capitalization and numbers, two of the various elements of writing called **mechanics**, are governed by the *Publication Manual of the American Psychological Association*. Please refer to it for specific information concerning those topics. The following rules are standard practice governed not only by the APA style manual but also by grammar textbooks.

Italics

- Like quotation marks, italics can be used to refer to words as words.

    EXAMPLE: The word *is* in the example demonstrates the use of a weak verb.

- Use italics to indicate the titles of books, magazines, journals, movies, works of art, and newspapers.

    EXAMPLE: Mark Twain's *The Adventures of Huckleberry Finn* was published in 1884.

- Italicize all foreign words that have not been accepted into the English language as common.

    EXAMPLE: I have nicknamed my hard drive *sine qua non.*

The Apostrophe

- Use an apostrophe to indicate possession.

    EXAMPLES

    Please hand me Tim's book.

    The book belongs to Tim.

    All of the boats' masts were bent by the wind.

    The masts belong to several boats.

- In compound constructions, use the apostrophe with the appropriate meaning.

    EXAMPLES

    Wordsworth and Coleridge's poetry mark the Romantic period.

    Indicates that Wordsworth and Coleridge wrote poetry together.

    Wordworth's and Coleridge's poetry mark the Romantic period.

    Indicates that Wordsworth's poems and Coleridge's poems were landmarks.

- Apostrophes are also used to form contractions (*can't, won't, shouldn't*) but only in informal settings or documents. When quoting someone else, use that person's contractions, but you should avoid using contractions in your professional work. Write out your words to avoid any confusion.

The Hyphen

Use a hyphen with the following constructions:

- Compound numbers, if required to write out: twenty-one

- Fractions: two-thirds

- Compound constructions that are not generally accepted as one word and to indicate prefixes: self-centered, Pre-Christian, ex-lover, pro-Republican, mother-in-law, great-grandfather

- Adjectival expressions in which two words serve one modifying purpose: Fifty-gallon drum; nineteenth-century literature

- To avoid awkward spellings or confusion: pre-emptive, re-creation, re-cover.

Other Rules of Punctuation

Refer to the earlier discussions on comma, semicolon, or colon usage. This section discusses the use of the dash, quotation marks, brackets, and parentheses.

The Dash

- Use a dash to indicate sharp breaks in thought.

    EXAMPLE: I decided not to go—you won't believe this—because the moon was full.

    Obviously, this type of writing is more informal or conversational and should be used sparingly, if at all, in formal writing assignments.

- A more appropriate use of the dash derives from sentences with complex punctuation. Use a dash to separate nonrestrictive phrases or clauses that have heavy internal punctuation.

    EXAMPLE: Her roommates—June, Alice, and Wanda—were late for the dinner.

    In this example, commas would normally replace the dashes to indicate a nonrestrictive appositive phrase, but the heavy use of commas could create confusion.

Quotation Marks

Use quotation marks to enclose direct quotations, either from a source or from spoken words.

EXAMPLE: He said, "Give me liberty or else."

In cases where you have a quote within a quote, use single quotation marks to separate the quoted material within the direct quote:

EXAMPLE: He said, "I'd like to begin with 'Give me liberty, or give me death.'"

Note: Notice that the terminal mark of punctuation is within the quotation marks. Semicolons or colons appear outside, unless they are part of the quoted material. Question marks also raise this concern:

EXAMPLE: He asked, "Can I use your restroom?"

In this example, the quoted material is a question; consequently, the question mark appears within the quotation marks.

EXAMPLE: Did he say, "I want to use your restroom"?

In this example, the whole sentence is the question, not the quoted material; consequently, the question mark appears outside the quotation marks.

Quotation marks also are used to enclose titles of short stories, short plays, poems, articles, and television programs.

EXAMPLES

Did you watch "One Time" on *ER* last night?

I read "Young Goodman Brown" over the weekend.

Finally, quotation marks are used to indicate words that are referred to as words or used as a special consideration in the sentence.

EXAMPLES

The word "their" does not modify "she" in the sentence.

They recruited the only "blue chip" player from Western New York.

With the use of word processing software, the use of quotation marks for this purpose is almost archaic. Try using the italics function and eliminating the quotation marks.

Parentheses

Parentheses, obviously, separate parenthetical arrangements in sentences, but we already have commas and dashes that can perform this function. Therefore, use parentheses for supplementary information that clarifies the sentence

but that is not imperative to the success of the sentence.

EXAMPLES

The Ardener Model (see appendix C) explains this phenomenon.

The co-pay is ten dollars ($10.00).

Many people will make the mistake of using parentheses for the purpose of clarifying an idea or adding supplemental information. Using parentheses for either of these purposes would be acceptable only in informal writing assignments. In formal writing, employ the rules of comma usage or revise the sentence to appropriately position this information.

Brackets

Use brackets to indicate that you have added information to quoted material for readability, for grammatical correctness, or for further explanation:

EXAMPLE: Jones explains that "aspirin [does not cause] blood coagulation and encorages [sic] blood flow."

Use brackets also if a parenthetical expression is necessary within another parenthetical reference.

EXAMPLE: The Ardener Model (see appendix C [under separate cover]) explains this phenomenon.

Exercises

GRAMMAR, MECHANICS, AND PUNCTUATION

■ Punctuation and the Four Major Errors

Directions: Correct the following sentences with punctuation or identify the error as a comma splice (CS), run-on sentence (RO), sentence fragment (SF), or subject-verb disagreement (SV). After identifying the error, correct the mistake. A sentence may have more than one error.

1. The patient complained of angina and the doctor administered nitroglycerin to make the patient more comfortable.

2. A list of the patient's allergies were posted in the chart that the nurse referenced.

3. The patient's current health, family history, and lifestyle suggests an increased risk of heart disease.

4. Blood tests revealed high clotting factor in the patient's blood. After I administered a heparin IV bolus.

5. Following the procedure, the doctor prepared the patient for recovery it became evident that the patient needed further care.

6. I changed the dressings on the abdominal wound, I found the dressings saturated with and the area irritated.

7. Although I found the patient had clear sputum, good breath sounds, and normal temperature. The patient's differential white blood cell count tested high.

8. I assigned the patient therapeutic exercises to aid in her discomfort, she benefited from the therapy.

9. The nurse practitioner prescribed a sulfa antibiotic for the patient's infection but the bacteria was resistant to the drug, the N.P. then prescribed Cipro to cure the infection.

10. Due to the severity of the trauma, the patient could not breath on his own, therefore, the physician inserts an endotracheal (ET) tube which was attached to a ventilator that the respiratory therapist maintained throughout the patient's stay in the hospital.

11. As a result of the surgery, the patient's right knee exhibit decreased range of motion in flexion and extension.

12. The woman began labor contractions in her seventh month of pregnancy, because of the early labor the obstetrician performed a cesarean section to ensure the safety of the mother and child.

13. The patient's blood tests reveals a high count of cancerous white blood cells, which lead his doctor to the diagnosis of leukemia.

14. Chest x-ray films of the patient demonstrated an accumulation of fluid within her pleural spaces and the doctor ordered a thoracentesis to relieve the pressure on her lungs and to enable to patient to breath with ease.

15. The patient, Mr. Smith, sustaining an infection in his right foot for 2 months. The undetected infection spread and induced secondary inguinal lymphadenopathy.

16. After complaining of bilateral knee pain, Mrs. Whitman's physician performed and arthro-scopy and determined that she had decreased cartilage in her knees and hypertrophy of her femur and for the pain and discomfort the doctor recommended aspirin, glucosamine, and chondroitin and then he recommended that she have total knee replacement if these treatments proved insufficient.

17. The radiologist performed an ultrasound on the patient and identified two cysts in her breast. Although the mammogram revealed no abnormalities.

18. Mrs. Banks, a 37 year-old office assistant, complained of wrist pain and a tingling sensation in her fingers, Dr. Sanki diagnoses her with carpal tunnel syndrome.

19. Although other dermatologists diagnosed Mary with eczema, Dr. Horn determine her problem to be psoriasis and the physician provided a prescription for a topical cream.

20. Hank suffering from noticeable anisocoria due to a massive head trauma, and the ophthalmologist offered no solution to improve his physical appearance.

■ Punctuation

Directions: Insert semicolons, colons, dashes or hyphens, quotation marks, and italics as needed in the following sentences.

1. The players on the Wall of Fame Jim Kelly, Kent Hull, and Cookie Gilchrist deserve awards.

2. Several cities participated in the clean-up effort Buffalo, Rochester, Syracuse, and Binghamton.

3. Give me liberty is one of my favorite quotes I cannot remember who said it, though.

4. In last week's New York Times, Larry Felser was quoted from his most recent book entitled The Glory Years.

5. He left us with one choice swim for the shore.

6. The word is is often considered weak in verb based writing strategies.

■ Grammar Rules and Word Choice

Directions: Correctly rewrite any sentences containing mistakes in mechanics, punctuation, or grammar or informality of language.

1. After her surgery, Mrs. Sanders complained of being hot, tired and in need of something to drink.

2. Dr. Francis intends either to operate on the patient, or instruct her to attend physical therapy.

3. After stocking all the rooms, weighing all the patients, and recording all the vital signs, Susie, the nurse's aid then distributed all the lunches, supplied the phlebotomy kit, and cleaned all the medical equipment.

4. The patient complained that his ankle was painful, swollen, and having problems while walking.

5. The therapist demonstrated appropriate exercises, answered the patient's questions and documents the patient's history.

6. For the procedure, the nurse prepared a multitude of sterile gauze, a suture kit, and anesthetized the area.

7. For a primary diagnosis, Dr. Davis believed the patients problem could be Crohn's disease, irritable bowel syndrome or a duodenal ulcer, but to solidify a diagnosis the physician requested a barium swallow, a barium enema, and possibly exploratory surgery.

8. When the nurse answered the call bell, the patient asked the nurse to help him to the chair and finding his glasses.

9. Months of occupational therapy enabled Mr. Appolito to walk, dress and eating independently.

10. While bathing the patient, the nurse noticed redness, poor capillary refill, and numbing to his coccygeal region.

■ Punctuation, Grammar, and Mechanics in an Essay Sample

Directions: Correct any mistakes in punctuation, grammar, or mechanics within the following paragraph.

Admitted to the ER on Thursday January 26, the patient complained of angina. A 60 year old man, he has an extensive history of heart problems. At the age of fifty-one the patient Mr Rouge, suffered from a minor heart attack. CHF (congestive heart failure) developed presumably as a result of this myocardial infarction: however, Mr. Rouge sustains a healthy lifestyle including; walking, gardening, and cross-country skiing. The patients family reports that he is a pillar of strength. Throughout his ER visit, the physician's monitor his pulse, heart rate, and taking his temperature. A blood test revealed high troponin levels indicating that the patient, again, suffered from a myocardial infarction. Following his diagnosis the patient was transported to the cardiac unit on the 3rd floor. While on the cardiac unit, Mr Rouge will remain on a cardiac monitor which will allow the nurses 24 hour monitoring of his heart.

3

Phase Three of the Writing Process: Using Precise Words and Developing a Professional Style

Key Terms

Active voice   Creating a WHO-DID-WHAT focus of sentences; allowing the subject to act as subject

Conversational language   The type of language people use when speaking, which is not appropriate for writing

Diction   Choosing the words appropriate to audience

Noun-based language   Focus of sentence action is on noun instead of verb; often called *nominalization*

Passive voice   Allowing the object to serve as the subject of the sentence

Verb-based language   Focus of sentence action is on verb, not nouns

Word choice   Choosing the exact word for precise meaning

chapter objectives

On completion of this chapter, the reader should be able to

1. Express the main action in a sentence in a verb, not a noun.
2. Use strong verbs that create an impact on the reader and that do not depend on adverb modifiers.
3. Write in active, not passive, voice.
4. Avoid *it* and *there* as subjects.
5. Limit the use of "to be" verbs.
6. Distinguish between formal and informal language as required by proper diction.
7. Choose the appropriate words to create exact meanings.
8. Eliminate excess words created by noun-based writing, poor diction, and weak choice of words.

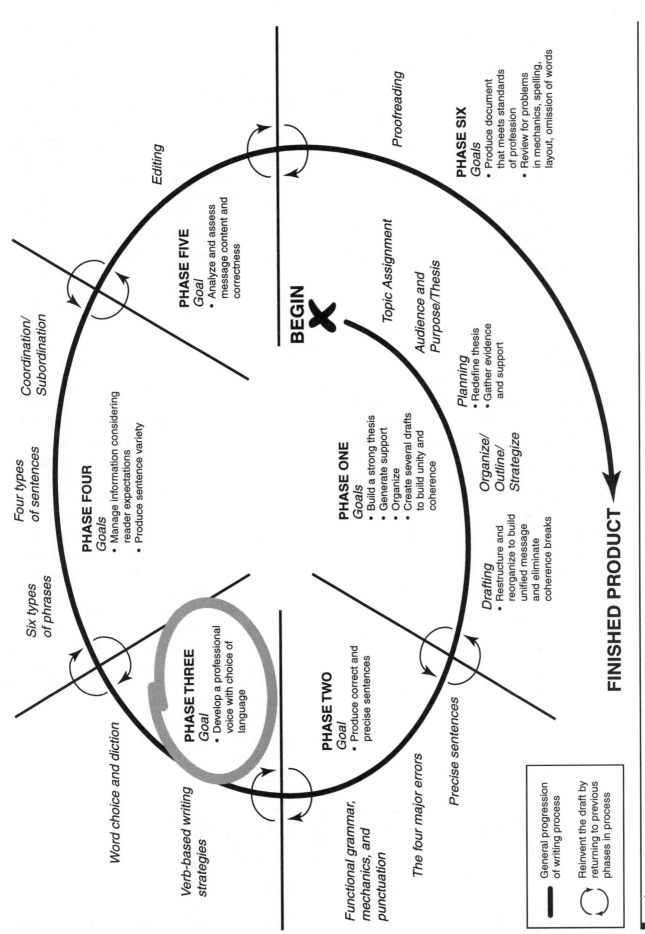

Figure 3-1   The Writing Process: Phase Three

When the sentence revision process is finished, plan to spend a few more hours working on word-level issues. You will assess your **diction** (audience-appropriate language) and **word choice** (to convey your exact meaning) for every mark on the paper, making sure that each word communicates its intended message. With that process completed (see Figure 3-1), you can begin altering your sentences to represent verb-based writing strategies instead of noun-based. This process will also help you eliminate **passive voice** (in which the object of the action serves as the subject of the sentence) and develop sentences that have a profound effect on your reader instead of simply being words on paper.

The point of applying the strategies presented at this stage is that words and sentences are an important component of writing well. You must be able to demonstrate your expertise in language appropriate to your profession and then be able to craft sentences that are grammatically and mechanically correct. Every mark on the paper is an element by which you can lead the reader to clearly understand your message or, instead, lead the reader into unintended confusion.

This section of the textbook allows you to move forward in the recursive writing process by addressing issues related to precise sentences and choice of words. Up to this point, your main focus has been to create an essay that supports a thesis statement and to then create paragraphs and sentences that represent unified and coherent ideas. Creating a logically connected set of ideas is only the first phase of writing well.

Your next task is to employ a professional writing style by eliminating excess words and phrases and using language that is concise, accurate, and appropriate to your profession. Your audience does not want to wade through a sea of words when only a few will suffice. Conversely, your audience must be led directly to your main argument or purpose without being misguided or distracted. This is a difficult process because your audience's needs may vary, but since you are a professional, you will be able to determine how best to communicate with your professional audience.

As you develop a concise writing style, you will also need to concentrate on creating sentences that are indeed sentences. You will damage your reputation and your standing as a professional if you demonstrate ignorance of the rules of grammar in standard written English. Consequently, you must identify incomplete sentences and major errors in grammar, as learned in Chapter 2. To understand the major errors in grammar, you must learn some of the rules of punctuation to create your sentences. You do not need to memorize jargon or diagram sentences. You will, however, need to understand the elements of a sentence and how these work together or how they are separated with punctuation.

Finally, in this chapter, you will be challenged to develop a professional voice through the words that you choose. Diction problems are indicative of laziness or an ineffective vocabulary. You will develop the language skills for communicating at a level that all professionals will expect. To do so, you will also learn how to change some of your weak sentence constructions into strong ones through verb-based writing strategies. You will no longer be able to depend on mental shortcuts to deliver your message. Such mental shortcuts derive from time constraints in the writing process. Immature writers will jot down words that come close to communicating their message, but the words they choose are not exact. As a result, the true intent of the message is lost. Mature writers will eliminate this weakness through the employment of several clarification strategies.

The purpose of this chapter is to help you develop a language that is precise, direct, and appropriate for your profession. You will find that employing these strategies is at first time-consuming and difficult, but once they are mastered, you are on your way to becoming a professional writer.

VERB-BASED WRITING STRATEGIES

Once you have chosen the exact words that indicate your precise meaning, your can begin altering your sentences to produce **verb-based**

language, instead of using weaker **noun-based language**. Verb-based writing strategies keep the focus of sentence action on verbs, rather than on nouns as in noun-based writing. This process will help you develop a professional voice and create sentences that make an impression on your reader.

Words and sentences are an important component of writing well. Obviously, you must be able to demonstrate your expertise in language and be able to craft sentences that are grammatically and mechanically correct, but every mark on the paper is an element by which you can lead the reader to clearly understand your message or lead the reader into unintended confusion. You will guide the reader with powerful language that is expertly tailored to your audience's needs.

Implement the following verb-based writing strategies as you edit your work to develop a professional voice and building precision in your writing:

Express the main action in a sentence in a verb, not a noun.

Use STRONG verbs that create an impact on the reader (no adverb modifiers).

Write in ACTIVE, not passive, voice.

Avoid *it* and *there* as subjects.

Limit your use of "to be" verbs.

Using Verbs Instead of Nouns to Express Action

Problem: Writers, failing to scrutinize the exact meanings of words, use nouns to represent the action in a sentence instead of using verbs.

The verb is the strongest part of speech, because readers are more likely to retain ideas presented through action. Experienced, professional writers craft their sentences around verbs because verbs produce an effective message. If used effectively, verbs will help a reader visualize the action of a sentence. Reading specialists and psychologists tell us that readers will remember an action or hold the image of an object performing that action in their minds more readily than simply visualizing a static

object. When we speak, however, we tend to use nouns as the focus of our sentences because nouns are easily identifiable, often by sight, and we can quickly scramble for and recall nouns because they are at the forefront of the limited vocabulary we use when we converse. As a result, we create sentences around nouns when we speak, and our sentences are not tightly constructed, nor are they crafted into powerful ideas presented through carefully chosen words. Instead, our sentences are filled with excess words, when we speak, that help us communicate our point about the noun we chose from our limited, conversational vocabulary. Ultimately, creating sentences with excess words is the result of our minds operating under time constraints. Wordiness gives us time to think and finish our thoughts verbally.

For these reasons, professional writers should not write as they would speak. (This issue is discussed later in the chapter under "Word Choice and Diction.") Instead of using such **conversational language**, a mature writer will rewrite, edit, and revise sentences that use informal language until the writer's intended function has been achieved: to communicate clearly and effectively.

Note: Attempting to write effective, verb-based sentences is impossible in a first draft. Review the first chapters of this text concerning drafting, and implement this strategy only after the essay has been edited for coherence and unity. Once the essay follows a logical and rational line of thinking, the writer can begin to attack specific sentences and specific language. This text suggests, then, that a writer approach the first draft by using whatever language available to complete the coherent and unified draft. When the message of the essay is clearly organized and rational, use these strategies to sharpen sentences and to communicate the intended message with precision and accuracy.

As a result of using nouns to express action instead of verbs, an inexperienced writer uses conversational diction or language that has not been scrutinized for exact meaning. Instead, the meanings of the sentences are lost or veiled in words that do not provide clarity and precision.

You are not throwing hand-grenades here — meaning that you cannot simply be *close* to your target to get results. You have to be a sniper with your words and mark your target with pinpoint accuracy.

Noun-based forms subvert the intended meanings of your sentences by bringing your reader close to your message but not setting the reader on target. A writer who uses noun-based language forms a noun out of the word that actually expresses the action of the sentence. Writers who use nouns to express action fail to communicate their message to the reader because they miss the opportunity to use powerful verbs, and they create sentences that use excessive words that further complicate the message or jeopardize the intended meaning.

Read the original sentences that use noun-based words as verbs. Then examine the accompanying revisions.

> **EXAMPLE:** We want you to give a discussion about the project at the next meeting.
>
> **REVISION:** We want you to discuss the project at the next meeting.

In the original example, the writer wants someone to perform an action, but the action suggested is to *give* something. The person who is intending to present information at a meeting is not "giving" anything. The use of the word *give* here represents a communication breakdown in that it asks for an action that is not required.

> **EXAMPLE:** When we do your tax preparation, we use a computer form for expense documentation.
>
> **REVISION:** When we prepare your tax returns, we document expenses on a computer form.

In both the independent and dependent clauses, the noun-based writing form interferes with communication of meaning. In the dependent clause, the verb is *do* and the noun is *preparation*. Any reader should recognize that *do* is a weak verb in that it is too general. Obviously, *prepare* is more precise. In the independent clause, the problem is the same. The word *documents* is a stronger, more effective verb in that it shows the actual action *we* will perform.

Observe the steps necessary to produce strong, verb-based sentences in the following examples:

> **EXAMPLE:** The CEO gave the indication that he would step down if the board asked him to do so.

Obviously, the CEO didn't *give* anyone anything here. However, the CEO did *indicate* his actions.

> **REVISION 1:** The CEO indicated that he would step down if the board asked him to do so.

We are not finished.

Although the main subject and verb combination is strong, the remainder of the sentence is filled with weak verbs. Consider the weaknesses in word combinations such as *step down* and *asked him to do so*. The CEO is not literally stepping, and as a result, this sentence is relying on conversational diction instead of providing precise language that creates precise meanings. Also, the last part of the sentence, *asked him to do so*, is wordy, and *do so* is a vague construction. Examine the following revision for suggested changes:

> **REVISION 2:** The CEO indicated that he would resign if the board asked him to do so.
>
> **REVISION 3:** The CEO indicated that he would resign if the board requested it.
>
> **EXAMPLE:** I offered my recommendation for Jones because he makes my job easy by getting his work done.

As in the previous example, this sentence is lethargic because *offered* is the verb, and this word distances the subject from the real action of the sentence: the "recommending." *Offered* is not a particularly weak verb, but it does not have the desired effect here.

> **REVISION 1:** I recommended Jones because he makes my job easy by getting his work done.

We are not finished.

Examine other parts of the sentence for weak or listless verbs. If you are aware of the weaknesses in language, you will immediately recognize that *makes*, *getting*, and *done* are all weak verbs because they do not provide precise meanings.

> **REVISION 2:** I recommended Jones because he works hard.

Although this revision solves the wordiness problem and eliminates the string of listless verbs, it produces another problem in accuracy. The term *hard* should represent an object opposite of soft. A rock is *hard*. A job is *hard* only in the conversational use of the word.

> REVISION 3: I recommended Jones because he produces results.

In this final revision, the two verbs, *recommended* and *produces*, create a specific meaning with powerful language showing action. This sentence will stay with the reader.

> EXAMPLE: Each month, we seem to be confronted with a sexual harassment charge against one of our chief executives.

In this example, the inexperienced writer will struggle to find the appropriate verb to attach with an appropriate subject. Obviously, verbs such as *seem* and *against* are weak and inappropriate, but *confronted* works; however, the only revision using *confronted* will create wordiness as well, with equally weak forms of "to be" verbs:

> REVISION 1: One of our chief executives is confronted with a sexual harassment charge each month.

This is a poor example because the actor, the person performing the action, is missing from the sentence. This problem is addressed later in this chapter under "Avoiding Passive Voice Verbs." However, this issue can be resolved here by naming in the sentence the party confronting the executives.

> REVISION 2: Each month, an employee confronts one of our chief executives with a sexual harassment charge.

Although this revision example solves the passive voice problem, it does not tighten the sentence to its logical end. Consider that the noun *charge* should be converted to a verb form since it is the operative word in this sentence.

> REVISION 3: Each month, an employee charges one of our chief executives with sexual harassment.

Learn this important lesson now: Writing for the profession will require time to rethink, reinvent, and revise every sentence that you create. Every revision will require you to write several drafts of each sentence.

> EXAMPLE: Any decision about increasing taxes will not be made by this administration until after consulting with leaders from both parties.

In this case, the actor, *this administration*, is easily identifiable as the actor.

> REVISION 1: This administration will not make any decision about increasing taxes until after consulting with leaders from both parties.

Although the passive voice construction is eliminated here, and consequently the weak "to be" verb, the sentence's main action rests with *make*. This is not an effective verb.

> REVISION 2: This administration will not decide about increasing taxes until after consulting with leaders from both parties.

This example seems to have a powerful verb, *decide*, but the sentence now seems convoluted—especially with the use of *until* and *after*, two prepositions, in such close proximity. The sentence still needs work. Examining the remainder of the sentence, the savvy writer will identify *consulting* as the operative word in the sentence. This should be the main verb.

> REVISION 3: This administration will consult with leaders from both parties before increasing taxes.

Using Strong Verbs

We established in the first section of this chapter that most of us tend to write as we speak, which means we rely on that limited vocabulary available to us under time constraints. As a result, when we write as we speak, we use only a small number of words that come quickly to mind. Our brains have not yet been trained to search for the exact words while we speak, and as a result, we choose language that is close to our intended meaning, not the intended meaning. This is often accomplished by using weak verbs, meaning verbs that have little meaning or vague meanings, or we recognize the inherent weaknesses in our conversational verb choice and attempt to supplement their meanings by adding words to modify or explain the verbs. Usually, this is accomplished by adding adverbs to verbs to clarify or enhance them because we do not allow ourselves the time to think of the exact verb that will convey a precise meaning.

When writing, unlike speaking, we have time to scrutinize our now-visible thoughts on paper and choose verbs that express ideas forcefully. In the following list, compare the weak (conversational) examples with the strong verb choice examples:

WEAK	STRONG
look over	review
run very quickly	sprint
spoke very clearly	articulated

As a general rule, eliminate unnecessary adverb-verb combinations and use one precise verb where two or three words attempt to create action.

The Revision Process Concerning Weak Verbs

EXAMPLE: The tour conductor said that we could not lean over the railing.

As was discussed in Chapter 2 in the section on four major errors, every conscientious writer should examine the subject-verb combinations in every sentence to ensure that these elements agree (grammatical correctness). Furthermore, while considering this task, examine the verbs for their meaning and the impact that meaning has on the sentence. In the example supplied, *said* is the verb that attaches itself to *The tour conductor. Said* used as a verb works but is not expressive. If the tour conductor was leading a group of elementary school children along a narrow walkway that is elevated 200 feet above the Niagara Gorge, the tour conductor will not simply *say* to these children that they cannot lean over the railing. Because these instructions are to be considered with their safety in mind, the verb should reflect such seriousness or importance.

REVISION 1: The tour conductor instructed the children to not lean over the railing.

REVISION 2: The tour conductor demanded that we not lean over the railing.

Depending on the urgency of this command, the verb will reflect the degree of importance.

Consider other words that will alter the meaning of this sentence. As you do, also consider that only one word should be used to express your point. Find the single word in your vocabulary that accurately demonstrates your point.

EXAMPLE: The painter came quickly down the shaky ladder and put his brush down in disgust.

In this example, the painter performs two actions: he *came quickly down* the ladder and he *put* his brush down. This construction is a compound verb, or two verbs attached to the same subject, but both verbs have weaknesses. If the painter was *disgusted*, he would not simply *come quickly down* the ladder. Instead, he *dropped* from the ladder, or he *scrambled* down the ladder. In either of these revisions, the sense of urgency is delivered without excessive words. Each of the terms *drop* and *scrambled* indicates, in descriptive terms, the action in one, powerful word choice. Additionally, no painter who scrambles down a ladder in disgust will simply *put* his or her brush down. To *put down* an object indicates that the action was completed deliberately and not necessarily in haste. This is not the case for the painter in our example.

REVISION 1: The painter *dropped* from the shaky ladder and *heaved* his brush down in disgust.

REVISION 2: The painter *scrambled* down the shaky ladder and *slammed* his brush down in disgust.

These revisions create visual images that have action. Your reader will respond by internalizing the action and remembering your message.

EXAMPLE: The girl cried softly when she learned that her bird had died.

In this example, *cried softly* is a weak verb with an adverb modifier—the verb itself did not complete the message for the writer. The girl could exhibit varying degrees of being upset—perhaps she *sobbed, blubbered, wept,* or *sniffled.* In any of these revision choices, the verb indicates a specific level of grief that can be described to the reader by using one powerful verb, instead of two weak words attempting to do the job of one.

To rectify this problem, use the adverb-verb combination sparingly in your writing and assess your reasons for doing so when you feel you are forced to use it. Study the adverb-verb combinations you use and scour your vocabulary for a one-word substitute.

Avoiding Passive Voice Verbs

Passive voice constructions create problems similar to those with noun-based language and weak verbs. Instead of thinking through the sentence and creating a clear connection between the doer of the action and the action, the passive voice hides the doer of the action from the reader. Furthermore, every sentence, when and where appropriate, should create a clear WHO-DID-WHAT relationship—the focus of the **active voice**. Passive voice disrupts this focus by hiding WHO from the action or allowing the object of the verb (WHAT) to take on the role of the noun.

Passive voice is also a weak writing tool because the passive voice emphasizes the noun instead of the verb and distances the subject from the verb with a helping verb—usually a form of "to be" (*is, are, was, were, be, been*). "To be" verbs literally create a sense of being or a static relationship between the noun and the verb. Good writers want a dynamic relationship, according to reading specialists and psychologists, because active (dynamic) verbs assist in our ability to encode information. When possible and appropriate, avoid the use of "to be" forms. They are weak and ineffective. Strong writers limit the use of "to be" verbs in their professional documents because they want to create stimulating sentences that show action.

PASSIVE: The tree was struck by lightning.

ACTIVE: Lightning struck the tree.

In this example, the passive voice literally creates a static relationship between the tree and the lightning. The helping verb *was* indicates that the tree simply existed and something was done to it. The tree is not acting, yet it is the subject of the sentence, and the reader will expect the subject to be the doer of the action. When the subject is not the doer of the action, the expectation of the reader is subverted, and the impact of the verb is displaced to another part of the sentence. The position of the words in the sentences compounds the problem by creating not a clear WHO-DID-WHAT focus but, instead, a WHAT-WAS-DONE-BY-SOMETHING focus. Examining the relationship of the words in this for-

mula demonstrates the convoluted nature of the passive voice. It asserts on the sentence an unnecessary act of convolution. Find the actor, or the doer of the action, in a sentence; make that word the subject; and then attach the appropriate verb to it.

Also, by creating a clear WHO-DID-WHAT focus, the weak helping verb, *was*, is eliminated, no longer creating that static relationship. Instead, because *lightning* is now the subject and therefore the actor, the sentence takes on a powerful verb in *struck*. The reader can now visualize the action being performed. In the passive voice example, the reader must consider the tree, a static object, and then associate the action with another word. This approach will weaken the impact of your sentences on your reader.

Think about ways in which you respond to the words on the page. Be an active reader. As you revise and reconsider your words, assess your reactions. If you feel that the words are not influencing you, the problem is not with you, the reader; the problem rests with the writer and the communication process that is breaking down. Consider your reactions to the following examples of passive and active voice:

PASSIVE: On the third strike, the ball was dropped by the catcher.

ACTIVE: On the third strike, the catcher dropped the ball.

The Revision Process Associated with Use of Passive Voice

EXAMPLE: Several new safety policies were mandated by OSHA.

This example is a straightforward representation of passive voice. It is easily corrected by identifying the problem and asking the appropriate questions. First, to identify passive voice, look for forms of the "to be" verb used in conjunction with another verb. In our example, *were mandated* is the passive voice culprit. To rectify this problem, the writer should ask, "WHO mandated WHAT?" Obviously, policies did not *mandate* anything. Policies are inanimate and cannot perform human functions. Instead, *OSHA* is the human force that performs this action. Therefore, *OSHA* is the subject of the sentence.

REVISION: OSHA mandated several new safety policies.

The "to be" verb has been eliminated to create a dynamic relationship between the doer of the action and the action itself, and the sentence now presents information through a clear WHO-DID-WHAT focus.

Many writers will not identify any problem with use of passive voice constructions because they seem acceptable—and they usually are acceptable in conversation. However, writing, as we know, is different from speaking and requires a new and different approach to language.

Remember that 50 percent of being a good writer is being able to identify the weaknesses in language and your writing. The other 50 percent derives from your ability to change these weaknesses to strengths.

EXAMPLE: The decision was made by management to look back over each bid before awarding the contract.

The first reaction in responding to this sentence is to fix the passive voice problem.

REVISION 1: Management made the decision to look back over each bid before awarding the contract.

Although the revision eliminates passive voice here, other verb problems exist. For example, the active voice revision allows *made* to be the verb. Primarily, *made* is a weak verb and should be scrutinized and replaced. However, this sentence is an example of noun-based writing that weakens the exact meaning. The term *decision* is used as a noun, but it is the operative word here and should be used as a verb.

REVISION 2: Management decided to look back over each bid before awarding the contract.

The main subject-verb combination is now acceptable, but other verbs in the sentence have not been scrutinized. Obviously, after we consider the previous discussion about weak verbs and using several words to express the action of one, the group *look back over* should be replaced.

REVISION 3: Management decided to reexamine each bid before awarding the contract.

This is now an acceptable sentence.

Exceptions to the Passive Voice Rule

Use passive voice under the following circumstances:

A. To express an action when the actor is unknown

   EXAMPLE: The pool had been emptied before we arrived.

B. To express an action when the writer does not want to disclose the actor.

   EXAMPLE: Mistakes were made and documents were shredded.

C. To emphasize the object instead of the actor.

   EXAMPLE: America was discovered in 1492.

   This last exception to the rule is the one that is most readily applied in scientific writing. In many cases, the writer is also the researcher and tires quickly of stating "I performed . . . ." "I then studied . . . ." "I then proposed . . . ." These examples indicate a sentence monotony that is boring for the reader. To counteract the effects of repetition or redundancy, the passive voice is often applied: "A study was performed . . . ." "The samples were studied . . . ." "The results were proposed . . . ." If anything, this use of passive voice has been accepted by the scientific community because it moves the focus of the study away from the scientist and onto the results and activities of the study itself.

EXAMPLE: The new access road will be completed before the end of the year.

To solve this passive voice dilemma, a savvy writer will ask, "WHO completed WHAT?" Given the information in the sentence, the writer cannot answer the question. The writer can assume that the doer of the action is a group of people who regularly perform this type of work.

REVISION: The construction company will complete the new access road before the end of the year.

Consider who actually performs the action in the following sentences:

EXAMPLE: We were assigned an extra chapter in the textbook.

REVISION: The teacher/professor/instructor assigned an extra chapter in the textbook.

EXAMPLE: The contract was eventually ruled invalid.

REVISION: The judge/jury/attorney eventually ruled the contract invalid.

Avoiding *It* and *There* as Subjects

In the following examples, *It* and *There* are used, seemingly, as subjects of the sentences. If we follow the instructions in the sections of this text about passive voice, we will want to create a clear WHO-DID-WHAT focus. This means starting sentences with the doers of the action and connecting a verb to them. However, in these cases, *It* and *There* are not the doers of action. In fact, *It* and *There* are pronouns, and pronouns take the place of nouns. What word or words do *It* and *There* replace in these examples? This question cannot be answered. The meanings of *It* and *There* in these examples are unclear. Actually, the words are meaningless. If writers use meaningless words as subjects or starters of sentences, they will reduce the impact of the verb and fail to communicate their point clearly. Sentences need a clear WHO-DID-WHAT focus in their structures. *It* and *There* weaken this focus and interfere with the meaning of the sentence.

EXAMPLE: *There is* no prior knowledge required for this job other than a general understanding of accounting principles.

Ideally, *There*, acting as a pronoun, should take the place of a noun. It does not, in this case, indicate a specific place. Ask, "To what does *There* refer?" In fact, it does not refer to or indicate a meaning for anything and should be eliminated.

REVISION: This job requires only a general understanding of accounting principles.

EXAMPLE: It has been indicated by our analysis that the new policies will cost millions.

In this example, the writer will ask the same question: "To what does *It* refer?" An inexperienced writer may quickly respond, *"Our analy-*

sis." This is not correct. Does this sentence make sense? *Our analysis has been indicated by our analysis that the new policies will cost millions.* The word *It* in this sentence, again, has no meaning and should be eliminated.

REVISION: Our analysis indicates that the new policies will cost millions.

Not only are *It* and *There* meaningless in these constructions, they also will require a form of the "to be" verb to finish the thought. Forms of the "to be" verbs are often considered weak or contribute to passive voice or wordiness problems. Limit your use of "to be" for precision.

The use of *It* and *There* as subjects or as sentence openers indicates that the writer is using a conversational form of diction instead of working to create exact and precise meanings. No one will react negatively to hearing this construction in conversation. Everyone should recognize that this construction, in the written form, is meaningless because the language of the author can be scrutinized and exact meanings should be elicited from the text.

EXAMPLE: *There have been* several occasions recently when the CEO has openly disagreed with the board of directors.

REVISION: The CEO has openly disagreed with the board of directors on several occasions.

EXAMPLE: *There were* several suggestions made by the designer about improving that model.

REVISION: The designer suggested several designs to improve that model.

EXAMPLE: I need to know when *it will be* possible for us to continue with the design project.

REVISION: I need to know when we can continue with the design project.

EXAMPLE: The foreman asked me if *there is* some way we could bypass the fused circuits on the discharger.

REVISION: The foreman asked me for suggestions on how to bypass the fused circuits on the discharger.

Limiting the Use of "To Be" Verbs

In many of the previous discussions concerning precision and accuracy, we have isolated a few types of words and made changes to them or found suitable substitutes. Add to your list the forms of the "to be" verb: *is*, *are*, *was*, *were*, *be*, and *been*. Limit your use of "to be" verbs because these are the culprits that make boring sentences. Literally, sentences using versions of "to be" create a static relationship between subject and verb. The subjects in the sentence are being described in a state of being; they are not acting in any other way except that *being* is an action—a bland one at that. Furthermore, not only are "to be" verbs the impetus for boring sentences, but they also lead writers into the passive voice.

Instead of depending on "to be" verbs to carry the weight of your sentences, find specific words that have more powerful meanings or that describe more accurately the action discussed.

Although you may find suitable substitutes for "to be," a replacement is not always necessary. In the event that you need to describe who a person is or a person's condition, you should consider using "to be" instead of creating an awkward combination.

EXAMPLE: Mr. Jones is 31 years old, and he is a diabetic.

You cannot find a reasonable substitute for the "to be" verb form in the first independent clause. For example, you could not reasonably write the following: *Mr. Jones exists as a 31-year-old*. You could, however, change the weak "to be" verb form in the second independent clause: *he suffers from diabetes*.

Examine the revisions performed on the following sentences and understand how to eliminate all "to be" verbs or weak verbs that serve as the main action of the sentence. Find powerful and meaningful words to substitute for these listless and vague verbs.

EXAMPLE: If we can complete the development of the project by 2010, we will again *be* able to compete for government contracts.

REVISION: If we develop the project by 2010, we will compete for government contracts in the future.

In the dependent clause, the noun-based form is used, and a single, strong verb, *develop*, serves as a suitable substitute. Additionally, the "to be" verb form is used in the independent clause.

The change to any verb will inevitably alter the meaning of the sentence. Be aware of any unintended changes in meaning.

Often, a writer will communicate in short, choppy sentences. Although they may be grammatically correct, the choppiness detracts from the continuity and flow of the document. This problem can easily be solved by combining sentences. Usually, the short, choppy sentences form that use "to be" verb forms are less important to the paragraph. If this is the case, subordinate these sentences by reducing them to a phrase that supports the independent clause. In doing so, you will eliminate the "to be" verb forms as well.

EXAMPLE: Acupuncture is the insertion of tiny needles into specific points on the body. Various types of acupuncture are used depending on the ailments.

This is an example of two sentences that diminish the flow of the paper because the sentences are short and choppy. They both begin with a similar format: subject-verb. Used frequently, this style becomes monotonous and boring. (See "Using the Four Types of Sentences to Avoid Sentence Monotony" in Chapter 4.) Furthermore, the actions of the sentences have been reduced to a static form because of the writer's dependence on the "to be" verb.

REVISION 1: Acupuncture, the insertion of tiny needles into specific points on the body, *uses* specific methods to treat various ailments.

In this first revision, the choppy sentence structure problem has been solved by combining sentences through an act of subordinating a less important element to a more important element. Additionally, the "to be" verb forms have been eliminated and a substitute has replaced the "to be" form. Although the "to be" has been successfully eliminated, the substitute, *uses*, is not strong. Consider the following revision:

REVISION 2: Acupuncture, the insertion of tiny needles into specific points on the body, *treats* various ailments with specific methods.

EXAMPLE: My steps were unsteady as I walked across the broken bridge.

In this example, the sentence is unnecessarily lengthy because of an excess of words and the use of the "to be" verb form. The simple message of this sentence is that the writer *walked across the broken bridge*. The fact that his or her steps were unsteady is important, but this fact can be made clear by using appropriate language. Notice, first, that the most useless part of this sentence is the element composed around a "to be" verb. Second, notice that *walked* is not a descriptive verb or one that demonstrates a strong action that the reader will remember. Consider the following revision:

REVISION 1: I *tip-toed* across the broken bridge.

Although *tip-toed* may send a particular message or create a suitable image, its use in formal writing assignments may be questioned, since it is a term more suitable for conversation.

REVISION 2: I *stole* across the broken bridge.

Words such as *traversed*, *leaped*, or *ran* do not demonstrate the precarious nature of this stunt —unless you want them to change the meaning of the sentence. The word *stole* provides a feeling of stealth or someone gingerly walking.

Conclusion

If you are not sure what you are trying to express, your writing will reflect that uncertainty. Uncertainty derives from not thinking clearly or thoroughly about your subject, and this is usually the result of using conversational diction. Writing as you speak leads to inaccurate and imprecise communication.

The lesson to be learned here is to REVISE. Put your ideas on paper and then scrutinize your words—several times. Challenge yourself to build strong sentences by frequently rewriting and revising each sentence to build exact meanings and to express your thoughts accurately. You have control over the power of words.

Easy reading comes from hard writing, and clear writing comes from clear thinking made visible. Consider how your audience will react to your words as you write and revise accordingly. You are not writing for communication with yourself but to communicate with others. Provide them with the tools to make your message clear.

Exercises

ADOPTING A VERB–BASED WRITING STYLE

Directions: Rewrite the following sentences into a verb-based writing style by reducing nominalization, eliminating weak verbs, eliminating "it" and "there" as subjects, eliminating passive voice, and limiting the use of "to be" verbs.

■ Exercise Set 1

1. There were many patients waiting to see the doctor.
2. The patient was feeling uncomfortable due to high temperatures and a pain in her arm.
3. The paramedic was providing oxygen to first the child and then to the mother in order to help them breath after the car accident.
4. There are many reasons why this 43-year-old patient could have suffered from a stroke including; his diet, the amount of exercise he did, his stress levels at work and home, and others.
5. After the nurse administered chest compressions, the doctor injected some dopamine which helped the situation because the patient's heart beat came back.
6. It became evident that the patient would need surgery to fix the damages from his skiing accident, so the nurse was preparing for the procedure.
7. No one was sure about the protocol for evacuation in the case of a bomb threat. It seemed that the problem had never before been faced.
8. Later the patients will be given their dinner trays and then the nurses will need to record the amount of food and liquids they had eaten.
9. Because of the fact that the nurses were very busy, the patients complained that they were not receiving the care that they deserved.
10. The physician became troubled over the patients status because the patient was looking jaundice and was recording a high temperature.

■ Exercise Set 2

1. Recently the recordings from John Doe's blood pressure has provided the nurses with reason to believe his days are numbered.

2. The patient is going to radiology, and he is receiving a CT scan to verify his doctor's diagnosis.

3. It seems that the doctor's are agreeing on the appropriate billing procedures regarding this procedure of a localized biopsy.

4. The nurse said to the aide to call for the doctor because it was an emergency.

5. The patient was examined in order to determine the problem that was causing her abdominal pain, and it was found to be from a weakness of the pyloric sphincter.

6. The patient is returning today for his final and third hepatitis B vaccine booster shot.

7. Following her stroke, Dr. Metting gave the indication to Mrs. Hinman that an EEG should be done to determine if any brain damage had occurred.

8. After piecing together the patient's history obtained from family and friends, it seemed that the patient may well have forgotten to take his insulin shot and was suffering from ketoacidosis.

9. The psychiatrist came to believe that Megan suffered from bipolar disease as indicated by her rapid mood changes.

10. The patient has presented with complaints of fatigue, sore throat, and swollen axillary lymph nodes, and the preliminary blood tests give an indication of mononucleosis.

Exercise

REVISING A SAMPLE STUDENT ESSAY

Directions: In this sample student essay, the overuse of the verb "to be," dependence on passive voice, use of weak verbs, unnecessary nominalization, and *It* and *There* used as subjects limit the effectiveness of the writing. The weak and ineffective verbs are italicized. Find ways to revise these sentences to create a more effective message. In some circumstances, the use of the "to be" verb forms is necessary, such as in the exceptions to the rules of passive voice and in describing a state of being. In most cases, however, the "to be" verb forms can be elimi-

nated by revising the sentences or subordinating "to be" constructions in phrases or nonessential elements.

Within the field of medicine, many treatments *are being found* from ancient remedies. Many remedies used in ancient societies *are* now being studied to *see* if *there is* any validity in using them as a treatment. A major area of the world *being sought after* is Asia. In many of the oriental cultures there, acupuncture *has been used* for thousands of years. Acupuncture *has been implemented* to aid in medical problems such as arthritis, pain management, addictions, and cancer. *There are* many reasons for using it.

Acupuncture *is* simply the insertion of extremely small needles into specific points in the body. Generally, moxibustion *is used* in association with acupuncture. Moxibustion *is* burning specific herbs while acupuncture is performed. Varying types of acupuncture *are used* depending on ailments. Electroacupuncture *is* a new technique in which small electrical impulses *are sent* through the needle. Electroacupuncture *is generally used* as a pain reliever. Another type of method *is* sonopuncture. Sonopuncture *is* the use of sound waves within the ear to reach other parts of the body. Ailments such as obesity *have been treated* with sonopuncture. Another treatment that is synonymous with acupuncture *would be* acupressure. The only difference between the two *is* that one *is based* on using needles while the other uses pressure.

Exceptions to the Rule

In many cases, the use of the "to be" verb is acceptable. Obviously, in discussing the state of being of a person or a condition, the "to be" verb is necessary.

EXAMPLE: Rhonda *is* a hypochondriac.

Many writers, understanding that the "to be" verb causes various problems with accuracy, try to eliminate it from their work entirely. For example, the foregoing example would be written in the following manner:

Rhonda *exists* as a hypochondriac.

Obviously, this is not effective writing.

Sample Student Essay
AWKWARD CONSTRUCTIONS CREATED BY AN ATTEMPT TO ELIMINATE THE "TO BE" VERBS

Directions: The following sample paper from a student is a rewrite of her original draft. She received feedback about her paper and was told that her verbs were weak. As a result, she attempted to eliminate all forms of the "to be" verb from her writing. The following is the result. Read the passage and identify solutions to the awkward verb usage.

A superior student *embodies* someone who receives good grades, *involves* themselves in extracurricular activities, and *works* hard to achieve his or her goals. Many *argue* that the GPA *defines* the superiority of a student. The definition of a superior student *includes* several different characteristics based on perceptions and opinions. A superior student *emits* certain qualities besides a high GPA that *define* them as an excellent student.

Students attending a college or university *can study* to ensure good grades on their homework and tests. Good grades *demonstrate* a student's understanding of the material. Existing as a conscientious student *enables* a person to *excel* in studies and *develop* learning skills. In school, students *illustrate* a certain learning style that they *apply* when completing homework and studying for tests. Each student's style *holds* a certain amount of strength.

Personal learning style along with homework completion *can help* students' comprehension of assignments. Completing homework assignments efficiently *enables* students to show an improvement in their overall attitude. Homework *can serve* as an important tool to *excel* students in many areas, and completing homework *shows* many positive results. Students *may develop* stronger comprehension of the information presented in class, and they *may improve* their study skills.

Involvement in extracurricular activities *helps* students become well-rounded. Joining a club or running for office in school *demonstrates* a student's superiority among peers. Sports also *serve* as a way to demonstrate leadership. A big part of school activities *focuses* on athletics. Participation in sports *helps* students become leaders and exposes them to authority.

COMMENTS
The foregoing passage unnecessarily removes "to be" verbs from sentences where they can be employed effectively. Not all "to be" verbs create problems. A writer should, however, scrutinize verbs for their exact meanings and effectiveness.

Exercise

WEAK VERBS
Directions: Examine the following sample student essay and identify the problems with weak verbs. This essay was used in an earlier chapter to represent coherence breaks and problems with unifying the essay. Consider how a strong use of verbs might help alleviate some of these problems as sentences are revised.

Punishing a child teaches children what is right and what is wrong. Many parents punish their children by talking to them or by reward and punishment. Child abuse consists of hurting a child physically, mentally, or emotionally. There have been parents beating their children for hundreds of years. Some punishments do consider spanking but do not hurt the children. Spanking a child is considered a soft slap to show the children that they did something wrong. Beating a child leaves bruises and psychological problems. Unfortunately, there are parents all over the world that deliberately hurt their children. Child abuse causes many unresolved issues that usually do not get explored. Discipline can often be used in different ways. In case a child does not relate to a certain way, the parent can approach them in different ways to teach them morals.

As hard as it is to punish children, it needs to be done. Our society focuses on parent-child relationships and specializes in natural parenting. Punishment gives children a sense of what proper behavior is. Children need to learn the difference between right and wrong. Punishing children can be done in many different ways. One example to discipline a child is isolation. When a child is left alone they get bored easily. When they are forced to pursue something they do not get motivated unless they want to do it. Then they realize what they did was wrong. Another way to discipline children is by reward and punishment. When children are young, they react well to this. They realize that when you take something that they want away, they did something wrong, but when they do well or if they do something that you ask them to do, they get a reward. People believe that reward and punishment works well with children. This creates problems because every time they do something right, they expect to get something in return. If they know that they are not going to get something in return, they may not do what you ask them to do. If this happens, you may have to approach the situation in a different way. Lastly, talking to children begins a great relationship and tells them what is right and what is wrong. In this case, punishment may not be the answer, but explaining to them what is wrong can create an image of what is right. Speaking to your children can be a powerful tool for explaining morals. A theme is created from experiments and it shows the relations between a parent who wants to raise their children properly and the society in which they live. If you talk to children, it teaches them to trust you and to respect you and the decisions you make. The examples you set for your children also teach them what is wrong and right by your actions.

Many parents do not understand the concept of talking to your children like they are human. This is when spanking gets too far. Child abuse creates mental, physical, and emotional problems. Children who are hurt constantly deal with numerous problems and side affects. Some examples include becoming sensitive to pain, destructive, and depressed. The child becomes unlovable and is likely that they will not be loved by anyone because of their behavior. Usually when there seems to be child abuse in a family, the parent is usually the one with the problem and they hit the child to blame someone else. As a society we project problems of child abuse and try to concentrate on helping the parents. They are usually dealing with mental health issues or they have expectations of their children to do unrealistic things. In many cases, the child gets stressed out and needs to take his or her aggression out on someone who won't fight back. Child abuse is used as a form of control but sometimes the child is left with destructive organs or even death.

Child abuse stems from stress or the parents' childhood. Changes have occurred by giving the parent therapy and treatments. The parent may think that beating a child is normal if they were hit as a child. The parents need to recognize what they are doing to their children and realize the relationship that they could have with them. It has been shown that the link between economic and social atmospheres affect families that are involved in child abuse. Physical abuse normally occurs with low-income families because they have too much stress keeping control in their life and to support their families. Evidence proves that there is a relationship between child abuse and low-income families. They get stressed easily because of poverty and become likely that they are unable to support their families. Emotion becomes very natural to a human being in how they respond to certain situations. In the past, it has been shown that people are embarrassed to deal with the poor. Emotional abuse usually takes place within a high income-tax family, because they don't seem to spend enough time with their children and they search for attention. Rich families create a life worth living but do not create time to spend with their children. Parents involved in this need to realize that they need to care for their children and give them guidance.

Children who are in an abused situation usually need psychological help. After a child is abused they suffer many side effects. These side effects include that they cannot trust, they have shame and doubt in anything they do, and they become destructive with people and property. It strains their brain and creates an image so they perceive themselves as not being good enough. Many abusive parents have low self-esteem and some do not even know who they are. Hitting a child is wrong and often enough parents who do this need mental and emotional help as well as the children. For some reason, the parents believe beating someone satisfies their urge to control something and forces them to believe that it is right. Child abusers form discipline into an extreme level. The parent's attention should be on the child and what they can do to help them, not what they can do to help themselves. Discipline creates morals and behavior, so telling them to do something right by doing something wrong and hurtful is not the right approach. Sadly, child abuse is done in many ways. They may not be hitting them, but child abuse can also be from not taking care of them. Some examples are leaving a baby in a hot car for hours, not cleaning up after the children, or even not feeding them. If these parents can't take care of themselves then they should not be taking care of children.

Control is an issue that needs to be resolved before the children are born. Control helps life and releases some stress. Control leads to a natural relationship between parents and their children. They can learn how to discipline them by finding out what their children react to and how they can learn. If a parent is stressed, they should seek help if they cannot control it. Control seems to be one of the main problems because if they can't control something in their life, they need to control something else. Lack of self-control usually leads to child abuse. Punishment deals with a child's behavior and teaches them what they did wrong. It does not physically harm them. Child abuse is not discipline. It controls the way a parent reacts to certain situations. When trying to discipline children, hurting them is not the point, teaching them a lesson is. Parents need to understand that and if they don't, they need psychological help. This will help parents deal with their problems and create new relationships with their children.

WORD CHOICE AND DICTION

When the sentence revision process is finished, plan to spend more time and another draft working on word-level issues. You will assess your diction and word choice at every mark on the paper, making sure that each word communicates its intended message. Additionally, at this phase of the revision process, concentrate on eliminating wordiness, paring down your sentences into short and exact sentences.

This phase of the writing process is most difficult because you are the author of the words that are on your documents, and since you wrote them, you may not see the inherent weaknesses in your choice of words or your use of language. At this stage, it is critical to use an editor, someone who can read your work objectively and challenge the words you have written.

In academic or professional writing, you should understand that you are not afforded the luxury of writing what you would normally say or speak. With the popularity of word recognition software packages, many writers claim that they would like to produce their documents with a microphone instead of a keyboard: "If only I could just say it and have someone type what I say, ..." This is a typical mistake in thinking from inexperienced writers.

Diction

Professional writing requires precision, and precision requires time to consider and reconsider what has been written. When you write what you would say, you do not have the time to consider carefully your choice of words. Consequently, you rely on a set of words or a vocabulary that your brain has readily available. Often, these are easiest to recall and have little meaning or create vague constructions because we do not have time to scour our vocabulary for the exact word. Using words you would normally use in conversation is called *weak diction*. Diction is as important to your writing success as any other element in the recursive writing process.

Many writing teachers use the following saying to indicate the importance of precise words: "Fuzzy writing comes from fuzzy thinking." Consider the following example:

The article states that the research was faulty.

In this example, the verb is *states* and *the article* is the subject. Does an article actually *state* anything? What is the exact meaning of *state*?

When we are not sure exactly what we are trying to express, our writing will reflect that uncertainty. Likewise, everyone will agree that unclear, imprecise writing can bring about results that are unintended. Your writing should be designed to help you think clearly and write precisely.

Without doubt, good writing is essential to your academic success, but good writing is not effortless to produce, because good writers struggle with the language to find the words that meet their exact needs. Consider another saying: "Easy reading comes from hard writing." The effective communicator's first task is to engage assertively in the act of writing. Committing thoughts to paper enables us to look critically at what we are trying to express, and this latter activity helps us to clarify our thinking by choosing the right words. The excuse "I know what I am trying to say, but I can't think of the right words" fails when we are forced to put words on paper and then to consider our message. Forced to think deeply about our ideas and how to articulate them, we can no longer rely on the mental shortcuts that allow fuzzy thinking to persist. We are able to scrutinize our now-visible thoughts and, with the exact words, to clarify any aspects or concepts that lack needed precision. Through thoughtful revision and challenging the meaning of every word in the text, we can reach our communication objective. Remember another saying: "Good writing is clear thinking made visible."

The use of appropriate words and phrases in academic or professional writing requires an understanding of the types of language from which a writer can choose. For example, you would not write a formal proposal to your employer asking for changes in your work place in the same voice and with the same language that you would use in an informal note to a friend or in conversation with a friend. Consequently, you have two camps of words from which to choose: formal and informal. These categories have varying degrees of formality and informality. When you write for the profession, you will avoid the conversational and adopt the formal. Conversational words and phrases will often borrow from "mental shortcuts" or they will derive from an individual's culture or experiences. You cannot be assured that every reader will share your experiences and will therefore understand your message. Formal words will assure you and your reader that no information is lost in the transfer of ideas through words. Every reader who understands English will understand the message if it is written in formal diction. Examine Figure 3-2 and determine the level of diction you use when you speak and the level you use when you write.

Examine the following list of conversational verbs and understand that the formal may be more effective in your work:

make easy	versus	facilitate
run fast	versus	sprint
make	versus	create
do	versus	facilitate
has	versus	presents

Vague or Meaningless Words and Phrases

Other conversational diction problems are the result of our inability to recognize them as a writing weakness. Read carefully for words with inexact meanings. For example, avoid conversational words such as *very*, *a lot*, and *so*. These words often can easily be eliminated because they are vague or meaningless, and you should be able to find a single word that serves as a substitute for the combination of words that these constructions require. Be precise and struggle with the language to increase your vocabulary, and as a result, your power with words.

EXAMPLES

I am very happy.
versus
I am excited (or ecstatic).

We must drive a lot further to reach our destination.
versus
We must drive 150 miles further to reach our destination.

Colloquialisms

Likewise, you should avoid using colloquial expressions as well; such expressions often are meaningless because they do not constitute

Formal	Popular	Conversational	Slang

$\longleftrightarrow$

More Professional   **Less Professional**

Figure 3-2 Diction Scale

exact language. A *colloquialism* is a word or phrase that borrows from informal speech and derives from an expression.

I've gotten into a *fix*.

"Fix" is colloquial for *predicament*.

I'm *kind of mad* about the test results.

Both "kind of" and "mad" are weak and colloquial. Try *somewhat* and *angry* or find the word that creates the specific message your writing intends: miffed, perturbed, or aggravated.

Slang

Obviously, slang is not formal diction, but some writers may be confused about weak diction that borders on the use of slang. Consider the following example:

The entire chapter *deals with* osteoarthritis.

In this example, the verb is *deals with*. What is the exact meaning of this combination of words? The answer to that question will reveal that this combination of words is not precise in its meaning for this sentence. Try substituting *covers* for *deals with* in this example, and as a general rule, find the exact meanings of your words before you decide that they are appropriate.

Trite Phrases and Clichés

Additionally, do not use trite phrases or clichés in your writing. These are often derived from euphemisms or from an inability to choose the precise terms over the mental shortcuts.

EXAMPLES

I was on pins and needles.

He didn't want to upset the apple cart.

Last but not least, . . .

They were having a ball at the party.

In the long run, . . .

Excessive Words That Create Confusion and Meaninglessness

Just as trite phases have no meaning, sometimes a writer can become confused by words and create meaninglessness with excess.

EXAMPLES

I regret to tell you the true facts about the necessity of your imminent travel.

Her work evidences a necessity to terminate her employment status.

Jargon and Pretentious Language

Do not try to impress your reader with excessive length or confusing words and phrases. Volume does not count. Precision and accuracy are important. Write to communicate, and this is best done using direct language that is not pompous or pretentious.

EXAMPLE: Implementation of the new, unique, and illustrious procedure will be accomplished on the administrative level prior to its implementation at the clinical level.

REVISION: Administrators will implement the procedure before clinicians.

Most inexperienced writers will think that they should "sound" like writers when they attempt to communicate. To that end, they will create lengthy sentences and use complex language forms that will keep the reader from following the message. Often, when inexperienced writers do not know what to communicate, they will create sentences intended to baffle and confuse the reader to conceal their ignorance. Experienced, professional writers will create short sentences, eliminate jargon, and be specific in their word choice to invite even a weakly educated reader into the communication process.

EXAMPLE

The primary and, indeed, mechanical function of the anterior cruciate ligament is to prevent hyperextension and anterior displacement of the tibia while also acting, secondarily, as a rotational guide during the "screw-home" mechanistic procedure of extension, and as the ligament performs its tertiary function, as a secondary restraint to varus and valgus stress, it is most vulnerable to trauma during recreational and noncompetitive sports and activities, although it is equally vulnerable during competitive sports as well as nonathletic activities.

In this example, a single sentence establishes four different points, of which the most important is difficult to ascertain. This single sentence could be divided into two or three shorter sentences that each helps to illustrate the main point. Furthermore, this lengthy sentence contains 78 words. Ideally, sentences should be short and powerful, and they should make meaningful connections to your other sentences as well as your main point. Sentences of this length will lose the reader in the complex maze of language and ultimately fail to communicate the most important point. Some authors of writing texts will claim that a single sentence should not contain more than 17 words and should not attempt to make more than one point. A crafter of the language can control his or her reader to establish a position without being limited by an arbitrary number. A word count is not necessary, but a writer should be aware of the difficulties presented by overly complex sentences.

Redundancy

Avoid redundancy, or unnecessary repetition, as well.

EXAMPLES

Repeat that again.

I, personally, will provide it.

Consider redundancy on the sentence level:

EXAMPLE

A big part of school activities focuses on athletics. Working with others in groups helps to expand the knowledge of students and results in forming strong leadership qualities. Participation in athletics helps students to concentrate on becoming strong leaders. Sports teams help students to learn to work with others and gain success in groups.

As you revise and redraft, look for language problems or issues with diction. Your goal is to create clarity and precision by presenting the exact words that trigger an understanding in your reader. Avoid the conversational and provide the formal or exact. You will eliminate slang, weak words, and meaninglessness from your text.

Word Choice

In professional or academic writing, your choice of words must be exact; otherwise, you risk a failure to communicate clearly—or worse, your miscommunication could be damaging to the health or wellness of others. Because good writing is an exact science, professional writers must have control of the words they choose to provide pinpoint accuracy to their messages.

Commonly Misused Words in Medical Writing

Consider the following words, highlighted in italics, and their meanings.

Utilize versus Use

INCORRECT: The children were tested *utilizing* a standard sight chart.

CORRECTION: The children were tested *using* a standard sight chart.

Utilize and *use* are not synonymous. *Utilize* has the following meaning: to turn to practical use. In other words, I would *use* a chair to sit down, but I would *utilize* the chair as a weapon to smash a window.

In other cases, weak writers will attempt to cover their inability to correctly choose words or will attempt to hide their ignorance by trying to *sound* like a writer. In the following examples, the italicized words make us sound like writers but are incorrect:

The treatment does not *impact* men over age 50.

Use *affect* or *effect* (see following). Also, *impact* should be used to demonstrate a force that buries or submerges an object. Meteorites hit the earth with an *impact*. Wisdom teeth are *impacted*.

The patient was *toxic* when he was admitted.

Patients are not toxic; their conditions can be, though.

How does diabetes *present*?

Patients *present*, not their conditions.

Biopsy the lump.

Biopsy is a noun, not a verb.

Review the following words and, as you write, refer to them often to check their meanings.

Affect versus Effect

Affect (v) = to influence.

The drug can affect balance and alertness.

Affect (n) = behavior, outward appearance.

The patient demonstrated an inappropriate affect when he laughed at his severed limb.

Effect (v) = to bring about.

This drug can effect changes to the tissue and reduce swelling.

Effect (n) = outcome.

Sleep is the desired effect of this drug.

Lay versus Lie

Lie = to recline, rest, or stay (does not take an object)

EXAMPLES

Lie (lying, lay, lain):

I like to lie on the sand.

My dog lies in the shade.

After she lay in the sun for hours, she was roasted.

The body had lain in the bog for centuries.

Lay = to put or place something; to put in a certain position (takes an object).

EXAMPLES

Lay (laying, laid, laid):

Lay down your weapons and I won't shoot.

A good education lays the foundation for future success.

The workers were laying bricks.

He laid the book on the desk.

The rain fell after the shingles had been laid on the roof.

i.e. and e.g.

The abbreviation *i.e.* stands for "that is." Use it before amplifications.

EXAMPLE: He has Parkinson's disease, i.e., a neuro-muscular dysfunction.

The abbreviation *e.g.* stands for "for example." Use it to introduce examples of what has been previously mentioned.

EXAMPLE: Choose any of the readily recognized style formats to write your paper, e.g., APA, MLA, Chicago, or CSE.

Eliminating Wordiness

Use the following strategies to craft your words into precise sentences instead of allowing mental shortcuts to take the place of exact meanings. To eliminate wordiness from your writing, consider all of the following issues, and dedicate a draft of your paper to implementing these strategies:

- Avoid passive voice

- Weed out needless repetition

- Replace weak verbs with precise, strong verbs

- Limit the use of the "to be" verb

- Limit your dependence on adverb (-ly words) + verb combinations

- Eliminate clichés and trite phrases

- Reduce lengthy dependent clauses to short, effective ones.

Sometimes, writers' vocabularies fail them. They know that a precise word exists to clearly present their idea, but they cannot think of the exact word or words when they write. Instead of struggling with the language, they allow themselves to choose the words or phrases that are part of their conversational vocabulary or they choose language that has a meaning but not a precise meaning. These are mental shortcuts. They simply add words that help describe a noun or verb because they know that the reader should focus on these two elements of the sentence. Actually, these words do little to create a clearer understanding for the reader. Instead, such shortcuts fill the paper with unnecessary words that slow down the process of comprehension. These "filler" words do not add meaning to the sentence and should be eliminated.

WORDY EXAMPLES

Any *particular type of* note pad works well.

Getting to Pittsburgh by Sunday is impossible without *some kind of* extra help.

I, *personally*, would like to know the answer.

He said he would *definitely* be there.

I am *really* mad.

I am *very* happy.

I buy *a lot* of shoes.

MORE CONCISE REVISIONS

Any note pad works well.

Getting to Pittsburgh by Sunday is impossible without extra help.

I would like to know the answer.

He said he would be there.

I am livid.

I am ecstatic.

I own 50 pairs of shoes.

Exercise

REVISING SENTENCES TO ELIMINATE WORDINESS

Directions: Revise these sentences to state their meaning in fewer words. Avoid passive voice, needless repetition, and wordy phrases and clauses. The first sentence has been completed as an example.

1. There are many nurses in the area who are planning to attend the meeting which is scheduled for next Friday.

   Many area nurses plan to attend next Friday's meeting.

2. Although Smithery Hall is regularly populated by the medical students, close study of the building as a structure is seldom undertaken by them.

3. He dropped out of nursing school on account of the fact that it was necessary for him to help support his family.

4. It is expected that the new dress code for the therapists will be announced by the hospital administrators within the next few days.

5. There are many ways in which a graduate student of physical therapy who is interested in meeting other physical therapists may come to know one.

6. It is very unusual to find a health professional who has never told a deliberate lie on purpose.

7. Trouble is caused when patients disobey rules that have been established for the safety of all.

8. A recent rally in front of a hospital was attended by more than a thousand nurses and residents of the local area. Six residents were arrested by hospital guards for disorderly conduct, while several other nurses are charged by hospital administrators with organizing a public meeting without being issued a permit to do so.

9. The courses that are considered most important by students pursuing a career in health science are those that have been shown to be useful to them after graduation.

10. Upon graduation, occupational therapists who have recently graduated from college must all become aware of the fact that there is a need for them to make contact with other health professionals in other health fields concerning the matter of a patient.

11. In our clinic there are wide-open opportunities for professional growth with a clinic that enjoys an enviable record for allowing our patients to get rid of walking problems as soon as possible.

12. Some people believe in direct access, while other people are against it; there are many opinions on this subject.

Sample Student Essay
ELIMINATING WORDINESS IN AN ESSAY

Directions: Revise the following two paragraphs, taken from a position paper. Focus closely on diction, word choices, and weak verb usage underlined throughout the paragraphs.

In February 1997, the first mammal clone from an adult sheep, Dolly, was made[1] from a mature ewe. A lot of[2] press interest was attracted[1] towards the scientists at the Roslin Institute in Edinburgh, Scotland who came through with[3] the creation of the theoretical possibility of cloning humans. Following this scientific advancement, there were[4] ethical concerns issuing from the process as both a moral and technical problem. The claim was made[1] that human cloning not only deprives humans of their uniqueness but also has to do with[3] the interference with the natural process of human development. In other words[5], by interfering with the natural process, opponents argue that scientists tamper with nature along the way[5]. Despite these oppositions to human cloning, however, there is[4] stronger evidence why scientists should do[6] human cloning. Using cloning, breakthroughs will be discovered[7] affecting the study of genetics, cell development, human growth, and obstetrics. Human cloning is[7] beneficial to infertile couples and also allows certain replacement organs to be cloned[7] for transplants. Because of all of the advancements that cloning creates for the scientific world, the technological benefits of cloning tends to be better than[3] the possible social consequences.

There are[4] a number of practical applications for human cloning. For instance, scientific engineering may come through for[3] infertile couples who do not wish to adopt to produce a biologically related child. In addition, cloning may also be used[7] to produce an offspring free of genetic diseases. For example, a variety of disorders affecting the brain, eyes, and muscles of a newborn are produced[7] by bad genes[2] found in the mitochondria, the energy-producing structures within the cytoplasm of a cell. If one of these bad genes[2] is[7] in a woman, a geneticist could take out[6] the nucleus of one of her cells, put in[6] new DNA from a healthy donor oocyte into the cell, and put in[6] the resulting embryo into the womb. As a result, a healthy child is born[7] free of the genetic defect. Furthermore, scientists working hand-in-hand[5] with other genetic engineers make cells different[6] using cloning to treat existing diseases. For example, reprogrammed insulin-producing cells from the pancreas could be taken[7] by a genetic engineer and switched with[6] the genetic material from skin cells of a diabetic. The bad material[2] of the pancreatic cells was switched[6] with new DNA from the skin cells and then put[6] the new cells back into the pancreas to produce insulin; consequently, the diabetic patient overcomes the disease.

Sample Corrections

Note: Revisions may vary.

In February 1997, a mature ewe gave birth to Dolly, the first mammal cloned from an adult sheep. This announcement from the scientists at the Roslin Institute in Edinburgh, Scotland, attracted massive press interest creating the theoretical possibility of cloning humans. Following this scientific advance, opponents of human cloning voiced ethical concerns issuing from the process as both a moral and technical problem. These opponents claim that human cloning not only deprives humans of their uniqueness but also interferes with the natural process of human development. By interfering with the natural process, opponents argue that scientists tamper with nature. Despite these oppositions to human cloning, however, proponents present stronger evidence why scientists should implement human cloning. Using cloning, scientists will discover breakthroughs affecting the study of genetics, cell development, human growth, and obstetrics. Human cloning not only provides bene-

fits to infertile couples but also allows scientists to clone only certain replacement organs for transplants. Because of all of the advancements that cloning creates for the scientific world, the technological benefits of cloning outweigh the possible social consequences.

Geneticists foresee a number of practical applications for human cloning. For instance, infertile couples who do not wish to adopt may use cloning to produce a biologically related child. In addition, genetic engineers may also employ cloning to produce an offspring free of genetic diseases. For example, flawed genes originating in mitochondria, the energy-producing structures within the cytoplasm of a cell, produce a variety of disorders affecting the brain, eyes, and muscles of a newborn. If a woman carries a gene for one of these disorders, a geneticist could extract the nucleus of one of her cells, insert new DNA from a healthy donor oocyte into the cell, and implant the resulting embryo into the womb. As a result, the woman bears a healthy child free of the genetic defect. Furthermore, scientists may also reprogram cells using cloning to treat existing diseases. For example, a genetic engineer could reprogram insulin-producing cells from the pancreas with the genetic material from skin cells of a diabetic. The geneticist would replace the defective material of the pancreatic cells with new DNA from the skin cells and then infuse the new cells back into the pancreas to produce insulin; consequently, the diabetic patient overcomes the disease.

Explanations for Revisions

1. In each of these cases, diction problems and weak verb usage are at fault. By using "was" as a verb makes the sentence weak. In this paragraph, the verbs become stronger by rearranging the sentence and eliminating the "was". For instance, instead of "The claim was made . . . ," the beginning of the new sentence read, "These opponents claim . . . ." The verb becomes stronger because a new subject for the sentence is created, thus eliminating the diction problem.

2. The words "a lot" and "bad" are all weak in nature. Instead, they can be substituted by descriptors such as "massive" or "flawed" to make a better word choice for the paper.

3. Here, the verb phrases "came through with" and "has to do with" should be eliminated from the paper and replaced with stronger verbs. In the first case, the whole sentence is rearranged to eliminate the phrase, creating a stronger sentence: "This announcement from the scientists at the Roslin Institute in Edinburgh, Scotland, attracted massive press interest creating the theoretical possibility of cloning humans."

4. In each of these cases, "there was" started the sentence. Not only is this weak, but what exactly does "there" refer to? By creating a subject and a new verb, the problem is eliminated. For example, " . . . opponents of human cloning voiced ethical concerns issuing the process as both a moral and technical problem" proves to be clearer and more distinct than " . . . there were ethical concerns issuing the process as both a moral and technical problem."

5. Clichés and trite phrases are other phrases that should be eliminated from professional papers. In this particular paper, "in other words" and "along the way" are just two examples. These types of phrases are conversational in nature and may not mean the same thing to all people. Therefore, they should be eliminated from the paragraphs. In some cases, the phrases can be deleted to eliminate the problem (as in this case), whereas in some cases, better words will need to be substituted.

6. The word "do" in this paper is very weak and is replaced in the second paper with "implement," which is much stronger, to prove a point in a opinion paper.

7. The "to be" verb in general is very weak too and should be replaced to create a more professional paper. For instance, in the second-to-last sentence in the first paragraph, the two "to be" verbs are eliminated and the following sentence results: "Human cloning not only provides benefits to infertile couples but also allows scientists to clone only certain replacement organs for transplants." As seen here, the sentence becomes much more professional-sounding.

Exercises

ELIMINATING WORDINESS

■ Rewriting Sentences to Correct Improper Usage, Diction, and Wordiness

Directions: Rewrite the following sentences, correcting any improper word usage, wordiness, or informality.

1. As a physician, I, personally, believe Mrs. Strom's health problems relate to her drinking.

2. After prescribing the antibiotic, the nurse practitioner was not aware of the fact that the patient was allergic to sulfa drugs.

3. On one hand, the patient required physical therapy after the intense surgery, but, on the other hand, he required rest.

4. Discussing the diagnosis, Mr. Fuller excepted the necessary treatment course and the risks involved.

5. Following the examination, Dr. Schlay determined the patient was in alright condition to continue participation on the basketball team.

6. Repeatedly, the nurse keeps taking the patient's temperature and checking my blood glucose to ensure that he doesn't go into diabetic shock.

7. For her stroke rehabilitation, Mrs. Adams believed that physical therapy was equally as important as speech therapy and that all the people she worked with were a fine bunch of fellows.

8. When choosing her physician's assistant, Dr. Knowles couldn't decide which candidate was more preferable.

9. The unproductive nature of the contract talks with the nurses' union made Carrie's blood boil.

10. With the advancement in research, Mrs. Collins explored lots of different treatment options.

■ Eliminating Wordiness Using Verb-Based Writing

Directions: Rewrite the following sentences into a verb-based writing style by reducing wordiness, replacing weak verbs, and replacing passive voice with active voice construction. Correct any other errors within the sentence.

1. There were many patients waiting to see the doctor.

2. The patient was feeling uncomfortable due to high temperatures and a pain in her arm.

3. The paramedic was providing oxygen to first the child and then to the mother in order to help them breath after the car accident.

4. There are many reasons why this 43-year-old patient could have suffered from a stroke including; his diet, the amount of exercise he did, his stress levels at work and home, and others.

5. After the nurse administered chest compressions, the doctor injected some dopamine which helped the situation because the patient's heart beat came back.

6. It became evident that the patient would need surgery to fix the damages from his skiing accident, so the nurse was preparing for the procedure.

7. No one was sure about the protocol for evacuation in the case of a bomb threat. It seemed that the problem had never before been faced.

8. Later the patients will be given their dinner trays and then the nurses will need to record the amount of food and liquids they had eaten.

9. Because of the fact that the nurses were very busy, the patients complained that they were not receiving the care that they deserved.

10. The physician became troubled over the patients status because the patient was looking jaundice and was recording a high temperature.

11. Recently the recordings from John Doe's blood pressure has provided the nurses with reason to believe his days are numbered.

12. The patient is going to radiology, and he is receiving a CT scan to verify his doctor's diagnosis.

13. It seems that the doctor's are agreeing on the appropriate billing procedures regarding this procedure of a localized biopsy.

14. The nurse said to the aid to call for the doctor because it was an emergency.

15. The patient was examined in order to determine the problem that was causing her abdominal pain, and it was found to be from a weakness of the pyloric sphincter.

16. The patient is returning today for his final and third hepatitis B vaccine booster shot.

17. Following her stroke, Dr. Metting gave the indication to Mrs. Hinman that an EEG should be done to determine if any brain damage had occurred.

18. After piecing together the patient's history obtained from family and friends, it seemed that the patient may well have forgotten to take his insulin shot and was suffering from ketoacidosis.

19. The psychiatrist came to believe that Megan suffered from bipolar disease as indicated by her rapid mood changes.

20. The patient has presented with complaints of fatigue, sore throat, and swollen axillary lymph nodes, and the preliminary blood tests give an indication of mononucleosis.

■ Sample Student Essay: Word Choice and Diction

Directions: In the following sample student paper, identify the word choice problems and offer suggestions for change. Eliminate wordiness and vague constructions as well, replacing them with precise and accurate terms or language.

Anorexia is an eating disorder that could be life threatening and cause seriously problematic health problems. A major symptom of the disease consists of a fear of becoming too heavy and gaining weight. Sufferers of the disease will count calories, exercise excessively, and eat little amounts of food. An increase in pressures from family members can result in a really unhealthy outcome. The media, and other forms of radio and television, send out negative and false images and messages about body images. A perfect body, defined as tall, thin, and beautiful in all ways, remains an impossible appearance to accomplish within today's society and leads to the idea of an unhealthy being. The reality of reaching such a body state or such a dream coming to life remains unreal.

Parents, especially mothers, add to the pressures of young adult life. Many mothers, unhappy with their own appearances and who suffer from eating disorders themselves, pass the grief onto their daughters. Recent studies fit well with this idea of eating disorders. Mothers who constantly influence daughters to lose weight and to become thin can lower self-esteem and lead a child to feel bad about herself, ultimately resulting in anorexia in order to halt the nasty comments. Words remain more powerful when compared to a mother simply loses a dramatic amount of weight and the daughter witnesses the success story. In the long run, the idea of negative comments from a parent can destroy someone internally and make one feel like less of a person. People desire to feel loved and accepted, but if others view a person as unattractive, especially parents' views on their children, the outcome may result in an eating disorder. Two people in a child's life are most important: mother and father, the parents. If parents criticize their children too much, a child may starve in order to feel beautiful in their parents' eyes. Teens are especially unstable about personal perceptions of self during adolescent years, so parents who comment negatively about the child can emotionally destroy a teen.

The researchers raise a good point because a lot of girls I associated with fear becoming heavy; overweight means a person is shunned from her surroundings. In society, fat associates with ugly and isolation, and thinness connects with beautiful and and popular. Personally, I am terrified of weight gain because people may not like me or reject me from the work place in the future. Dieting consumes my mind and literally drives me crazy because I can never lose enough weight.

How to Edit for Word Choice, Diction, and Verb-Based Writing Strategies: Sample Student Essays with Comments

EXAMPLE 1

. . . **It seems** [1] that the author **does not grab the reader's attention** [2] in the first paragraph. The article is supposedly **speaking about** [3] homosexuals, but the first paragraph **has to do** [4] with heterosexuals. The author is comparing and contrasting homosexual marriages to heterosexual marriages. In my opinion, **there is** [5] no logical way that one can compare the two . . . .

. . . The author **makes a comment** [6] that discriminates against homosexuals in the last paragraph. The author does not **have** [7] sufficient sources to gather this information. **He is not supposed to ask questions when writing an article of any sort. It is really not the author's business anyway to say that homosexual couples will tire of each other.** [8] He is **being prejudice to homosexuals** . . . .[9]

COMMENTS

1. "It" does not refer to anything. The writer must modify the sentence to clarify its meaning.

2. REVISION: "The author loses the reader's interest in the first paragraph."

3. This phrase is conversational. REVISION: "The article supposedly discusses homosexuals . . . ."

4. REVISION: " . . . but the first paragraph actually discusses heterosexuals."

5. Writers should not begin a sentence with "there is" or "there are" because the subject is not clear.

6. "Makes a comment" exemplifies a weak verb phrase. The writer needs to change the entire sentence to avoid using that phrase.

7. "To have" is a weak verb. REVISION: "The author has not used enough sources . . . ."

8. Word choice problems in this sentence lead to an overly conversational tone. REVISION 1: "As a journalist, the author should not ask questions when writing an objective news article." REVISION 2: "This question should not concern the journalist because it lacks significance when considering the article's objective."

9. This phrase contains an incorrect use of a preposition. REVISION: "In this article, I think that the author showed his prejudices against homosexuals . . . ."

EXAMPLE 2

. . . Throughout high school, many students know the courses in which they need to enroll. **That is why students prepare themselves ahead of time so they will not encounter any problems.** [1] **When you enter a college or a university, you are given a curriculum according to your major** . . . .[2] . . . The author **feels** [3] that the math classes are irrelevant to his goals. **Every major needs to have some sort of creative thinking, especially for law majors, and math derives from creativity.** [4] In order for Adams to graduate, he must take this **math class and pass it.** [5] I do not see why **anyone** would want to jeopardize **their** [6] career by trying to change something that has existed for many years . . . .

. . . I would be convinced of the author's well-organized argument, but **I am totally against breaking requirements.** [7] **It is not necessary for him** [8] to argue with the committee if he says that he already has a well-rounded education . . . .

COMMENTS

1. "That is why," "that is when," "that is because," and "that is where" are all examples of improper predication.

REVISION: "With this knowledge, students can prepare for college and avoid most academic problems."

2. Writers must avoid using "you" or "your" in academic papers.
REVISION: "When students enter a college or university, they receive a curriculum that suits their major . . . ."

3. "Feels" is conversational. "Thinks" or "believes" is more appropriate.

4. This is a generalized statement that the writer has failed to support with any factual information.

5. REVISION: "To graduate, Adams must enroll in . . . ."

6. The pronoun ("anyone") must agree with the antecedent ("their"). "Anyone" is singular, and "their" is plural.
REVISION 1: "I do not see why students would want to jeopardize their career . . . ."
REVISION 2: "I do not see why anyone would want to jeopardize his or her career . . . ."

7. People use the word "totally" so frequently that it has lost its meaning.
REVISION: ". . . I do not think that universities should exempt students from degree requirements."

8. REVISION: "He should not argue . . . ."

EXAMPLE 3

. . . Sexual harassment is **very** [1] popular in the United States of America. It is nothing to consider **unserious**. [2] **Sexual harassment is a criminal offense, even if the person is a minor** . . . .[3]

. . . **Surveys prove that there is sexual harassment going on in junior high.** [4] When adolescents become the victims of sexual harassment, they are being **disrespected** [5] and their self-esteem can sometimes **take a turn for the worse** . . . .[6]

. . . Sexual harassment is a **major** [7] problem that exists in school systems, **but school officials are not opening up their eyes enough to see it going on so they can put a stop to it.** [8] When adolescents start junior high, they are old enough to know the difference between right and wrong. Parents or guardians should occasionally remind them that **you should not touch someone in a sexual nature. Then you list some examples of sexual harassment** . . . .[9]

COMMENTS

1. People use "very" so frequently that it has lost its meaning.
REVISION: "Sexual harassment frequently occurs in the United States of America."

2. This phrase uses a nonexistent word, "unserious."
REVISION: "People should consider sexual harassment a serious problem."

3. REVISION: "Sexual harassment is a criminal offense, even if the person who commits the crime is a minor . . . ."

4. This phrase uses informal language.
REVISION: "Surveys prove that sexual harassment occurs in junior high."

5. "Disrespected" is inappropriate in academic writing because it is a slang term.

6. "Take a turn for the worse" is a trite phrase.
REVISION: "Their self-esteem can sometimes suffer . . . ."

7. People use "major" so frequently that it has lost its meaning.

8. REVISION: ". . . but school officials generally ignore the problem and, therefore, it still affects students."

9. These phrases contain pronoun-antecedent problems. The first "you" refers to adolescents, not the reader.
REVISION: ". . . they should not touch someone in a sexual nature." The second "you" refers to "parents or guardians."
REVISION: ". . . then the parents or guardians should list some examples . . . ."

EXAMPLE 4

. . . Low self-esteem is **extremely** [1] common **throughout** [2] most young women. They **get their misleading information** [3] from television and Hollywood . . . .

. . . **Many young women feel that they would fit in if they were slim.** [4] Television shows can also lower a young woman's self-esteem. **The television show** Beverly Hills 90210 **portrays females on the show to be pretty looking girls who are popular.** [5] This can result in **young women** [6] becoming anorexic or even suicidal . . . .

. . . Most young women think that if men are **not in pursuit for them,** [7] then they are not popular . . . .

Young women read magazines that feature gorgeous women and mimic the actresses and models **that** [8] are featured . . . .

A young women's self-esteem can also be lowered if she is smart. [9] Peer pressure can lead to low self-esteem because friends tend to influence **someone to do many things.** They think that if they **don't do it**, then they will not **be cool** [10] and they will not be able to socialize with popular cliques . . . .

COMMENTS

1. People use "extremely" so frequently that it has lost its meaning. Limit your use of adverb-verb combinations.

2. This exemplifies wrong use of a preposition. REVISION: "Many young women experience low self-esteem."

3. "Get" is a weak verb.

4. REVISION: "Many young women think that they would become popular if they were slim."

5. This phrase uses the verb "to portray" incorrectly. REVISION: " . . . *Beverly Hills 90210* features actresses who portray beautiful, popular girls."

6. The reader cannot tell to what "young women" refers. As written, it may refer to either the audience of young women or the young women who act on the show.

7. This phrase does not exist in either standard or colloquial English.

8. Because "actresses and models" refer to people, the proper relative pronoun is "who," not "that," which normally refers to things.

9. "Women" is plural, but the writer wants to use the singular form as indicated by "self-esteem," which is a singular noun. REVISION: "Peers can lower a young woman's self-esteem if she is smart."

10. These are all examples of clichéd language resulting from weak verbs.

4

Phase Four of the Writing Process: Creating Essays That Flow

Key Terms

Appositive phrase A group of words renaming the noun before it

Complex sentence One or more dependent clauses added to an independent clause

Compound sentence Two or more independent clauses

Compound-complex sentence One or more dependent clauses added to two or more independent clauses

Coordination Making elements of equal importance equivalent in grammatical structure

Dependent clause A group of words that contain a subject and a verb but does not make a complete thought

Essential elements Elements that a sentence requires to maintain its meaning

Gerund phrase A group of words beginning with a word that ends in *ing* and acting as a noun in the sentence

Independent clause A group of words that contains a subject and a verb and makes a complete thought (a sentence)

Infinitive phrase A group of words beginning with a root form (*to + verb* construction) and acting as a modifier

Nonessential elements Elements that a sentence does not require and therefore can be set off with commas

Participial phrase A group of words beginning with a word ending in *ing*, *t*, *d*, *ed*, or *n* and acting as an adjective describing the subject of the sentence

Prepositional phrase A group of words showing relationship (*in*, *on*, *under*, *of*, *to*, *at*, and so on)

Simple sentence A single independent clause

Subordination Making information less important in a sentence by reducing it to a phrase or dependent clause

chapter objectives

On completion of this chapter, the reader should be able to

1. Identify, create, and implement the five types of phrases to avoid sentence monotony.
2. Identify, create, and implement the four types of sentences.
3. Eliminate sentence monotony and subordinate less important information using sentence types.
4. Control the dissemination of information to a reader by determining what is important and what is less important.
5. Control the reactions of the reader by moving less important information into phrases and dependent clauses.
6. Control the reactions of the reader by maintaining equivalent grammatical structures for equally important information.

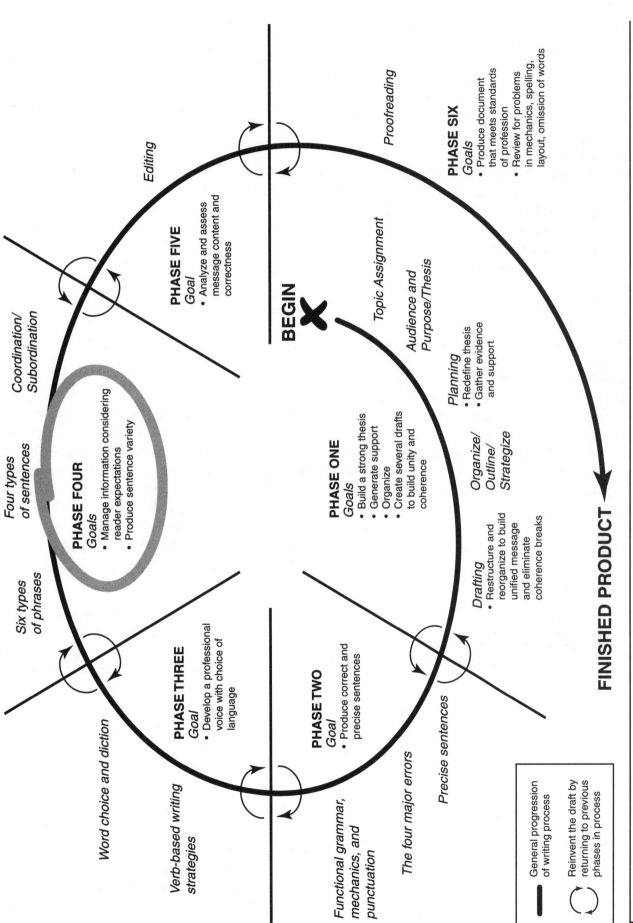

Editing

Proofreading

*Coordination/
Subordination*

PHASE SIX
Goals
• Produce document
  that meets standards
  of profession
• Review for problems
  in mechanics, spelling,
  layout, omission of words

PHASE FIVE
Goal
• Analyze and assess
  message content and
  correctness

*Four types
of sentences*

BEGIN
✗

Topic Assignment

*Audience and
Purpose/Thesis*

Planning
• Redefine thesis
• Gather evidence
  and support

PHASE FOUR
Goals
• Manage information considering
  reader expectations
• Produce sentence variety

PHASE ONE
Goals
• Build a strong thesis
• Generate support
• Organize
• Create several drafts
  to build unity and
  coherence

*Organize/
Outline/
Strategize*

*Six types
of phrases*

Drafting
• Restructure and
  reorganize to build
  unified message
  and eliminate
  coherence breaks

Word choice and diction

PHASE THREE
Goal
• Develop a professional
  voice with choice of
  language

PHASE TWO
Goal
• Produce correct and
  precise sentences

FINISHED PRODUCT

*Verb-based writing
strategies*

*Functional grammar,
mechanics, and
punctuation*

The four major errors

Precise sentences

— General progression
  of writing process

↻ Reinvent the draft by
  returning to previous
  phases in process

Figure 4–1 The Writing Process: Phase Four

*A*s you begin to see that your document is close to completion (see Figure 4-1), begin focusing on your reader again. Recognize that what you have written may not be completely clear to your reader. Sometimes, as writers, we can get too close to our work, and we cannot see the obvious problems in grammar, sentences, wording, or any other issue of writing ("Can't see the forest because of the trees"). For this reason, we all need editors and proofreaders to help us see our mistakes.

An educated editor can be pivotal in helping you create a document or paper that engages the reader well. Often, as we get too close to our subject, we tend to forget that we have an audience of people who need to be guided, informed, or entertained. An editor may be able to tell you when your writing has turned stale, has become boring, or has deviated from its intended purpose. Your goal is to put your reader on a set of tracks and push him or her down the line. You cannot afford to provide any "exits" from that line. If your reader gets off track, you have failed to guide him or her appropriately. When a reader cannot understand the message, the problem rests on the writer, not the reader. Your job as a writer is to communicate the message. If the message is not clear, *you* are at fault, and *you* need to clarify the message to your audience by revising your work.

AVOIDING SENTENCE MONOTONY

Running together several sentences that begin with the same grammatical structure creates sentence monotony. Consider the following example:

> Sarah is a good student. Sarah studies in the library.

Notice that these two sentences have the same grammatical structure of subject-verb-object (S-V-O):

> S-V-O. S-V-O.

Any writer will recognize the way to fix this problem: Combine the sentences into one. To do so requires the use of some grammatical elements.

> **ORIGINAL:** Sarah is a good student. Sarah studies in the library.

> REVISIONS:

> Sarah, a good student, studies in the library.

> In the library, Sarah studies to become a good student.

> Studying in the library helps Sarah to become a good student.

> Studying in the library, Sarah has become a good student.

> To become a good student, Sarah studies in the library.

> Sarah is a good student, and she studies in the library.

> Although Sarah studies in the library, she is a good student.

Everyone who has ever written will recognize the various forms that create sentences with essentially the same meaning. These forms, however, have names, and good writers will understand how to use these elements and why they use them. This chapter will help you understand these mechanisms.

Consider the original example again:

> Sarah is a good student. Sarah studies in the library.

Anyone will quickly recognize that this writing sounds like the work of a third grader. Each short sentence may or may not be related to the other. With more sophisticated writing techniques, however, the words you use and the sentences you craft will develop a rhythm or flow that will allow your reader to follow your line of reasoning. Consider a paragraph that is filled with the kind of short, choppy sentences in the preceding example.

> Many rivers flow out to sea. They take the most direct route. They flow quickly down the sides of mountains. They flow more slowly on flat terrain. Rapidly moving water wears away the land. The wearing-away process is called erosion. The planting of trees, shrubs, and grasses can prevent erosion.

This style of writing is boring. The writing sounds more like a list than like an essay. Grammatically, every sentence begins with a subject-verb combination, and every sentence is short. Writers in the sciences and the health professions struggle with this problem often because they are managing large amounts of information, and their intention is to simply spill the information onto the page. Although this short and choppy style is acceptable for a first draft, it is not acceptable in the final stages of the writing process because the reader will become bored with the monotonous style or simply will be lost in the overload of information in a list form. Remember that documents are written for the benefit of the *reader*, not the writer. Write to communicate and not to simply toss out facts. Likewise, many writers will combine sentences, burying the reader with information instead of supplying a communication link with the words. In other words, they will use long sentences that address several issues or make several points. This type of writing is as damaging as the short and choppy style, and the result is often the same: failure to communicate. Write to communicate, not to impress.

To fix the problem of monotony, employ sentence variation techniques; however, to employ sentence variation techniques, you need to know where to create such sentences. Examine your document or draft, and look for sentences that have similar grammatical elements serving as sentence openers. In other words, look for sentences that start with the subject-verb combination that created the previous boring example.

As you begin implementing sentence variation techniques, consider again the effect on your readers. You can control the readers' emotions and attention by varying sentence structure. For example, if you create a paragraph of longer sentences, your readers will expect more of the same because they have "caught on" to the rhythm. However, if you insert a short sentence into the mix of longer sentences, your readers' attention will be drawn to the short sentence because it stands out from the rest. This short sentence, then, creates emphasis. Use this technique strategically to highlight important messages or astute conclusions in your papers.

Not only are these sentence variation techniques useful for creating emphasis in a paragraph, but they can also help the reader identify the more important information in a sentence. For example, when combining sentences, you have some choices. You can put some information into a phrase or a **dependent clause** (a group of words containing a subject and a verb that nevertheless cannot stand alone) and other, often more important information into an **independent clause** (a clause that makes a complete thought).

Consider the example again.

ORIGINAL: Sarah is a good student. Sarah studies in the library.

REVISION: Sarah, a good student, studies in the library.

In the revised sentence, the independent clause is the following: *Sarah studies in the library*. The supplemental information in this sentence, *a good student*, is placed in an appositive phrase. Placing less important information in a phrase (or in a dependent clause) is called **subordination**.

Consider this example:

ORIGINAL: Sarah is a good student. Sarah studies in the library.

REVISION: Sarah is a good student, and she studies in the library.

In the revised sentence, the information about Sarah is that she *is a good student* and that *she studies in the library*. These elements that describe her both are placed in independent clauses. In doing so, the writer tells the reader that these descriptive elements are equal in importance. This is the process of **coordination**. Elements of equal strength should be placed in grammatically equivalent sentence types.

Furthermore, as you consider subordination and coordination techniques, examine the emphasis that each sentence creates. Writers and reading specialists tell us that the most important part of a sentence to a reader is the information that comes at the end of the sentence. Good writers, then, will place important information at the end of a sentence and at the end of the independent clauses. Less important information will be used in phrases and dependent clauses at the front end of the sentences.

Sentence variation techniques use different types of phrases as sentence openers or different types of sentences that break up an unnecessary monotony. A good editor will help you see the parts of your paper where these problems occur. Additionally, you can also act as your own editor by distancing yourself from your paper and subject. (Spend some time doing something else. Stop writing and revising, go for a walk, or simply take a break. Try not to think about your paper. Then, after you have refreshed your brain, go back to the paper and read it as if you are the intended audience. This will awaken your senses to monotonous sentences, poor word choice, awkward sentence constructions, or even grammar problems and coherence issues. A sense of objectivity is your goal when you review and refashion sentences with variety.) Once you have reached a stage of objectivity, attack your draft by looking for unintended consistencies in sentence openers. The easiest technique to employ here is to look for a series of sentences that begin with the subject-verb combination. Find ways to combine these sentences or to create phrases and clauses that will break up such monotony. Furthermore, as you add these elements, be aware of the impact of your choices on the message you intend to send. Keep your important points in the independent clauses, and put less important information in phrases and clauses at the front end of your sentences.

While you manipulate your sentences and words, you are manipulating your reader. Understand how the changes you make will create meaning for your audience.

USING PHRASES TO AVOID SENTENCE MONOTONY

A *phrase* is a group of words that contains an object or a predicate but not both. Variation of sentence structure can occur with the use of

phrases, as well as what we already know about creating different types of sentences by using independent and dependent clauses. The English language contains six types of phrases, and of these, one has become archaic and is used sparingly: the absolute phrase. The other five—appositive, infinitive, prepositional, gerund, and participial phrases—should be employed regularly by any writer attempting to create sentence variations in professional writing. The goal here is not to use the phrases for the sake of using phrases but to avoid monotonous subject-verb-object constructions that make paragraphs boring.

Each of the following sentences is written in S-V-O form, or as a **simple sentence** (a single independent clause).

> Sarah studies often in the library. Sarah is an exceptional student.

The addition of phrases, however, will provide specific meaning changes and build continuity. These sentences now can be combined by using specific types of phrases:

> **GERUND:** Studying often in the library allows Sarah to be an exceptional student.

> **PARTICIPIAL:** Studying often in the library, Sarah has become an exceptional student.

> **INFINITIVE:** To become an exceptional student, Sarah studies often in the library.

> **PREPOSITIONAL:** In the library, Sarah studies often and has become a better student.

> **APPOSITIVE:** Sarah, an exceptional student, studies often in the library.

Keep in mind that these phrases can appear in any position in the sentence, although the appositive typically follows the noun it modifies. Using these phrases as sentence openers provides the variety writers seek.

Note: Placing information in a phrase subordinates that information to the information in the independent clause, making it nonessential. Use of **nonessential elements** *will require attention to the rules of comma usage.*

Of the five phrases listed, three are also considered verbal phrases: infinitive, participial, and gerund. These are made from verbs but function as nouns, adjectives, or adverbs. If you identify a word that looks like a verb but is not the main verb in the sentence, then you have probably found a verbal. You should recognize verbals as such, but our emphasis here is on verbal phrases, of which these are also a part.

The Prepositional Phrase

The **prepositional phrase** shows relationship. Such phrases are easily recognized by the use of introductory words such as *on*, *in*, *under*, *over*, *beyond*, *through*, *before*, *after*, and so on. Other words such as *for*, *of*, *as*, and *to* also serve as prepositions, because they too show relationship.

In the house, I left my tools.

For breakfast, I would like eggs and bacon.

Through the fields, the river twisted and turned.

Obviously, not every prepositional phrase begins a sentence. Look through old papers and you will find them frequently used in many positions in the sentence. They are used here as introductory elements to demonstrate that all sentences can begin with a mechanism of sentence variety by employing them as introductory elements.

ORIGINAL: Sarah is a good student. Sarah studies in the library.

REVISION USING PREPOSITIONAL PHRASE: *In the library*, Sarah studies to be a good student.

When prepositional phrases begin a sentence, however, grammarians disagree about the use of commas to separate them from the independent clause (see "Rules of Comma Usage" in Chapter 2). You will never be wrong if you separate any introductory prepositional phrase from the independent clause. Some textbooks will require that you eliminate the comma from short prepositional phrases (three words or less), and others provide the option of including or excluding it. In my experiences as a writer, I have found that consistency works best. The rules for other introductory phrases call for a comma. Use the comma here as well, if for nothing more than consistency.

The Appositive Phrase

The **appositive phrase** renames the noun it modifies in the sentence. Typically, an appositive follows its noun.

ORIGINAL: Sarah is a good student. Sarah studies in the library.

REVISION USING APPOSITIVE PHRASE: Sarah, *a good student*, studies in the library.

The appositive is used as a mechanism that explains or provides additional information. It is used here as a mechanism to provide internal variety to your sentences.

Dave, *my friend*, is a good mechanic.

In this case, the phrase in italics simply renames or redescribes the noun *Dave*. Notice that, in this case, the phrase is set off by commas from the remainder of the sentence. The information within the commas is not necessary for the sentence to maintain its integrity or message; therefore, it is considered nonrestrictive (see the section on "That versus Which" in Chapter 2). This group of words can be eliminated and the sentence still makes sense.

However, not all appositives are nonrestrictive. Consider the following sentence:

My friend *Dave* is a good mechanic.

In this sentence, "Dave" is still an appositive because it renames the subject "My friend," but it is restrictive in this case, meaning that it must be there for the sentence to make sense. If the word "Dave" is surrounded by commas, making it nonrestrictive, the sentence means: "I have only one friend, and by the way, his name is Dave." Because the speaker has more than one friend, however, "Dave" is an essential part of the sentence because it answers the question "which friend?" Such restrictive appositives are examples of **essential elements** of sentences.

The Gerund Phrase

The **gerund phrase** functions as a noun in the sentence. The gerund is identified easily because it always ends in *-ing*. Be sure to differentiate between gerund phrases and participial phrases, because both can end in *-ing*, but the participle acts as an adjective, not a noun or subject of the sentence.

> **EXAMPLE**: *Planning* his route took serious concentration.

Notice that the gerund phrase, because it holds the grammatical function of subject of the sentence, requires no marks of punctuation to separate it from the remainder of the sentence. We have no rules that indicate that subjects and verbs should be separated by commas, and hence, the rules apply here: No comma is used.

> **ORIGINAL:** Sarah is a good student. Sarah studies in the library.
>
> **REVISION USING GERUND PHRASE:** Studying in the library allows Sarah to be a good student.

The Participial Phrase

The **participial phrase** acts as an adjective describing the subject of the sentence. The present participle ends in *-ing*, and the past participle ends in *-ed, -d, -t,* or *-n*.

> *Falling* into the water, he tossed me his keys and wallet.
>
> (Present participle)
>
> *Known* for his intelligence, Steve received a perfect score.
>
> (Past participle)
>
> *Disappointed* with her grade, she confronted her professor.
>
> *Hurt* by his comments, she dropped the class.
>
> *Heard* across the water, the foghorn is still a useful tool on lighthouses.

These phrases can appear in any part of the sentence. In these examples, they serve as introductory elements to show one means of providing sentence variation.

The participial phrase acts as an adjective describing the noun it refers to. If it serves as an introductory element (see "Rules of Comma Usage" in Chapter 2), it must be set off with a comma.

> **ORIGINAL:** Sarah is a good student. Sarah studies in the library.
>
> **REVISION USING PARTICIPIAL PHRASE:** *Studying in the library*, Sarah is a good student.

The Infinitive Phrase

The **infinitive phrase** consists of *to* + the base form of the verb and can appear in any part of the sentence. It is used here as an introductory element to provide sentence variety.

> **ORIGINAL:** Sarah is a good student. Sarah studies in the library.
>
> **REVISION USING INFINITIVE PHRASE:** To become a better student, Sarah studies in the library.

To identify the infinitive, think about early grammar or foreign language classes. Whenever you would conjugate verbs, you would start with the base form of the verb. (I think of my first day of Spanish class when we conjugated *hablar*: to speak.) Be sure that the infinitive phrase uses the *to + base verb* combination; do not confuse them with prepositional phrases beginning with *to*.

Infinitive Phrases

> *To avoid* the crowds, we stayed at home all weekend.
>
> *To be* a good writer, you must be able to demonstrate sentence variety.

Compare with prepositional phrases that start with *to*:

> *To the pool*, the children ran.

In these examples, the infinitive phrases serve as introductory elements and should be set off from the independent clause with a comma (see "Rules of Comma Usage" in Chapter 2).

Exercises

USING PHRASES FOR SENTENCE VARIETY

■ Combining Sentences Using Phrases

Directions: Work through these monotonous, simple sentences and rewrite each one five times using all of the five commonly used types of phrases.

1. Alabama was organized as a territory in 1817. It was admitted to the Union in 1819.
2. Virginia is nicknamed "The Old Dominion." It was the oldest of the English colonies.

It remained loyal to the king during the English Civil War.

3. Rhode Island is the smallest state in the Union. It has played a great part in American history. It was a haven for individuals seeking religious freedom.

4. Dr. Jones is a professor of comparative literature. He believes that Wordsworth is the founder of modern literary criticism.

5. Professor Holland is our soccer coach. She also teaches American literature.

6. My father graduated from USC. He is now a professor at Tufts.

■ Revising for Sentence Variety

Directions: Revise the following paragraph using phrases to create variation.

Many rivers flow out to sea. They take the most direct route. They flow quickly down the sides of mountains. They flow more slowly on flat terrain. Rapidly moving water wears away the land. The wearing-away process is called erosion. The planting of trees, shrubs, and grasses can prevent erosion.

USING THE FOUR TYPES OF SENTENCES TO AVOID SENTENCE MONOTONY

Writers often search for ways to manipulate sentence structure to break the monotony of reading similarly constructed sentences. If all sentences were written in a simple S-V-O style, the document would be boring. We already know how to subordinate and coordinate different elements of sentences, and these strategies can be employed to build sentence variety as well. Examine the different types of sentences presented and find ways to incorporate these variations into your documents to avoid unnecessary monotony.

A boring paragraph has the following structure. Most sentences begin with the subject-verb combination, and all are simple sentences.

S-V-O

S-V-O

S-V-O

Phrase-S-V-O

A more sophisticated arrangement would allow for different sentence types that are interspersed among and around the simple sentences. Undoubtedly, most of your sentences will be simple. Use the other sentence types—compound (CP), complex (CX), and compound-complex (CP-CX), as described later—to break the monotony, as in the following example:

Phrase-S-V-O

S-V-O (S)

CP (S-V-O, and S-V-O)

CX (dependent clause, S-V-O)

S-V-O

CP-CX (dependent clause, S-V-O, and S-V-O)

Use a variety of sentences in order to provide continuity and flow to your work.

Simple Sentence

A simple sentence consists of a single independent clause and *no* dependent clauses.

EXAMPLES:
Hawthorne writes "Young Goodman Brown" in 1835.
In 1835, Hawthorne writes "Young Goodman Brown."
Hawthorne writes and edits "Young Goodman Brown" in 1835.
Hawthorne writes "Young Goodman Brown" in 1835 and edits it in 1836.

In each of these examples, the structure is the same. The group of words forms a single independent clause. The first two examples are obvious: S-V-O-prepositional phrase. The last two, however, may not be obvious for the beginning writer. These two examples contain two verbs, and many writers will automatically assume that since a second verb operates in the sentence, the sentence must contain two independent clauses. This is not the case. In these two examples, the verbs *writes* and *edits* connect with the subject *Hawthorne*. This is one independent clause, and this can be determined by employing a test. A simple sentence is one complete thought. Therefore, cover the language before the coordinating conjunction and the conjunction. Do the same for the language after the coordinating conjunction. If the words showing do not make a complete sentence, then the words are not independent.

> **EXAMPLE:** Hawthorne writes "Young Goodman Brown" in 1835 ~~and edits it in 1836~~.

In this case, the language before the coordinating conjunction creates a sentence. You can identify this as an independent clause. However, examine the remainder of the sentence by performing the same test:

> **EXAMPLE:** ~~Hawthorne writes "Young Goodman Brown" in 1835 and~~ edits it in 1836.

Notice that *edits it in 1836* is not a sentence. Therefore, the verb belongs to the subject in the first independent clause. This sentence, then, is one independent clause.

Compound Sentence

A **compound sentence** is made up of two or more independent clauses. This type of sentence is created by using two (or more) simple sentences of equal weight and combining them with the proper use of the coordinating conjunction and the rules of comma usage.

> **EXAMPLE:** Hawthorne writes "Young Goodman Brown" in 1835, but he did not edit it until 1836.

Notice the rules of comma usage employed here. Furthermore, employ the test as discussed previously.

> **EXAMPLE:** ~~Hawthorne writes "Young Goodman Brown" in 1835, but~~ he did not edit it until 1836.

The remaining words create an independent clause. They are a complete thought containing a subject and a verb.

> **EXAMPLE:** Hawthorne writes "Young Goodman Brown" in 1835, ~~but he did not edit it until 1836.~~

The remaining words create a complete sentence here as well.

Since both groups of words are a complete thought containing a subject and a verb, they can be joined by a comma and a coordinating conjunction.

Complex Sentence

A **complex sentence** is composed of one independent clause and one or more dependent clauses.

> **EXAMPLE:** When Hawthorne writes "Young Goodman Brown" in 1835, he does not understand its importance to American literary history.

In this example, the first group of words, *When Hawthorne writes "Young Goodman Brown" in 1835*, is a dependent clause. It contains a subject and a verb, but it cannot stand on its own because of the word *when*. *When* makes this group of words dependent on another sentence. As a result, this group of words depends on the independent clause to create a full and complete thought.

The independent clause, then, is *he does not understand its importance to American literary history*. This group of words contains a subject and a verb, and it can stand on its own to make a complete thought.

In the following example, words in *italics* indicate dependent clauses. Words in **bold** indicate the independent clauses.

> *When Hawthorne writes "Young Goodman Brown" in 1835*, **he does not understand its importance to American literary history**, *although Emerson realizes its worth*.

Compound-Complex Sentence

A **compound-complex sentence** contains two or more independent clauses and one or more dependent clauses. Use the same scheme to identify the *dependent* and **independent** clauses.

> *When Hawthorne writes "Young Goodman Brown" in 1835*, **he does not understand its importance to American literary history**, but **Emerson realizes its worth immediately**.

> **Hawthorne writes "Young Goodman Brown" in 1835**, but **he does not understand its importance to American literary history**, *although Emerson realizes its worth*.

Conclusion

Search your paper for different sentence types and look for unnecessary repetitions. You may want to consider highlighting sentence types in a draft and examining your use or over-use of one particular sentence type. Many writers find, through this exercise, that they use simple sentences throughout their papers and that they use compound or complex sentences rarely. Others will find that they use compound sentences frequently, and they will rarely use complex sentences. Most writers will not use compound-complex sentences with much frequency.

Since you now know that these sentence types exist, use them to effectively provide variety to your work. Also, by using dependent clauses effectively, you can subordinate less important information to the more important information, which should be housed in your independent clauses.

Exercises

USING THE FOUR TYPES OF SENTENCES

■ Combining Sentences Using Different Sentence Types

Directions: These are the same sentences that appeared in the section about phrases. Work through these monotonous, simple sentences and rewrite each one four times using all four types of sentences.

1. Alabama was organized as a territory in 1817. It was admitted to the Union in 1819.
2. Virginia is nicknamed "The Old Dominion." It was the oldest of the English colonies. It remained loyal to the king during the English Civil War.
3. Rhode Island is the smallest state in the Union. It has played a great part in American history. It was a haven for individuals seeking religious freedom.
4. Dr. Jones is a professor of comparative literature. He believes that Wordsworth is the founder of modern literary criticism.
5. Professor Holland is our soccer coach. She also teaches American literature.
6. My father graduated from USC. He is now a professor at Tufts.

■ Revising for Sentence Variation

Directions: Revise this entire passage using sentence variation techniques. When finished, rewrite it again using combinations of the four types of sentences and the five commonly used types of phrases:

Many rivers flow out to sea. They take the most direct route. They flow quickly down the sides of mountains. They flow more slowly on flat terrain. Rapidly moving water wears away the land. The wearing-away process is called erosion. The planting of trees, shrubs, and grasses can prevent erosion.

SUBORDINATION AND COORDINATION OF IDEAS

As you know, when you join independent clauses, you use coordinating conjunctions to do so. The independent clauses, then, are equal in weight, meaning that since they are used in coordination, they deserve equal consideration from the reader. Likewise, parallelism allows a writer to coordinate like or equal ideas or parts of sentences; however, not all parts of a sentence or ideas are equal. Some should not take on as much emphasis as other parts. As a result, writers subordinate some ideas or sentence parts to the main part of the sentence. Subordination allows a writer to indicate degrees of importance without writing separate sentences.

As a writer, you should follow this general rule: Keep the important information of your sentence in the independent clause. Use less important information in dependent clauses or phrases, or in introductory words and phrases.

Consider some examples derived from the following two sentences:

She is an exceptional student. She studies frequently.

To combine and coordinate the sentences, you would use a coordinating conjunction:

> She is an exceptional student, and she studies frequently.

You could also subordinate either of these ideas to create different impacts:

> Because she studies frequently, she is an exceptional student.

> Although she is an exceptional student, she studies frequently.

Consider how subordination of some thoughts and sentence parts changes the meaning of your sentences. Try subordinating and coordinating various elements of these sentences. You should become familiar with the different types of phrases and types of sentences in order to vary your sentence structure, for continuity and flow, and to protect the exact meaning of your paragraphs.

Explanations for Sentence Variation Strategies: Subordination and Coordination

EXAMPLE: Rhode Island is the smallest state in the Union. It played an important part in American history. It was a haven for political and religious freedom seekers.

REVISION: Rhode Island, the smallest state in the Union, played an important part in American history, and it was a haven for political and religious freedom seekers.

In the first phase of revision, the unimportant information is taken out of the form of an independent clause. The fact that Rhode Island is the smallest state in the Union is insignificant when compared with the thrust of the other two sentences. Consequently, the first independent clause can be reduced to an appositive phrase to demonstrate its less important role.

The remaining sentences can be combined to form one independent clause:

> Rhode Island, the smallest state in the Union, played an important part in American history and was a haven for political and religious freedom seekers.

This form may not be the most effective form to use. The verbs, *played* and *was*, are in parallel structure, but they do not have the same effect on the reader. Consider the differences in the strength of the two: *played* creates action; *was* is weak and creates inaction. Also, since these elements are used within the same independent clause, they may be taken together to mean that one causes the other. This may not be the case.

To help fix this sentence, set out the information as two independent clauses joined by a coordinating conjunction.

> Rhode Island, the smallest state in the Union, played an important part in American history, and it was a haven for political and religious freedom seekers.

This form will dictate to your reader that both independent clauses are to be considered equally. Rhode Island played an important role AND it was a political and religious haven. Your reader cannot be confused about the exact meaning here.

Exercise

SUBORDINATION AND COORDINATION

Directions: Combine the following sentences using the four types of sentences and appropriately subordinating relevant parts of the original in your reconstruction.

1. Professor Jones teaches English. She is also our rugby coach. Her coaching duties are part of her job.

2. Many colleges in New York are private. Most students attend the public colleges and universities. Many of these students do not live in New York State.

3. My English professor for composition was good. He taught me how to formulate coherent essays. He also taught me how to recognize grammatical problems.

4. The buildings on campus are old. Some are still useful and have character. Others are outdated and need to be demolished.

Exercises

SENTENCE VARIATION

■ Combining Simple Sentences for Sentence Variety

Directions: Combine the following groups of sentences into one effective simple or complex sentence.

1. The nurse prepared the sterile tray. The physician intended to perform a lumbar puncture.
2. A woman went into labor. Her family waited nervously. They were to be informed of any new details.
3. The patient in room 341 window has pancreatitis. His blood count is low as a result.
4. The patient is a 3-year-old boy. He was jumping on the bed. There was a pencil on the bed. The boy fell. The pencil went into his eye.
5. Dr. Gutman referred Ted Brimes to our office. Dr. Gutman diagnosed Mr. Brimes with rotator cuff tendonitis.
6. The nurse's aide transported the patient from the emergency room to the intensive care unit. The patient, Mr. White, began to arrest in atrial fibrillation. The nurse's aide began CPR in the middle of the hallway.
7. The radiologist detected an abnormality on the patient's mammogram. The ultrasound exam of the patient's breast revealed a mass. The physician performed a biopsy.
8. Samantha Green complained of sharp pain in her lower right quadrant. Her physician believed she had appendicitis. Ultrasound examination identified her problem as ovarian cysts.
9. The patient arrived in the emergency room at 6:30 A.M. complaining of a migraine. By 6:40 A.M., the patient developed a temperature of 103° Fahrenheit. He began to have seizures at 6:45 A.M. His condition worsened rapidly.
10. Margaret Levett had a stroke 6 months ago. She visits the speech therapist, physical therapist, and occupational therapist daily. Her functional skills are recovering quickly with the therapy.

■ Identifying the Four Types of Sentences

Directions: Identify the following sentences as simple (**S**), compound (**CP**), complex (**CX**), or compound-complex (**CP-CX**).

1. Although the emergency room was full, the unit maintained strict schedule and tended to patients quickly.
2. The physical therapist recommends 6 weeks of therapy three times a week.
3. When a patient visits the office complaining of chest pain, the nurses automatically record an ECG on the patient, and, if the doctor finds any problems, an ambulance rapidly transports the patient to the emergency room.
4. Being a pediatric neurosurgeon requires immense dexterity, and it also demands extreme patience.
5. The patient prepared with physical therapy for 3 weeks prior to the surgery.
6. The physician explained the traditional treatment for the patient's disease, but the patient decided to seek an unconventional intervention.

■ Combining Simple Sentences

Directions: Combine the following groups of simple sentences to form a compound, complex, or compound-complex sentence.

1. Dr. Hoffmann practices ophthalmology. He specializes in macular degeneration.
2. The doctor diagnosed Mr. Whitman with dermatitis. He referred the patient to a local dermatologist.
3. All blood tests done on the patient returned normal. He was discharged in good health.
4. The Emergency Medical Technician administered the Ambu bag. The victim suffered from heat exhaustion and collapsed.

Exercises

PHRASES

■ Identifying Types of Phrases

Directions: In the following examples, identify the italicized phrases as participial, gerund, prepositional, or infinitive phrases.

1. *Reading the mammogram* proved more difficult than the radiologist expected.
2. *To begin the day*, the nurse recorded the vital signs of his 30 patients.

3. The doctor informed the patient, *Mrs. Grouse*, *about the diagnosis, Raynaud's phenomenon, and the possible course of treatment.*

4. **Under the supervision of a faculty physician,** the resident correctly diagnosed over one hundred cases **throughout the year.**

5. ***Distracted by the activity in the emergency room,*** the patient answered the doctor's questions incorrectly.

6. The patient and the doctor jointly decided **to continue the chemotherapy treatment.**

7. ***Talking*** remains the most effective therapy **for the families of the ill.**

8. **Through extended discourse with other physicians,** Dr. Link determined the patient's diagnosis: gastric cancer.

■ Using Phrases to Combine Sentences

Directions: Combine the following sentences to create a participial, gerund, prepositional, appositive, or infinitive phrase.

1. The hospital specializes in trauma cases. It receives hundreds of trauma cases a week.

2. The patient is a 45-year-old woman. She complains of abdominal pain and back pain.

3. The physician was not sure about the diagnosis. He discussed the case with other physicians.

4. The patient underwent total knee replacement yesterday. She began physical therapy today. The therapist visited the patient in her room.

5. The patient visited the lab to have blood drawn. He must have blood tests done weekly. His physician requires the tests to monitor his blood coagulation.

6. Tanya Brass has diabetes. The nurse checks her blood sugar every 2 hours. The patient required further testing to confirm a diagnosis. The podiatrist requested another appointment.

Sample Student Essay:

SENTENCE VARIATION TECHNIQUES AND USE OF PHRASES IN ACTION

Directions: Read the following essay and observe sentence variations in techniques used.

Use the following key to recognize sentence types:

Double underline = simple sentence

Underline = complex sentence

Dash underline = compound sentence

Dotted underline = compound-complex sentence

Use the following key to recognize phrase types:

Italic text = *appositive phrase*

Bold text = **infinitive phrase**

Shadowed text = prepositional phrase

Bold italic text = ***participial phrase***

Bold shadowed = **gerund phrase**

Although lymphedema has received significant medical attention in recent years, medical records reveal that, throughout history, as many as 300 million people worldwide suffered from the disease (Wozniewski, Jasinski, Pilch, & Dabrowska, 2001). Unstandardized care for lymphedema results in a variety of treatment options: manual lymphatic drainage (MLD), skin care, exercises, compression pump, multilayer bandaging, compression garments, pneumatic compression, elevation, laser treatment, pharmacological management, psychosocial support, and surgical treatment. Caregivers alter the treatment based on the individual's needs and personal preferences, but most therapy programs include MLD, exercise, and compression produced by bandages, garments, or sleeves. Physical therapists all over the world employ these same treatments, which, provided adequate research, should become standard protocol.

The lymphatic system, *a network of lymphatic vessels, lymph, lymphoid tissues, and lymphoid organs*, functions to maintain normal blood volume by transporting lymph from peripheral tissues to the circulatory system (Silverthorn, 2001). A patient may experience improper re-absorption of lymph from the tissues, which causes a dysfunction in capillary-lymph exchange, and it may lead to edema (Silverthorn, 2001). The presence of parasites or cancer; the growth of fibrotic tissue; or the removal of lymph nodes, often a result of cancer treatment, leads to a decrease in the flow of lymph, which may also cause edema (Silverthorn, 2001).

The medical community arranged lymphedema into two classes: primary and secondary (Gillham, 1994). A person diagnosed with primary lymphedema, a result of a genetic abnormality, may lack sufficient valves in the lymphatic vessels, or they might possess vessels either too large or small for the existing valves (Gillham, 1994; Reynolds, 1996). Unlike primary lymphedema, secondary lymphedema derives from the removal of lymph nodes and vessels, infection, paralysis or immobilization, scars or burns from surgery, or other diseases (Buren & Linton, 2000; Reynolds, 1996).

To determine the effectiveness of complex decongestive therapy, which includes MLD, bandaging or garments, exercises, and a compression pump, Lydia Gillham completed a case study referred to as "Lymphedema and physiotherapists: Control not cure." Physicians diagnosed Mrs. Smith, a 51-year-old woman, with primary lymphedema of both legs and mild secondary lymphedema of the arm. While she used a weighted measuring tape and a pre-programmed computer, Gillman plotted a graph of the measurements, and she estimated retention of 11 pints of excess fluid in Smith's legs. Smith's treatments consisted of massage, multi-layered graduated compression bandaging left on for 24 hours, exercises, compression pump applied for 2 hours every visit, and skin care. After 2 weeks of this intense treatment regimen, a graph of new measurements revealed a loss of 3½ pints of fluid from Smith's left leg and 4½ pints from her right leg.

Weiss conducted a study identified as "Treatment of leg edema and wounds in a patient with musculoskeletal injuries." Following an injury and several surgeries, the patient developed edema of the lower limb and two sores and required physical therapy. The patient participated in a therapy program consisting of manual lymphatic drainage, compressive bandages, exercise, and skin care. Throughout the 7 weeks of therapy, 89% of the patient's wounds healed and the edema in the leg decreased by 74%.

Determining the efficiency of the complex physical therapy method in treating patients with lymphedema of the extremities, Wozniewski, Jasinski, Pilch, and Dabrowska conducted a study titled "Complex physical therapy for lymphedema of the limbs." Complex physical therapy consists of intermittent pneumatic compression, exercises,

and MLD. The study comprised 208 women between the ages of 17 and 83 years of age: 188 enduring lymphedema of the upper limb and 20 suffering from lymphedema of the lower limb. **Completing calculations both before and after complex physical therapy** allowed Wozniewski to determine the decrease in lymph volume in the limbs of the affected individuals. Lymphedema resolved completely in the upper extremity of 32 patients, the lower extremity of four patients with primary lymphedema, and the lower extremity of four patients with secondary lymphedema. Wozniewski calculated an average decrease of 43% in patients with slight edema, 33% in those with moderate edema, and 19% in individuals with severe edema.

No surgical or conservative methods currently available possess the capability of curing lymphedema. Health professionals caring for patients with lymphedema must accept the inability to treat the disease and instead try to control the effects of lymphedema (Gillham, 1994). In the past, medical professions refused to treat lymphedema, but now the debilitating disease gains more attention than ever from physical therapists (Reynolds, 1996). The unavailability of continuing education programs encompassing lymphedema prohibited interested physical therapists from attaining the necessary information for deliverance of treatment (Reynolds, 1996). Seeking out new treatment options, physical therapists found that traditional methods produced unsatisfactory results (Reynolds, 1996). Abandoning these traditional techniques, such as the compression pump and elevation, therapists develop new treatment programs that often include MLD, exercise, and compression (Reynolds, 1996).

The decline in skin elasticity, range of motion, and overall mobility resulting from edema necessitates the inclusion of exercise in the treatment plan (Reynolds, 1996). In the treatment of lymphedema, the use of exercise assists patients by producing enhanced lymph movement, muscle contraction, and deep breathing (Gillham, 1994). Activating the venous and lymphatic pumps, muscle activity contributes to the drainage of excess fluid from the tissues (Gillham, 1994). Exercising requires careful supervision because an increase in vasodilation, heart rate, and temperature, due to excessive exercise, escalates lymph production (Buren & Linton, 2000).

Compression bandages, garments and sleeves, used during the exercise period, maintain the progress made during the program period (Gillham, 1994). Patients wear compression garments and sleeves, as in intermittent pneumatic compression, to prevent the return of fluid to the limb (Gillham, 1994). Low stretch bandages, applied with padding, create low pressure during rest, which provides comfort, and high pressure during activity, which improves the function of deep vessels.

To maintain the effects of the various treatments, like MLD, physical therapists fit patients with compression garments. Applied in conjunction with other techniques, MLD, *a type of gentle massage*, directs lymphatic fluid away from damaged vessels and into healthy axilla (Gillham, 1994). The massage creates an augmentation in the uptake of lymph in superficial lymphatic vessels (Gillham, 1994).

Apart from the care provided by physical therapists and other healthcare professionals, physical therapists advise lymphedema sufferers on the importance of proper skin care. Patients dealing with lymphedema may experience transformations in the skin and underlying tissues due to the abundance of protein found in lymph fluid (Gillham, 1994). **To reduce the threat of infection**, one must adequately care for their skin. Physicians may recommend the use of nonallergenic soaps and moisturizers (Gillham, 1994). Daily moisturizing and protective clothing, such as gloves, help to prevent sores and cracking, both of which open the body up to infection (Gillham, 1994). Lymphedema also necessitates the evasion of trauma to the affected limb, as further injury could cause an increase in swelling and eventually scarring, which causes additional damage to the superficial lymphatic vessels (Gillham, 1994).

Although no standard treatment for lymphedema currently exists, most physical therapists create treatment plans including most, if not all, of the aforementioned techniques. The studies performed by Gillham, Weiss, and Wozniewski and coworkers all involved MLD, a form of compression, and exercise. The techniques employed produced desired outcomes in all of the studies mentioned above. **Proving their methods effective**, medical personnel must conduct additional research and provide a positive outcome. MLD, compression, exercises, and skin care should become the standard practice for lymphedema.

Reynolds believes that "[t]o bring lymphoedema treatment into the 21st century, the health care community must focus their attention on this condition and work as a team to develop better prevention and treatment options" (Reynolds, 1996). Despite the lack of research and standard procedures, the combination of MLD, compression, and exercise proves effective. **Combining skin care precautions** should become the protocol when treating patients with lymphedema.

References

Buren, J. M., & Linton, C. (2000). The role of exercise in treating lymphoedema. *Rehab Management: The Interdisciplinary Journal of Rehabilitation, 13,* 26–31.

Gillham, L. (1994). Lymphoedema and physiotherapists: Control not cure. *Physiotherapy, 80,* 835–842.

Reynolds, J. P. (Ed.). (1996). Lymphoedema: An "orphan" disease. *PT Magazine, 4,* 54–63.

Silverthorn, D. U. (2001). Blood flow and the control of blood pressure. In *Human physiology: An integrated approach* (pp. 461–462). Upper Saddle River, NJ: Prentice-Hall.

Weiss, J. M. (1998). Treatment of leg edema and wounds in a patient with severe musculoskeletal injuries. *Physical Therapy, 78,* 1104–1113.

Wozniewski, M., Jasinski, R., Pilch, U., & Dabrowska, G. (2001). Complex physical therapy for lymphoedema of the limbs. *Physiotherapy, 87,* 252–255.

Exercises

SENTENCE VARIETY IN THE ESSAY

■ Creating Sentence Variety

Directions: Change the sentence structure in the following passage to create continuity and flow and to eliminate choppiness and/or wordiness.

The new manager of Buffalo Allied Health has submitted a report in which she has outlined several problems that she feels are responsible for the low production that has been plaguing her facility. The first problem that she identifies is that employees and therapists are working with equipment that they have not been specifically trained to use. There are often significant differences that she has identified between the preparation workers have and the actual tasks that they are expected to perform. She feels that this is the primary reason for poor productivity. Her report also indicates that absenteeism in the Therapy Clinic is 15% higher than that which is experienced by the surrounding clinics and hospital facilities. It is also noted in her report that she can find no reason for the higher absenteeism. She is willing to speculate that there is a relationship between poor training and low morale. This can cause employees to be absent from work. The third problem in the clinic noted in her report is that because the Clinic operates some of the company's oldest equipment, down time and a lack of spare parts leave many workers idle for what she calls "extended periods." The manager speculates that these three problems could be the causes for low productivity. She adds that until the Clinic has newer equipment and better training for its personnel, productivity will continue to be a problem.

■ Sample Student Essay: Identifying and Correcting Sentence Variation Problems

Directions: Examine the following sample student essay and identify the problems in sentence variation. All sentences begin with the same format: S-V-O. Look for ways to combine sentences, coordinate, subordinate, or use the phrases and sentence types to make this work a readable piece.

MTV is a popular television station among teenagers. The videos MTV plays expose young people to unnecessary material. The material teens view in the videos is highly influential. Teens begin to duplicate the actions they see. Many people consider the material in music videos obscene. Something obscene is offensive to a group or person, includes indecent gestures, and contains degrading or immoral material.

In some music videos, artists make offensive references to different groups of people. The groups most referred to are gays and minorities. Videos offend the gay community by portraying gay relationships as being inappropriate. Teens viewing videos of this nature receive the impression that same-sex relationships are disgusting. The most offensive videos toward minorities are rap videos. Rap videos depict gang activity between groups. This offends minority groups because the videos give the impression that the groups portrayed are uncivilized. MTV makes no attempt to censor its material. It does blur some activities. These activities, however, are no secret. Young people will conclude that the images being hidden are exciting. They will want to replicate them even more.

The music videos played on MTV are obscene. They are obscene to many people for different reasons. The videos offend gays and minorities by portraying their lifestyles as wrong. The material in videos gives teenagers the wrong impression, teaches disrespect, and influences teens to follow in the same obscene behavior.

5

Phases Five and Six

of the Writing

Process: Editing

and Proofreading

Key Terms

Critical analysis Reading and thinking about a subject to discover errors in reasoning or presentation; also called *critical reasoning*

Drafting Reinventing the text according to a plan or formula addressing specific issues of the writing process

chapter objectives

On completion of this chapter, the reader should be able to

1. Identify a drafting scheme by which to revise documents in progress.

2. Develop effective writing by reinventing text according to the stages of the writing process.

3. Read his or her own work and the works of others critically to determine errors in reasoning and logic.

4. Ask a series of appropriate questions or propose issues that challenge content of the text and its place in the dialogue of the profession.

5. Perform final revisions as required to address problems identified by these types of questions and/or analyses.

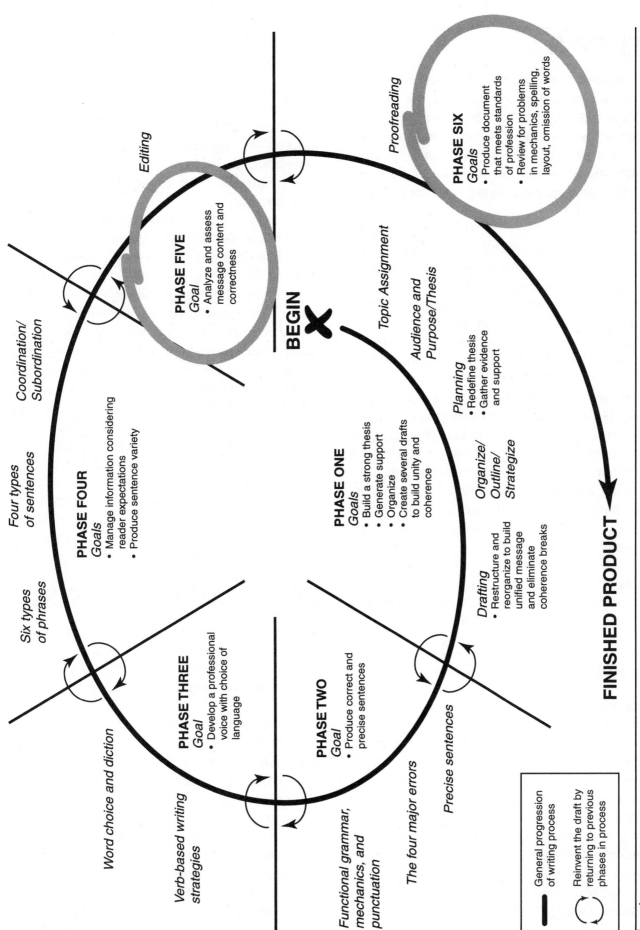

Proofreading

PHASE SIX
Goals
• Produce document that meets standards of profession
• Review for problems in mechanics, spelling, layout, omission of words

Editing

PHASE FIVE
Goal
• Analyze and assess message content and correctness

Coordination/
Subordination

BEGIN

Topic Assignment

Audience and
Purpose/Thesis

Planning
• Redefine thesis
• Gather evidence and support

Four types
of sentences

PHASE FOUR
Goals
• Manage information considering reader expectations
• Produce sentence variety

PHASE ONE
Goals
• Build a strong thesis
• Generate support
• Organize
• Create several drafts to build unity and coherence

Organize/
Outline/
Strategize

Drafting
• Restructure and reorganize to build unified message and eliminate coherence breaks

Six types
of phrases

Word choice and diction

PHASE THREE
Goal
• Develop a professional voice with choice of language

PHASE TWO
Goal
• Produce correct and precise sentences

FINISHED PRODUCT

Verb-based writing
strategies

Precise sentences

Functional grammar,
mechanics, and
punctuation

The four major errors

General progression
of writing process

Reinvent the draft by
returning to previous
phases in process

Figure 5-1 The Writing Process: Phases Five and Six

EDITING

The process of editing requires a different focus from any of the other steps in the writing process (see Figure 5-1). Here, you will make sure that the document is correct in format and not in meaning. Check grammar, spelling, punctuation, and mechanics (the correct use of capitalization, numbering, italicization, and abbreviations).

If you do not know the rules or if you are unsure, take the necessary time to look up the rules of correct writing. Incorrect usage of punctuation, grammar, or mechanics will distract your reader and damage your authority as a writer and professional in the field.

Notice that addressing issues of correctness is one of the last stages of the writing process. Do not distract yourself with issues of correctness when you are **drafting**, and do not distract yourself with issues of meaning while editing for correctness here. As a result, you can only begin editing for correctness when you have a draft that is in its final form; therefore, issues of meaning, messaging, communication, and coherence have all been addressed and appropriate changes have been made. However, you should approach the document one last time as an objective reader. Read the work with a **critical analysis**, asking questions and challenging the information on the page to check its validity.

PROOFREADING

After editing your work, proofread it for errors in typing or problems with the presentation.

Some people proofread by reading the text in reverse. This method allows the author to see each word clearly to make an assessment of its correctness; such a process keeps the message or content of the sentence or paper from interfering with the process of searching for more mechanical errors.

Also, try reading the final draft aloud. Hearing your words can often allow you to "see" the mistakes clearly. A better solution is to use a good editor.

Additionally, many writers depend on computer-generated help mechanisms such as spell-check and grammar-check to correct their work. Be aware of the limitations of spell-check and grammar-check in your word processing programs. When in doubt, look it up. Do not depend on software producers to provide expert writing advice or to guide you through the writing process to achieve grammatical correctness.

Ultimately, you are proofreading for inadvertent mistakes such as punctuation or words that have been left out. *Typographical errors do not exist at this level of your education.* You cannot expect your reader to allow you to submit a paper that has various mistakes and problems. As an instructor, I do not accept works that are littered with careless mistakes. I simply return the essay, and the opportunity for resubmitting it does not always exist. Essentially, when you submit a paper to your instructor, you are saying, "This is the best representation of my academic ability." Littering your paper with mistakes or carelessly proofreading will indicate that you do not care about the correctness of your work. Your colleagues, instructors, or contemporaries may surmise that you do not belong at this level of study or profession.

CREATING CHECKLISTS

Mature writers understand their limitations. Once those limitations are identified, they can analyze their work and apply strategies to overcome their weaknesses and create a better document.

This is an important lesson to learn. I tell my students that 50 percent of being a good writer is knowing how to identify what is bad or weak. The other 50 percent is fixing the problems and clarifying the ideas presented. To help you identify your weaknesses, make a list of the problems you often create or the problems that your instructor frequently addresses on your papers. You can also list your strengths. Then, check your work against both lists. If you recognize that a problem may exist, you can now devote time and energy to attack it. If you do not understand that your work may be incomplete or that your ideas are not clear, you will have no incentive to hunt for problems and fix them. No writer can write well in one or two drafts. Dedicate a separate reading for each of the problems you identify. This will take much of your time, but the result will be outstanding work.

Sample "Checklists"

The following sample error "checklists" created by students highlight problems experienced on a consistent basis.

Make a similar "checklist" to remind you of the details and subjects you should look for when you edit your work. You cannot expect to find all of these in one sitting or in one editorial session. You should plan to attack each of these subjects or groups of subjects in separate readings.

Student Sample "Checklist" 1

The Introduction—be clear with thesis and provide background information

Hotels use many different types of reservation systems. Although their names may be different, they all serve the same purpose. This purpose is to service customers quickly and efficiently. *(Combine these three sentences to break up monotony of sentence types and to create flow.)* One such system is known as MARSHA. MARSHA is used at all Marriott-owned properties. This system is fairly easy *(vague)* to use and once learned *(commas? also, words missing here?)* makes it even easier to learn another. *(Who is your audience? informed or not? This suggests that audience is informed. Be sure to indicate to your audience that some knowledge of the subject is expected.)*

Using Pronouns in Text Immediately Following Heading

Phase One

This *(do not start with pronouns that refer to the heading)* is the first stage of the test.

Examples of Weak Word Choice/Diction

The only thing *(vague)* that separates these three functions is order.

These instructions are very easy to follow and they are very effective. *Let your reader be the judge of this.*

What you could do *(informal)* is look at any product out there, and . . . .

It/There and Pronouns

Once a consumer is happy with what they are buying, it is very tough to change their minds.

Although ideas for products initially come from a variety of sources, it is *(it has no meaning or direct antecedent)* up to you to expand these ideas into more complete product concepts.

Once you have evidence that there is *(there has no meaning or direct antecedent)* a market for your product, you . . . .

Parallelism

The criteria may be cost, food, size of the room, or it could be location. *(Make each item in a series parallel to the others by creating each element in the same grammatical form.)*

Informal Voice

Examine how these conversational terms lead to inaccuracies. Such informality will allow the writer to lose authority over readers.

It is sort of like saying "Here it is."

Let's look at the following example.

Major Errors

Sentence fragment:

Read each section carefully. More than once if needed.

Comma splices:

The formula is the main element, however the components need explanation.

This is something that cannot be understood overnight, it takes time and practice.

Inconsistency with Commas

In column one, do not place the data. In column two do not tabulate the data.

Student Sample "Checklist" 2

1. **Introduction/conclusion**
   No place for evidence.

2. **Improper comma usage**
   Such a test determines that supplements are ineffective, and worthless.

   Items in a series:
   Consumers sees a quick fix, cheap drugs and save money.

Introductory prepositional phrases (optional):

Upon seeing this they still buy them.

Independent clauses:

PTs want to do what they can but the patient lives his or her own life.

Scientists study these drugs, however, they are not reliable.

Appositive phrases:

They are better in body, but not in mind.

Wenske a reporter is not reliable.

3. **Cliché**

There is one thing that just gets right under my skin. They are not preparing for the long road.

4. **D = Diction**

The article said that . . . . There is/are. It seems. They'll do whatever it takes.

5. **Trans = rough transition**

The daily dosage is 1500 mg a day. People pay $40 for a bottle of 100.

6. **AWK = awkward**

Despite restrictions, physical therapists must give them what they want anyway.

7. **WC = word choice**

Pills can be destructible. *(ive?)*

8. **Vague terms**

People think pills will cure something. This is a thing that . . .

9. **Coherence:** Connect sentences

10. **Passive voice** versus active voice

11. **Shift in verb tense**

The pills caused her pain, but she has taken them anyway.

12. **Dangling modifiers**

Dissecting the quote, the author describes the problem . . .

13. **Pred = improper predication**

This practice is where they see the problems.

14. **Spelling**

15. **Proofread**

16. **Four major errors**

Sentence fragment:

Which anyone should be freely allowed to have.

This will detroy the system; parts of the larger economy.

Comma splice:

Her weakness is not caused by her dependence, it is her lack of understanding of herself.

Run-on sentence:

The author does not really lie it was only speculation.

Subject-verb disagreement:

Readers learn how use of supplements in their lives have caused them to reach this state.

Others

Asking questions: Do not ask questions—give answers

RELATE POINTS TO THESIS

Citing information that is borrowed

Student Sample "Checklist" 3

1. **Comma usage problems:** These are mistakes!

Such a test determines that technology is ineffective, and worthless.

Items in a series: Students see a quick fix, cheap access to the Web and save money.

Upon seeing this they still buy them.

Jones a reporter is not reliable.

Students want to do what they can but the instructors must do what they can also.

2. **Clichés**

The article said that this is pie in the sky thinking.

3. *It* and *There*

There are fourteen kidneys for sale on the street.

It seems we can do nothing right.

They'll do whatever it takes.

4. **Transitions**

Technology advances more quickly every day. People are not comfortable with computers and modern advancements.

5. **Passive**

   The patient was prescribed medication by the doctor.

6. **Weak verbs**

   The patient demonstrates poor mobility, and she had weak muscle activity.

7. **Dangling modifiers**

   Turning on the computer, the program described the problem.

8. **Improper Predication**

   This is where the problems occur.

9. **Do not ask questions**

   How can this type of research be published in a respectable journal?

10. **Four major errors**

    Which anyone should be freely allowed to have.

    This is a convenience, but not effective.

    This will destroy the system; parts of the larger economy.

    This weakness is not caused by dependence, it is a lack of understanding of the impact.

    In the article the author does not really lie it was only speculation.

    The reader learns how technologies in their life has caused them to reach this state.

Student Sample "Checklist" 4

INITIAL EVALUATION

Wording

The therapists in this department are going to work with patient to get his ROM and strength back to where it needs to be to function properly in everyday activities.

It is important to have early motion because it decreases effusion, pain, and inhibition. Weights should also be used early, but in small amounts and little by little.

It is essential for Chris to attend physical therapy to repair his range of motion of the patellofemoral joint (knee) and strength of the quadriceps and hamstring muscles.

She was able to handle 25 lb of weights.

The onset began when . . .

The left biceps and triceps had 5 out of 5.

Patient's ability to perform daily activities should show a little improvement.

She has problems going from wheelchair to shower. The use of crutches is a must.

APA rule: Use figures to express numbers 10 and above; use words to express numbers below 10. Exceptions: 3 of 21 analyses; 5-mg dose; 2½ times; 4 on a 7-point scale; grade 8.

Choppy sentences and shift in verb tense

The patient receives treatment for her right shoulder. The treatment consists of electrical stimulation, ultrasound, joint mobilization, and exercises from active assisted and active free range of motion (ROM) to active resisted. The exercises include using pulleys and pendulum. The exercises were used to strengthen the patient's strength and ROM.

Combine: Edna Smith fractured her right radius on August 3, 2000. She injured her radius by slipping on ice.

Cliché: On the other hand, she will be receiving treatment . . .

Passive: No specific action was recalled that may have caused this pain.

Parallelism: The patient was requested to participate in exercises and attending therapy.

Dangling modifier: In evaluating the information obtained during the examination, it can be organized and interpreted in the following way.

Grammar

The patient is not allowed to put weight on leg, no coordination can be measured.

The pain can be intense at time, on a scale of 1 to 10, she says it can vary from 8-9.

The stairs will be slow going, however she will have a ramp to help these things.

Although the therapy proved unsuccessful because the patient still experiences problems.

Patient will be able to increase his movement and strength ability back to it's original status.

Patient <u>demonstrates</u> normal range of motion for his injury with his active range of motion (AROM) at 140° for extension and for flexion, he <u>demonstrated</u> his AROM to be 90°.

Predication: This section <u>is where</u> the therapist can . . .

Commas

He will be encouraged to continue those exercises when he is not in the clinic and he will also be given some additional exercises that can be done strictly at home.

Good posture is essential for him because it will help with his aerobic capacity for sports, and it will benefit treatment because posture affects joint integrity and mobility which <u>is what we are trying to get the most out of.</u>

Dr. Myers diagnosed patient on September 8, 2000 with a torn ACL and on the 15th of Sep-

tember, reconstructive surgery was performed *(who performed? = passive voice)* on patient's knee.

The treatment that Ms. Smith receives on a regular basis would improve her range of motion, and strengthen her muscles gradually.

The patient being an avid basketball star has experienced many problems.

Mechanics

The patient will attend 5 sessions for three to four weeks. *(Most style manuals, including APA, specify to spell out one to ten in running text and to use numerals for time and other units.)*

Some of the injuries are listed below:
1. Torn ACL
2. Dislocated knee
3. Sprain to knee *(need end period)*

The patient engages in strenuous exercises such as; running, jumping, and swimming.

Self-Assessment Inventory

Directions: Use this checklist to help you create a strategy for assessing your work and editing it. When you receive a paper from your instructor, highlight the positive comments and the negative. Then focus your editorial energies on the areas where you need the most help.

STRENGTHS

OVERALL ESSAY:
- ☐ argument persuasive
- ☐ clear thesis
- ☐ coherence
- ☐ conciseness
- ☐ creative/imaginative
- ☐ details
- ☐ development
- ☐ engaging style
- ☐ formal tone
- ☐ focus
- ☐ organization
- ☐ purpose
- ☐ revision
- ☐ sense of audience
- ☐ voice

PARAGRAPH LEVEL:
- ☐ introduction
- ☐ cohesion
- ☐ conclusion
- ☐ details/ support
- ☐ organization
- ☐ transitions

SENTENCE LEVEL:
- ☐ active voice
- ☐ clarity
- ☐ transitions
- ☐ variety
- ☐ verb-based

DICTION:
- ☐ conciseness
- ☐ word choice

FORMALITIES:
- ☐ rules of usage
- ☐ punctuation
- ☐ mechanics

NEEDS IMPROVEMENT

OVERALL ESSAY:
- ☐ audience
- ☐ clarity/ coherence
- ☐ depth/ details
- ☐ informal tone
- ☐ organization
- ☐ purpose
- ☐ redundancy
- ☐ thesis development

PARAGRAPH LEVEL:
- ☐ introduction
- ☐ cohesion
- ☐ conclusion
- ☐ paragraphing
- ☐ transitions
- ☐ verb tense shifts

SENTENCE LEVEL:
- ☐ object-based
- ☐ passive voice
- ☐ structure: parallelism, modifiers, mixed
- ☐ sharp transitions
- ☐ variation

DICTION:
- ☐ wordiness
- ☐ vagueness
- ☐ trite phrases and clichés
- ☐ idiomatic expressions
- ☐ slang
- ☐ word confusion
- ☐ words missing

GRAMMAR:
- ☐ comma splices
- ☐ run-on sentences
- ☐ sentence fragments
- ☐ disagreement: subject-verb
- ☐ disagreement: pronoun-antecedent

PUNCTUATION:
- ☐ commas
- ☐ semicolon
- ☐ colon
- ☐ dash
- ☐ quotation marks

MECHANICS:
- ☐ capitalization
- ☐ apostrophe
- ☐ hyphen
- ☐ numbers
- ☐ spelling
- ☐ proofreading and editing needed

Conclusion

The writing process is indeed a formula for writing success, but it is not a rigid formula. Try the steps in the process first, and adopt the strategies that work well for you. Then, recognizing your weaknesses, omit those strategies that do not.

Understanding that we all need editors and that we all need help clarifying our ideas is a sign of a mature writer. No one who writes professionally or for a living sends anything to be published unless it is read by someone who can give feedback and constructive criticism. We cannot realistically know everything about writing well, but we can know where to look for answers, and we can know whom to ask for help.

▌CRITICAL THINKING AND READING FOR REVISION

The quality of our professional lives depends on the quality of our thinking. The ability to store facts does not make a professional; the ability to rationalize, think, and then act appropriately, however, will lead to success. The process of thinking applies to your writing and to the reading of your writing as well, because "good writing is clear thinking made visible." If you do not present your ideas in a fashion that is rational and logical, no reader will understand your message. Think about critical thinking and its effect on the writing process in this way: You must be able to put words on your paper (rationalize), read those words and rip them apart looking for inconsistencies and errors in logic and reasoning (thinking), and then make appropriate changes to solve your errors in reasoning (acting). Poor thinkers are usually poor writers.

What does it mean to be a quality thinker? Although many people do not realize it, standards for rational thinking exist. Few people at this stage of their academic careers have actually sat down and created a list of ideas or principles that define for them the elements of quality thinking or well-reasoned writing. Instead, they read an article or paper, and they know, when they finish, that the piece is rational and logical by instinct. They want to gain some type of knowledge or information from the paper, and in doing so, they challenge the writer's assertions and compare them with what they already know. In a well-written paper, as readers challenge the writer's assertions while they read, the writer will anticipate their questions and meet their demands. This is the craft of writing: meeting the needs of the reader.

The following list provides the concepts that govern critical reasoning. Be aware of these concepts as a writer and as a reader of your own work and the work of others, as they are often considered by most strong thinkers to be the foundations of clear communication. These concepts can be used to help any reader, and writer, determine standards for quality thinking and, as a result, clear communication pathways. Critical readers examine every text for the following principles of reasoning:

- *Clarity and precision:* Every sentence and word must make an exact point. Vague words or incomplete thoughts create gaps in reasoning and destroy rational thought.

- *Accuracy:* Every conclusion must support the author's claim with verifiable evidence. Evidence that does not support the claim is not relevant; evidence that supports something other than the claim is not accurate. Be sure to form a clear purpose, as this will control the type of evidence you gather.

- *Relevance:* Every idea and conclusion should relate back to the thesis/purpose. At the end of every paragraph, a reader should ask if the information provided supports the purpose of the paper. Writers can add sentences that clarify the principles of the information provided in terms of the thesis. A critical reader should also focus on the issue of relevance when considering the organizational strategy of the paper. Examine the concluding paragraph and then compare it with the introduction. Look for inconsistencies. If the paper started out to prove one issue but concludes by proving another, the work is faulty and must be revised.

- *Depth:* Take into account the questions or issues that are created by the author's position or ideas. Writers who address the topic superficially open themselves to criticism from various angles or points of view. Make sure that all categories of influence have been addressed and explained.

- *Logic:* Any and all conclusions should be clearly derived from the stated purpose and the evidence presented. When you finish reading your own work or the work of others, ask this simple question: Does it all make sense?

Writers should read their own work while taking these ideas into consideration and should edit their work according to these principles.

Can anyone be a critical reader and a well-reasoned writer? Many people feel that critical reasoning is the same as innate intelligence. It is true that people are born with varying degrees of intelligence or intellectual ability; however, the principles of critical thinking, and therefore of critical writing and critical reading, are not issues of intelligence. They are merely the foundations of thinking that everyone uses to establish reason. As a health care professional, you should recognize that all writers in the professions communicate in the forms of standard written English and apply the standard rules of grammar and punctuation in order to communicate on a level that anyone, regardless of academic preparation, will understand. The elements of critical thinking are like the rules of grammar. No one will understand your intended message if you cannot supply the information in a form that others will understand. As a result, you must adopt these principles; otherwise, few people, or even no one, will understand your message. These elements of critical thinking are the basic boundaries that we expect from all people in the profession.

These elements of critical thinking are not innate, however, nor do the super-intelligent people of the world control them. Instead, they are available to anyone who is willing to put forth the time and effort to scrutinize the words on the page for meaning. Quality critical thinking is nothing more than a skill. Like writing, it must be honed.

Assessing Your Own Work: Being a Critical Reader

The following items are elements of thinking that can influence a writer's writing. These must be studied, through critical reasoning, to assess the quality of the work.

- *Purpose:* The purpose of any writing is established in the work's thesis. As explained in the first section of this text, the thesis guides the reader's thinking. As a writer, ask yourself, "What am I, ultimately, trying to accomplish?" Sometimes the thesis is in the form of a question or a debatable statement, and the writer intends to answer the question or prove an element of the debate. In any case or form, be sure that the purpose of the work is clearly stated and in a logical location. The most important element of the work should be easily found.

- *Point of view:* Everything we write is influenced by the emotional or intellectual baggage we bring with us to the discussion. As a result, the written word often mirrors our emotional or intellectual baggage without our realizing it. Consider any and all angles of the subject, and compare your point of view with the alternatives. A good writer asks,

    Am I being fair to my reader? Am I providing this information in an objective fashion? Have I considered that a reader could interpret this information differently? If so, how? How did I conclude my information?

Ultimately, the writer needs to understand the audience. Write to meet the demands of your reader.

- *Evidence:* We cannot expect our readers to understand our positions as writers and researchers if we do not supply the reader with reasons for our thinking. We need to supply evidence to prove our point. Good writers provide relevant and sufficient support to prove the purpose. A critical thinker should ask,

    How did I gather this information?

    Does it come from a legitimate source?

    How else can this information be interpreted?

- *Interpretations:* Most of our conclusions in our written work derive from concepts or ideas implied from the evidence. Ultimately, writers supply facts, data, and formulas, but these pieces of evidence need to be interpreted to make conclusions that will effect the purpose of the document. Ask,

    Are interpretations logical? consistent?

    Are these the result of my point of view?

    Are these assumptions grounded in rational thought?

- *Theories and laws:* The rational thoughts writers use to make conclusions are often based in the work of others. Scientists, researchers, and critical thinkers have established principles of reasoning to make interpretations. These are often in the form of absolute mechanisms called *laws*. Others are educated guesses and are called *theories*. However, nothing can be concluded accurately if the laws or theories are not fully understood by the writer and the reader.

    Have I explained these theories/laws thoroughly?

    Have I defined them?

    Can I explain all of this logically?

Read your work and the work of others as if solving a puzzle. Find the direction the author intends, and assess whether the author succeeds in directing the reader to that end. Address the following issues and ask the following questions when you read critically.

1. **Find the author's intended purpose.** Is the thesis regularly reinforced? Does the author keep the purpose at the front of the discussion? Is the problem or issue to be discussed clearly presented and in a logical location within the document?

2. **Assess the problem to be solved by figuring out what tools you will need to answer the question or issue.** Does the author follow the same path of reasoning that you do? Or does the author use information tools that you did not suspect? What or whose is the more logical approach?

3. **Challenge the information collected.** Are the sources legitimate? authoritative? Can the experiments be reproduced, or is this a one-time event that the writer assumes all other cases will follow exactly?

4. **Assess how to revise the ideas presented if the reasoning breaks down.** How can I solve the dilemma? Should the author let the reader know about the alternatives? How can the author discuss the options without making his or her case look weak?

Conclusion

Critical reading and writing, as we have seen, is the process of asking questions and searching for problems to solve. When applied to writing, critical thinking is nothing more than a detailed process of self-correction. By constantly looking for ways to make his or her writing better, the critical thinker attacks the words and ideas of others, looking for inconsistencies and faulty reasoning. The critical thinker (reader and writer)

assesses information, tests it against principles of logic, develops conclusions and solutions to the problems, and communicates those findings clearly with others.

These basic principles constitute the foundation of thinking that all professionals will expect from any writer.

THE PROCESS OF DRAFTING: CASE STUDIES AND SAMPLE STUDENT PAPERS

The central concept of this text is that writing is a skill, and any skill can be improved and made more effective. The application of this concept involves a variety of skills. Obviously, certain mechanical aspects of standard written English must be addressed: grammar, mechanics, and stylistic elements. However, effective communication goes far beyond these elements. It involves the ability to generate ideas, to clarify one's purpose, to analyze an audience, to arrange ideas in a rational format, to select words appropriate for the target readers and specified purpose, and to construct paragraphs that develop ideas clearly and thoroughly. Consideration and application of all these elements equal the writing process, and the implementation of this process will produce a document that expresses ideas clearly and concisely to the intended audience.

The following samples delineate the drafting process. These papers were created by students who revised their papers according to stages of development in the writing process, as discussed in the previous chapters. Each edition or draft signifies a new editorial advancement. Note that some of these papers required up to six drafts to complete.

Case Study 1
From Idea to Final Draft

TOPIC

How I feel about limitations/restrictions placed on me as a medical professional (i.e., a physical therapist) dealing with reimbursement for new and innovative procedures?

INTRODUCTION

Currently it is unlawful for physical therapists to practice interventions for which there is no medical practice–based evidence. This means that if physical therapists decided to step out of their scope of practice, insurance companies would not reimburse them for their procedures. The law should allow physical therapists to perform interventions on willing patients and receive reimbursement for doing so.

BODY

- A PT's job is to provide rehabilitation to patients.
- Scope of practice dictates what can and cannot be done.
- Stepping outside means breaking the law set forth by the government.
- Stepping outside of scope of practice for research reasons should be legalized.
- Breaking the law results in suspension of license.
- Advances are made in the physical therapy field by trial and error.
- Legalizing stepping out of scope allows advances.
- Such interventions should be allowed only if patient has consented.
- Advances are a necessity to prevent stagnancy within the physical therapy field.
- PTs cannot try new interventions for free, or else they will not have money to pay their bills.

- Patient must choose to receive new procedure.
- PT's job is to present both sides.
- Explain standard rehab procedure and include that medical practice–based research shows positive effects exist and it works.
- Explain new procedure and include its being new with no medical evidence to back it up.
- If a patient decides on the new procedure, get written consent.
- Signed form includes
  1. their decision
  2. realization that it is new
  3. agreement to not sue for malpractice
  4. knowledge of no medical evidence.
- If and only if signed form—signed by guardian if patient under 18—then new procedure can be done.

CLOSING

Once all criteria are met concerning the patient's acceptance to receive the new intervention, the rehabilitation process can begin. If the PT has written permission from the patient, then insurance companies should be required by law to reimburse the PT. If there is no written consent from the patient, then the PT is not allowed to step outside scope of practice. Doing so would result in not being reimbursed and the suspension of PT's license.

First Draft

How do I feel about limitations/restrictions placed on me as a medical professional (i.e., a physical therapist) dealing with reimbursement for new and innovative procedures?

Currently, it is unlawful for physical therapists to practice interventions for which there is no medical based evidence[1]. This[2] means that if physical therapists decided to step outside[3] of their scope of practice, that[4] insurance companies would not reimburse them for their procedures. The law should allow physical therapists to intervene on willing patients and to receive reimbursement for doing so.

A physical therapist's job is to provide rehabilitation[5] to patients. Guidelines that physical therapists follow are set up by[6] the physical therapy scope of practice. The scope of practice dictates what can and cannot be done[7] within the physical therapy field. Stepping outside[3] of this scope of practice, for research-based reasons, should be legalized. Presently, stepping outside[3] of the scope of practice results in the therapist breaking the law, which the government has set up[6]; consequently; suspension of the therapist's license will take place[8]. Fear of the consequences of breaking the law, along with morals, prevent physical therapists from stepping outside[3] their scope of practice and breaking the law.

Advances are made within the physical therapy field by trial and error. Trial and error can occur only if a therapist legally steps out[3] of the scope of practice which is currently illegal[9]. Legalization of stepping outside[3] the scope of practice allows advancements to happen[10]. Advancements become a necessity to prevent stagnancy within the physical therapy field.

If stepping outside[3] of the scope of practice became legal for research reasons, the patient must provide written consent[11] for the procedure to begin. This[12] ensures that it is[13] the patient's decision, not the therapist's decision[14], to try the new procedure. In order for a patient to make an educated decision, the physical therapist must present the patient with both options. The therapist must explain the standard rehabilitation procedure including that the procedure is[15] based upon medical research showing positive effects exist. An explanation of the new procedure would follow, including educating the patient that this new intervention is new and has no medical evidence to back it up[16]. If the patient decides to receive the standard rehabilitation procedure, then therapy progresses, and the insurance company reimburses the therapist for services rendered. However, if the patients selects[17] the new and innovative treatment plan, the therapist must obtain a written consent form from the patient. As with all legal signatures, if the patient's age falls below 18[18], then a guardian's signature needs to also accompany the child's[19]. A signed consent

form would include the patient is aware of that he or she has decided to receive this therapy, that the procedure is new, that he or she will not sue for malpractice, and that he or she knows their is no medical evidence for the treatment[20]. Once the patient signs the consent form, the new procedure can be implemented.

Once all criteria are met concerning the patient's acceptance to review[21] the new intervention, the rehabilitation process can begin. If the physical therapist obtained[22] written permission, then law requires insurance companies to reimburse the therapist. If the patient does not provide written consent[11], then stepping outside[3] of the scope of practice by the physical therapist is prohibited. Stepping outside[3] would result in not getting reimbursed[23] and the suspension of their[24] license.

COMMENTS

1. To avoid using "it is," in which the *it* does not refer to any subject, recast (reorganize the wording of) the sentence.

   REVISION: Currently, physical therapists are prohibited by law from performing interventions . . .

2. The use of "this" presents ambiguity. A simple reference to the topic of the previous statement provides proper explanation.

   REVISION: This limitation

3. The use of "step outside" incorporates conversational language into a formal paper. Taken literally, the wording means that the physical therapist would move one foot out of the scope of practice; obviously, this interpretation does not express the intent of the writer.

   REVISION: practice without regard to the scope of practice

4. "That" is unnecessary. The sentence should read

   If . . . , insurance companies . . .

5. Physical therapists cannot provide rehabilitation. Rehabilitation is a process. Also, rearranging the sentence eliminates the use of a form of the "to be" verb.

   REVISION: Physical therapists provide rehabilitative services to patients.

6. Again, conversational language decreases the integrity of the paper and should be avoided. Also, the scope of practice cannot "set up" guidelines. This action is accomplished by a committee of people.

   REVISION: Physical therapists follow guidelines outlined in the physical therapy scope of practice.

7. The word choice in this sentence requires improvement. "Done" sounds informal and does not accurately express the intention of the writer.

   REVISION: The scope of practice dictates which interventions can and cannot be performed within the physical therapy field.

8. This sentence exhibits wordiness. The phrase "will take place" can be avoided altogether by rearranging the preceding portion of the sentence.

   REVISION: Consequently, the therapist will have his or her license suspended.

9. Without any internal punctuation, the sentence is confusing. The use of "legally" and "illegal" in such close proximity creates confusion. The use of a semicolon and a simple sentence including the explanation of the "illegal" portion provides greater clarity.

   REVISION: Trial and error can occur only if a therapist legally practices outside of the scope of practice; however, this process is currently illegal.

10. This wording uses weak verbs. Elimination of "to happen" increases the effect of the wording within the sentence.

    REVISION: . . . provides opportunities for advancement.

11. "Concent" is a spelling error. The correct spelling is *consent*.

12. The "this" presents ambiguity. The reader must be aware of what "this" refers to.

    REVISION: This written consent form . . .

13. The use of "it is" should be avoided because the "to be" verb is a weak verb, and the *it* does not refer to any particular subject.

    REVISION: . . . the patient makes the decision . . .

14. The use of the word "decision" again becomes redundant.

    REVISION: . . . , not the therapist, . . .

15. The use of the word "including" is misleading. The standard rehabilitation procedure does not include the fact that medical research exists.

    REVISION: . . . and mention that the procedure is based upon . . .

16. "To back it up" represents poor diction. Taken literally, the meaning does not make sense in the sentence.

    REVISION: . . . has no supporting medical evidence.

17. "Patients selects" has subject-verb disagreement. Patients is a plural subject while selects is a verb for a singular subject.

    REVISION: Patients select . . .

18. This expression is wordy and could be simplified.

    REVISION: . . . if the patient is a minor, . . .

19. The "also" is unnecessary. By using the verb "accompany," the reader understands that both signatures are included.

    REVISION: . . . must accompany the child's.

20. This sentence is confusing and unclear in how it reads. Elimination of many words can simplify the sentence.

21. "To review" is not the appropriate verb for the sentence. The patient has already reviewed the practice and has now consented to its implementation.

    REVISION: . . . to undergo . . .

22. Within this sentence, the verb tense shifts. "Obtained" is past tense, whereas the remaining sections are in the present tense.

    REVISION: . . . obtains . . .

23. This verb combination is too wordy and can be simplified.

    REVISION: . . . denial of reimbursement . . .

24. The use of the pronoun *their* is inconsistent with the previous statement of physical therapist (singular).

    REVISION: . . . his or her . . .

Case Study 2
Six Drafts to Success

Draft #1

Electrical Stimulation Therapy and Its Effects on Muscular Rehabilitation

The Therapeutic Effect of Electrical Stimulation[1]

In rehabilitating patients with immobilizing injuries, maintaining the strength, range of motion, and muscle mass of the injured limbs proves difficult, but necessary[2]. Loss of these functions increases the time of rehabilitation and decreases the probability of a complete recovery. Muscle weakness and atrophy remains a common problem[3] in treating patients lacking movement in their limbs due to spinal cord injuries (SCIs), stroke, or injuries causing a loss of muscle control and/or a decrease in the use of certain muscles. In patients[4] with partial paralysis or loss of muscle control, regaining normal gait patterns, balance control, and stride length requires a lengthy, strenuous rehabilitation. Electrical stimulation (ES) proved effective, in several studies, for use in increasing the muscle mass, strength, and control of unutilized limbs.[5] By decreasing the time the muscles remain inactive, ES increases the likelihood of a full recovery. Consisting of a series of programmed electrical stimuli generated by a stimulator and conducted to the nerves and muscles through electrodes attached to the skin, ES produces movement in the initially immobile muscle.[6] The electrical stimuli used in ES act as impulses from the brain. Although experts have proved ES effective in conjunction with traditional therapy, therapists still classify ES as an experimental treatment. Electrical stimulation in combination with traditional therapy, increases the muscle mass in unutilized limbs, allowing the patient to regain control over gait patterns and balance more rapidly and more easily when performed with conventional therapy.

METHODS

[7]Wieler, Stein, Ladouceur, and others completed a study measuring the effects of ES on the walking ability of patients with SCIs and cerebral impairments. The experimenters accepted only participants who were able to walk[8] and stand with[9] an assistive device without the need for ES. Thirty-one of the 40 participants chosen for the study had experienced a partial SCI, and 9 participants suffered from cerebral impairments. Conducted over a 3-month period, this study involved placement of electrodes to areas where the patient exhibited the most instability when walking. The therapist then applies[10] the electrical stimuli using the 1-channel Unistim, Walkaide, or 4-channel Quadstim stimulating devices. The supervising therapist monitored and videotaped each patient while walking with and without ES to review and examine the patient's gait patterns as therapy progressed. This study included four trials, each trial consisting of a rapid 5-meter walk with and without ES, during which the therapist measured the stride lengths and cycle times.

[11]Lewek, Stevens, and Snyder-Mackler organized a case study involving a 66-year-old man with osteoporosis recovering from a total knee arthroplasty on his left knee. The therapists assigned a range of motion exercise program that the patient performed 3 times a week in the clinic.[12] The patient continued with his regular rehabilitative therapy including range of motion, bicycle, strength, and resistance exercises, in addition to daily ice and elevation of the injured knee. Every session also included[13] 10 minutes of neuromuscular ES applied to the left knee. With the leg bent at a 60° angle, the therapist attached electrodes over the distal vastus medialis muscle and the proximal vastus lateralis muscle. Volitional isometric contractions were performed[14] three times to obtain the needed dose of ES. After programming the Versa-Stim 380 for 10 contractions, the therapist increased the stimulation amplitude to the maximum toleration.[15] After this treatment, the patient performed volitional strengthening exercises with weights. After 18 sessions, the patient achieved all the goals established, and the therapist discharged him.[16]

[17]Bircan, Senicak, Kaya, Tamci, Gulbahar, and Akalin investigated the effect of ES on healthy patients. For this study, the experimenters recruited 30 healthy medical students and separated them into three groups of ten. Group A and group B both received varying levels of ES, while group C remained the control group receiving no ES at all. The supervising therapist applied ES for 15 minutes, five days a week, at the maximum tolerated intensity with the knee fully extended. This[18] study continued for three weeks.

Scremin conducted an experiment that measured the amount of change in the muscle mass in the lower extremities due to ES.[19, 20] Thirteen men with complete SCI performed a 3-phase exercise program. The first phase consisted of quadriceps strengthening. The second phase consisted of progressive sequential stimulation to achieve a pedaling motion, with electrodes placed on the quadriceps, hamstrings, and gluteal muscles. The third phase included thirty minutes of ES-induced cycling. Only when the patients met the objectives in one phase did they progress to the next phase. Therapists progressively measured the muscle mass of the quadriceps throughout the study.

[21]Bogataj, Gros, Kljajic Acimovic, and Malezic performed a comparative study of the effects of conventional therapy versus those of functional ES therapy. Each patient participating in the study executed conventional therapy and ES therapy for half the total duration of the experiment, three weeks.[22] The patient attended therapy once a day, five days a week.[23] This study consisted of twenty patients suffering from severe hemiplegia, or partial paralysis of a certain side of the body, due to cerebrovascular accident.[24] The participants needed certain standards of health and wellness before experts accepted them into the study.[25] Experimenters then randomly assigned ten patients to one of the two groups. Group 1 consisted of five males and five females who started the experiment with the conventional therapy. Group 2 consisted of six males and four females who all started with ES therapy and finished the experiment performing conventional therapies. The conventional therapy included gait and balance training, strength exercises, and range of motion exercises. The therapists applied ES to the peroneal nerve and soleus muscle for ankle movement, the hamstring muscles and quadriceps femoris musculature for knee movement, the gluteus maximus muscle for hip extension, and the triceps brachii muscle for the arm swings. The therapist applied ES as the patient walked along the 100-meter pathway. A stride analyzer measures certain aspects of the patient's gait to compare in tabular form. As therapy progressed, the distance walked increased for each patient. Because the ES therapy applies only to gait training, all results represented the effect of ES in conjunction with conventional therapy.

Experimental Results[26, 27]

[28]Walking speeds increased by 0.14 meter per second (m/s) with the use of the ES in Wieler's, Stein's, and Ladouceur's study. After calculations, the mean walking speed of the participants measured at a 45% total increase. Among the participants with SCI, the mean walking speed increased by 55%, while increasing only by 19% in the participants with cerebral impairments. Similar studies revealed comparable results. The case study organized by Lewek, Stevens, and Snyder-Mackler, indicated a net increase of 36% muscle mass in the quadriceps femoris muscle of the patient who returned to work after only 10 weeks of therapy. The net gains of muscle mass the patient experiences exceeded those of previous experiments.[29] The study performed by Bircan and his colleagues produced results in which groups A and B, after receiving varying degrees of ES, experienced a large change in the isokinetic strength of the treated quadriceps femoris muscles. Group C experienced no increase in strength at all.[30]

[31]The results of Scremin's experiment agreed with the above-mentioned statement.[32] The rectus femoris increased in mass by 31%, the sartorius increased by 22%, the adductor magnus-hamstrings increased by 26%, the vastus lateralis increased by 39%, and the vastus medialis-intermedius increased by 31%. There was also a significant increase in the muscle mass of the calves and thighs of the patients. These results prove that a program including ES increases the muscle mass in unused limbs.

[33]Bogataj and his associates achieved similar results in their experiment. Measurements and data showed that in conjunction with conventional therapy, ES greatly increases the progress of rehabilitation.

Experimental Conclusions[34, 35]

The experiments performed show evidence that electrical stimulation (ES) increases the muscle mass in immobile limbs when performed in addition to conventional therapy. ES proved effective when performed by patients with hemiplegia, SCIs, and musculoskeletal injuries.[36] Rehabilitation proved to be faster and more effective with the use of ES.[37] As research into the possibilities of ES continues, experts will reveal more uses for ES.

Already, researchers have begun testing the use of ES with speech and breathing impairments, bladder control, and pain relief.

COMMENTS

1. Use main-level headings only in this paper (same as for "Methods" later).

2. No comma is needed here, as " . . . but necessary" is not an independent clause.

3. Subject-verb disagreement

4. Awkward wording

5. Awkward sentence

6. Awkward transition—make a new paragraph beginning with this sentence.

7. Introductory sentences are needed to ensure coherence and smooth transitions between paragraphs.

8. Passive voice

9. Incorrect word choice

10. Incorrect tense

11. Introduction and transitional sentences are needed.

12. This sentence needs to be more specific.

13. Repetition of the verb "included"

14. Passive voice

15. This sentence needs to be more specific.

16. The results of the experiments do not belong in the "Methods" section.

17. Introduction and transitional sentences are needed.

18. The word "this" is vague.

19. Introduction and transitional sentences are needed.

20. Many of the paragraphs have been moved to increase the flow and coherence of the paper.

21. Introduction and transitional sentences are needed.

22. Unclear sentence

23. Short, choppy sentence

24. Awkward sentence

25. Awkward sentence

26. Use main-level headings only in this paper.

27. The "Results" section consists of the combined results from all of the separate experiments.

28. Introduction and transitional sentences are needed.

29. Awkward sentence

30. Awkward sentence

31. Introduction and transitional sentences are needed.

32. Awkward sentence

33. Introduction and transitional sentences are needed.

34. Use main-level headings only.

35. The "Conclusions" section should tie in all of the paragraphs.

36. Awkward sentence

37. Transitional sentences are needed.

Draft #2

Electrical Stimulation Therapy and Its Effects on Muscular Rehabilitation

INTRODUCTION

In rehabilitating patients with immobilizing injuries, maintaining the strength, range of motion, and muscle mass of the injured limbs proves difficult but necessary[1]. Loss of these functions increases the time of rehabilitation and decreases the probability of a complete recovery. Muscle weakening and atrophy remain common problems when treating patients lacking movement in their limbs due to spinal cord injuries (SCIs), stroke, or injuries causing a loss of muscle control and/or a decrease in the use of certain muscles. For patients with partial paralysis or loss of muscle control, regaining normal gait patterns, balance control, and stride length requires a lengthy, strenuous rehabilitation. In recent studies, electrical stimulation (ES) proved effective for increasing the muscle mass, strength, and control of the unutilized limbs. By decreasing the time the muscles remain inactive, ES increases the likelihood of a full recovery. Because the therapists perform ES while the patients are immobile, rehabilitation starts immediately after surgical recovery.[2]

Consisting of a series of programmed electrical stimuli generated by a stimulator and conducted to the nerves and muscles through electrodes attached to the skin, ES produces movement in the initially immobile muscle. The electrical stimuli used in ES act as impulses from the brain.[3] Although experts have proved ES effective in conjunction with traditional therapy, therapists still classify ES as an experimental treatment.[4] ES in combination with traditional therapy increases the muscle mass in unutilized limbs, allowing the patient to regain control over gait patterns and balance more rapidly and more easily.[5]

METHODS

Recently, therapists and medical experts organized and conducted experiments to determine the effects of ES on healthy, injured, and diseased patients. Wieler, Stein, Ladouceur, and others[6] completed a study measuring the effects of ES on the walking ability of patients with SCIs and cerebral impairments.[7] The experimenters accepted only participants that were able to walk and stand with an assistive device without the need for ES. Thirty-one of the 40 participants chosen for the study had experienced a partial SCI, and 9 participants suffered from cerebral impairments. Conducted over a 3-month period, this study involved placement of electrodes to the areas where the patient exhibited the most instability when walking. The therapists then applied the electrical stimuli using the 1-channel Unistim, Walkaide, or 4-channel Quadstim stimulating devices. The supervising therapist monitored and videotaped each patient while walking with and without ES to review and examine the patient's gait patterns as therapy progressed.[8] This study included four trials, each trial consisting of a rapid 5-meter walk with and without ES, from which the therapist measured the stride lengths and cycle times.

Scremin also conducted an experiment in which the participants suffered from SCIs. Scremin's experiment measured the change in the muscle mass of the lower extremities due to ES.[9] The study included thirteen men with complete SCI performed a 3-phase exercise program. The first phase consisted[10] of quadriceps strengthening. The second phase consisted of progressive sequential stimulation to achieve a pedaling motion, with the electrodes place[11] on the quadriceps, hamstrings, and gluteal muscles. The third phase included thirty minutes of ES-induced cycling[12]. Only when the patients met the objectives in one phase did they progress to the next phase. Therapists progressively measured the muscle mass of the quadriceps throughout the study.

Bogataj's study did not consist of patients with SCI, but with severe hemiplegia, or partial paralysis of a certain side of the body.[13] This experiment compared the effects of conventional therapy and those of functional ES therapy. Each one of the twenty patients participating in the study performed conventional therapy and ES therapy for 3 weeks, half the duration of the experiment.[14] The patient attended therapy once a day, five days a week. Before experts accepted patients into the study, the participants needed to meet certain standards of health and wellness.[15] Experimenters then randomly assigned ten patients to one of the two groups. Group 1 consisted of five males and five females who started the experiment with the conventional therapy. Group 2 consisted of six males and four females who all started with ES therapy and finished the experiment performing the conventional therapies. The conventional therapy included gait and balance training, strength exercises, and range of motion exercises. The therapists applied the electric stimulation to the peroneal nerve and soleus muscle for ankle movement, the hamstring muscles and quadriceps femoris musculature for knee movement, the gluteus maximus muscles for hip extension, and the triceps brachii muscle for arm movement. The therapist applied this electrical stimulation as the patient walked along a 100-meter pathway. A stride analyzer measured certain aspects of the patient's gait as they walked, to compare later in the study. As therapy progressed, the distance walked increased for each patient. Because the ES therapy applied only to gait training with each participant, all results represented the effect of ES in conjunction with conventional therapy.

An experiment by Lewek, Stevens, and Snyder-Mackler studied the effect of ES on a patient with a musculoskeletal injury as opposed to a patient with a neuromuscular injury as in the previous experiments.[16] This experiment investigated the effect of ES on a 66-year-old man recovering from a total knee arthroplasty on his left knee. The therapist assigned a range of motion exercise program that the patient performed 3 times a week for 6 weeks.[17] The patient continued with his regular rehabilitative therapy including range of motion, bicycle, strength, and resistance exercises, in addition to daily ice and elevation of the injured knee. Included in every therapy session was 10 minutes of neuromuscular ES applied to the left knee.[18] The therapist attached the electrodes over the distal vastus medialis muscle and the proximal vastus lateralis muscle. To determine the needed dose of ES, the patient performed volitional isometric contractions three times. After programming the Versa-Stim 380 for 10 contractions, the therapist increased the stimulation amplitude to the maximum toleration for each session. After the ES treatment, the patient performed volitional strengthening exercises with weights.

ES proved effective on several types of injuries. Muscle mass increased, duration of therapy decreased, and strength increased in all the cases of ES mentioned above.[19] In order to prove that ES is effective in all patients, Bircan, Senocak, Kaya, Tamci, Gulbahar, and Akalin investigated the effect of ES on healthy patients. For this study, the experimenters recruited 30 healthy students and separated them into three groups of ten. Group A and group B both received varying levels of stimulation, while group C remained the control group receiving no ES at all. The supervising therapist applied ES for 15 minutes a day at the maximum tolerated intensity. Patients received this ES regimen five days a week, for three weeks.

RESULTS

Used in conjunction with traditional therapies, ES promotes faster rehabilitation, an increase in the muscle mass of unused limbs, and an increase in the likelihood of a full recovery from injury. The case study completed by Lewek, Stevens, and Snyder-Mackler[20] proved that ES, when performed in addition to conventional therapies, decreased the time necessary for rehabilitation. A 66-year-old man with a total knee arthroplasty, when treated by both ES and traditional therapies, acquired a force gain greater than 86% quadriceps femoris muscle index, in only 18 sessions of therapy.[21] Such results surpassed other recorded in literature, although no literature was written about this man's age group.[22] This study, however, was not designed[23] to measure the increase in strength due to ES (Lewek, Stevens, and Snyder-Mackler).[24] To answer this question, Bircan, etc[25] (2002) designed an experiment showing the effect of ES on a healthy patient. Data collected before and after the 3-week study showed a significant increase in the isokinetic strength of the quadriceps femoris muscles in two groups receiving varying degrees of ES.[26] The group denied the use of ES showed no improvement in isokinetic strength.

Scremin's[27] experiment measured not only strength increase but also the increase in muscle mass due to ES. The participants of this study suffered from complete SCI, indicating total immobility of the lower extremities. The calves and thighs showed signs of significant increase in muscle to fat ratio, and the muscle mass of the legs and thighs increased by approximately 24%.[28] Unlike Scremin's study, Bogataj[29] created a study in which the participants receive both traditional and ES therapies. After 6 weeks of research, Bogataj[30] concluded that ES therapy is an effective treatment when used in conjunction with conventional treatments. The ES allows patients to begin gait rehabilitation at the start of therapy and without training or strengthening beforehand. Bogataj[31] stresses[32] that ES should not and cannot replace conventional therapies. It is effective only when used in conjunction with conventional therapies.[33]

A study organized by Wieler, and reported on by Gawronski,[34] measured the effects of ES on walking ability and gait patterns but in patients with SCIs and cerebral impairments. After the application of ES, walking speeds of the participants increased by 0.14 meter per second (m/s).[35] After calculations, the mean walking speed of the participants measures[36] at a 45% total increase. Among the participants with SCIs, the mean walking speed increased by 55%, while increasing by 19% in the participants with cerebral impairments.[37]

CONCLUSIONS

The experiments performed show evidence that ES[38] increases the muscle mass in immobile limbs when performed in addition to conventional therapy. Data shows that ES is effective for patients with neuromuscular and musculoskeletal injuries. Rehabilitation proved to be faster and more effective with the use of ES. All of the research discussed pertains only to the lower extremities of the body. To determine the effect of ES on the upper extremities of the body, researchers need to perform more experiments. <u>As research into the possibilities of ES continues, new uses of ES.</u>[39] Already, researchers have begun testing the use of ES with speech and breathing impairments, bladder control, and pain relief.[40]

COMMENTS

1. By changing the dependent clause to an independent clause and adding a comma, a compound-complex sentence is created.

2. Awkward

3. Unnecessary sentence

4. Coherence issues

5. These words are vague. A transitional sentence is also needed here.

6. Replace with "et al."

7. It must be noted that the author of this article is not the original experimenters. Transitional sentences will then be needed.

8. This sentence needs to be rearranged to create sentence variation.

9. These sentences need to be combined to create a coherent transitional sentence.

10. Repetitive verb

11. "placed"

12. This phrase needs to be changed because it is too similar to that used by the author of the article.

13. Awkward

14. These sentences need to be combined.

15. The previous sentence needs to be explained further.

16. A comma needs to be added, and the sentence needs to be rearranged.

17. Awkward sentence

18. Awkward sentence

19. These sentences need to be combined to form a coherent transitional sentence.

20. A citation is needed in the "Results" section.

21. A citation is needed here.

22. Awkward sentence

23. Passive voice

24. Incorrect citation

25. The comma is not necessary. The words "et al." should replace the "etc."

26–29. A citation is needed here.

30. The words "et al." are needed here.

31. The words "et al." are needed here.

32. stressed

33. This sentence is unnecessary.

34. A citation is needed.

35. A citation is needed.

36. measured

37. A citation is needed here. A transitional sentence is also needed to tie in with the next paragraph.

38. Because it is a separate section, the words should be written out before the abbreviation.

39. Sentence fragment

40. Sentences are needed to tie together the whole paper.

Draft #3

Electrical Stimulation Therapy and Its Effects on Muscular Rehabilitation

INTRODUCTION

In rehabilitating patients with immobilizing injuries, maintaining the strength, range of motion, and muscle mass of the injured limb proves difficult, but <u>they are</u>[1] necessary. Loss of these functions increases the time of rehabilitation and decreases the probability of a complete recovery.[2] Muscle weakening and atrophy remain common problems when treating patients lacking movement in their limbs due to spinal cord injuries (SCIs), stroke, or injuries causing a loss of muscle control and/or a decrease in the use of certain muscles. For patients with partial paralysis or loss of muscle control, regaining normal gait patterns, balance control, and stride length requires a lengthy, strenuous rehabilitation. In recent studies, electrical stimulation (ES) proved effective for increasing the muscle mass, strength, and control of unutilized limbs.[3] By decreasing the time muscles remain inactive, ES increases the likelihood of a full recovery. Applying ES while patients are immobile enables rehabilitation to start immediately after surgical recovery.

Consisting of a series of programmed electrical stimuli generated by a stimulator and conducted to the nerves and muscles through electrodes attached to the skin, ES produces movement in the initially immobile muscle. The stimuli produce movement in the muscles that injured and disabled patients cannot exercise. Although experts have proved ES effective for use on these unutilized muscles, many therapists do not perform ES at all. Studies show that ES in combination with traditional therapy increases the muscle mass in unutilized limbs, allowing the patient to regain control over gait patterns and balance faster and easier than with conventional therapy alone. It is necessary that therapists review such findings to ensure that patients receive the most efficient care possible.

METHODS

Recently, therapists and medical experts organized and conducted experiments to determine the effects of ES on healthy, injured, and diseased patients. Wieler, Stein, Ladouceur, et al. completed a study measuring the effects of ES on the walking ability of patients with SCIs and cerebral impairments. Gawronski, a certified physical therapist in New York, reported[4] on this experiment. Gawronski noted that before the experiment began, the therapists accepted only the participants who were able[5] to walk and stand with the use of an assistive device or ES. Thirty-one of the 40 participants chosen for the study had experienced a partial SCI, and 9 participants suffered from cerebral impairments. Conducted over a 3-month period, this study involved placement of electrodes to the areas where the patients exhibited the most instability when walking. The therapists then applied the electrical stimuli through the electrodes using the 1-channel Unistim, Walkaide, or 4-channel Quadstim stimulating devices. Monitoring and videotaping each patient while walking with and without the aid of ES allowed the therapists to review and examine the patients' gait patterns as therapy progressed. This study included the four trials, each trial consisting of a rapid 5-meter walk with and without the application of the ES, during which the therapists measured the stride lengths and cycle times of each patient.

Scremin also conducted an experiment in which the participants suffered from spinal cord injuries, but it[6] measured the change in the muscle mass of unexercised limbs due to ES. Consisting of thirteen men with SCI, the study involved a 3-phase exercise program. The first phase of the program concentrated on strengthening the quadriceps. The second phase focused on achieving a pedaling motion,[7] through progressive sequential stimulation via electrodes placed on the quadriceps, hamstrings, and gluteal muscles. The third phase included a 30-minute exercise program in which the therapist applied ES to produce a motion of the legs similar to that in riding a bicycle. Only when the patients met the objectives in the previous phase did they progress to the next phase.[8] Therapists progressively measured the muscle mass of the quadriceps throughout the study.

[9]Bogataj's[10] experiment studied the effect of ES on different neuromuscular disabilities and included twenty patients suffering from the severe hemiplegia, or partial paralysis of a certain side of the body. Because this experiment compared the effects of conventional therapy and those of ES therapy, participants performed conventional therapy and ES therapy for only three weeks, half the duration of the entire experiment. The patient attended therapy once a day, five days a week, for a full 6 weeks. Before experts accepted patients into the study, the participants needed to meet certain standards of health and wellness. Therapists examined each patient to ensure each had a healthy cardiovascular system, and adequate reflex response, full cognitive ability, and the motor abilities to stand alone or with moderate support. Experimenters, then, randomly assigned the chosen participants into two groups. Group 1 consisted of five males and five females who began the experiment performing conventional therapies. Group 2 consisted of six males and four females who all began therapy receiving ES therapy and finished the experiment performing conventional therapies. The conventional therapy within the experiment consisted of gait and balance training, strength exercises, and range of motion exercises. When participants received ES, the therapists applied the electrical stimuli to the peroneal nerve and soleus muscle for ankle movement, the hamstring muscles and quadriceps femoris musculature for knee movement, the gluteus maximus muscle for hip extension, and the triceps brachii muscle for arm extension. The therapist applied ES as the

patient walked along a 100-meter pathway. To compare later in the study, a stride analyzer measured certain aspects of the patients' gait as they walked. As therapy progressed, the distance walked increased for each patient. Because the ES therapy applied only to gait training with each participant, all results represented the effect of ES in conjunction with conventional therapy.

An experiment by Lewek, Stevens, and Snyder-Mackler studied the effect of ES on a patient with musculoskeletal injuries, while the previous experiments included only patients with neuromuscular injuries. This experiment investigated the effect of ES on a 66-year-old man recovering from a total knee arthroplasty on his left knee. As in previous experiments, the patient performed a conventional therapy program containing range of motion exercises 3 times a week for 6 weeks. The patient continued with his regular rehabilitative therapy including range of motion, bicycle, strength, and resistance exercises,[11] in addition to daily ice and elevation of the injured knee. Applying 10 minutes of neuromuscular ES every session, the therapist attached the electrodes over the distal vastus medialis and proximal vastus lateralis muscles. To determine the needed dose of ES, the patient performed isometric contractions three times. After programming the Versa-Stim 380 for 10 contractions, the therapist increased the stimulation to the maximum toleration for each session. To ensure a fast recovery, the patient also performed volitional strengthening exercises with weights.

ES proved effective for several types of injuries by increasing muscle mass, decreasing the duration of therapy, and increasing muscle strength. Unlike previous experiments, Bircan, Senocak, Peker, Kaya, Tamci, Gulbahar, and Akalin[12] investigated the effect of ES on healthy patients. For this study, the experimenters recruited 30 healthy medical students and separated them into three groups of ten. Group A and group B received varying levels of ES, while group C remained the control group receiving no ES at all. The supervising therapist applied ES for 15 minutes a day at the maximum tolerated intensity. Patients received this ES regimen five days a week, for three weeks.

RESULTS

Used in conjunction with traditional therapies, ES promotes faster rehabilitation, an increase in the muscle mass of unused limbs, and an increase in

the likelihood of a full recovery from injury. The case study completed by Lewek, Stevens, and Snyder-Mackler (2001) proved that ES, when performed in addition to conventional therapies, decreased the time necessary for rehabilitation. A 66-year-old man with a total knee arthroplasty, when treated by both ES and traditional therapies, acquired a force gain greater than 86% quadriceps femoris muscle index in only 18 sessions of therapy (Lewek, et al. 2001).[13] According to Lewek et al., such results exceeded the expectations noted in other studies reported in the medical literature. The study completed by Lewek et al., however, did not measure the increase in strength due to ES. To answer this question, Bircan et al. (2002) designed an experiment showing the effect of ES on a healthy patient. Data collected before and after the 3-week study showed a significant increase in the isokinetic strength of the quadriceps femoris muscles in two groups receiving varying degrees of ES (Bircan et al. 2002).[14] The group denied the use of ES in the study organized by Bircan et al. (2002) showed no improvement in isokinetic strength.

Scremin (2000) prepared an experiment that measured not only muscular strength increases in participating patients but also the increases in the muscle mass of their[15] unutilized limbs due to ES. The participants in Scremin's (2000) study suffered from complete SCI, indicating[16] total immobility of the lower extremities. The calves and thighs showed signs of significant increase in muscle to fat ratio and the muscle mass of the legs and thighs increased by approximately 24% after ES therapy (Scremin, 2000). Unlike Scremin's study, Bogataj, Gros, Kljajic, Acimovic, and Malezic (1995) created a study in which the participants receive both traditional and ES therapies. After 6 weeks of research, Bogataj et al. concluded that ES therapy is an effective treatment when used in conjunction with conventional therapies.[17]

A study organized by Wieler, Stein, Ladouceur, et al., and reported on by Gawronski (2000), measured the effects of ES on the walking ability and gait patterns, but with patients with SCIs and cerebral impairments. After the application of the ES, walking speeds of the participants increased by 0.14 meter per second (m/s) (Gawronski, 2000)[18] After calculations, the mean walking speed of the participants measured at a 45% total increase. Among the participants with SCI, the mean walking speed increased by 55%, while increasing by 19% in the participants with cerebral impairments (Gawronski, 2000). This study showed how different injuries and disabilities respond to ES therapy in varying degrees (Gawronski, 2000).

CONCLUSIONS

The experiments performed show[19] evidence that ES increases the muscle mass and strength of immobile limbs. Data show that ES is effective for patients with neuromuscular and musculoskeletal injuries. Rehabilitation proved to be faster and more effective with the use of ES. All of the research discusses pertains to the lower extremities of the body. To determine the effects of ES on the upper extremities of the body, researchers need to perform more experiments.[20] As research into the possibilities of ES continues, new uses of ES are uncovered, and researchers have already begun testing the use of ES for speech and breathing impairments, bladder control, and pain relief. Although most of the reports stress that ES therapy is effective only when used as a collaborative method of treatment for all injuries, medical experts need to determine the most effective uses for ES through highly accurate and controlled experiments.

References

Gawronski, S. (2000). Multicenter evaluation of electrical stimulation systems for walking [Electronic version]. *Physical Therapy, 80,* 198. Retrieved November 11, 2002, from Health Reference Center Academic database.

Lewek, M., Stevens, J., & Snyder-Mackler, L. (2001). The use of electrical stimulation to increase quadriceps femoris muscle force in all[21] elderly patient following a total knee arthroplasty [Electronic version]. *Physical Therapy, 81,* 1565–1573. Retrieved November 11, 2002, from Health Reference Center Academic database.

Scremin, E. (2000). Increasing muscle mass in spinal cord injured persons with a functional electric stimulation exercise program [Electronic version]. *The Journal of the American Medical Association, 283,* 719. Abstract retrieved November 11, 2002, from Health Reference Center Academic database.[22]

Bogataj, U., Gros, N., Kljajic, M., Acimovic, R., & Malezic, M. (1995). The rehabilitation of gait in patients with hemiplegia: A comparison between conventional therapy and multichan-

nel functional electrical stimulation therapy [Electronic version]. *Physical Therapy, 75,* 40–53. Retrieved November 11, 2002, from Health Reference Center Academic database.

Bircan, C., Senocak, O., Peker, O., Kaya, A., Tamci, S. A., Gulbahar, S., et al. (2002). Efficacy of two forms of electrical stimulation in increasing quadriceps strength: A randomized controlled trial [Electronic version]. *Clinical Rehabilitation, 16,* 194–203. Retrieved November 11, 2002, from MEDLINE.[23]

COMMENTS

1. it is
2. Some of the sentences within this paragraph need to be rearranged to make the paragraph more coherent.
3. These sentences are moved to the beginning of the paragraph to improve the coherence.
4. Incorrect word choice
5. Passive voice
6. Vague word choice
7. No comma is needed here.
8. Coherence problem
9. A transitional sentence is needed here.
10. Correct citation is needed here.
11. The comma is not needed here.
12. The correct citation is needed here.
13. The correct citation is needed here.
14. A comma is needed here.
15. Vague word choice
16. Incorrect word choice
17. More information about this experiment is needed.
18. A period is needed after the closing parenthesis.
19. Awkward word choice
20. Unnecessary sentences
21. This is a mistake by the author and it needs to be noted by "[sic]."
22. This line needs to be moved up.
23. These references need to be put in alphabetical order.

Draft #4

Electrical Stimulation Therapy and Its Effects on Muscular Rehabilitation

INTRODUCTION

In rehabilitating patients with immobilizing injuries, maintaining strength, range of motion, and muscle mass of the injured limb proves difficult, but it is necessary. Loss of these functions increases the time of rehabilitation and decreases the probability of a complete recovery. Applying ES[1] while patients are immobile enables rehabilitation to start immediately after surgical recovery. By decreasing the time the muscles remain inactive, ES increases the likelihood of a full recovery. Muscle weakening and atrophy remain common problems when treating patients lacking movement in their limbs due to spinal cord injuries (SCIs), stroke, or injuries causing a loss of muscle control and/or a decrease in the use of certain muscles. For patients with partial paralysis or loss of muscle control, regaining normal gait patterns, balance control, and stride length requires a lengthy, strenuous rehabilitation. In recent studies, electrical stimulation (ES)[2] proved effective for increasing the muscle mass, strength, and control of unutilized limbs.

Consisting of a series of programmed electrical stimuli produced by a stimulator and conducted to the nerves and muscles through electrodes attached to the skin, ES produces movement in the initially immobile muscle. The stimuli produce movement in the muscles that injured and disabled patients cannot exercise. Although experts have proved ES effective for use on these unutilized muscles, many therapists do not perform ES therapy at all. Studies show that ES, in combination with traditional therapy,[3] increases the muscle mass in unutilized limbs, allowing the patient to regain control over gait patterns and balance faster and easier than with conventional therapy alone. It is necessary that therapists review such findings to ensure that patients receive the most efficient care possible.

METHODS

Recently, therapists and medical experts organized and conducted experiments to determine the effects of ES on healthy, injured, and diseased patients. Wieler, Stein, Ladouceur, et al. completed a study measuring the effects of ES on the walking ability of patients with SCIs and cerebral impairments. Gawronski, a certified physical therapist in New York, wrote about this experiment. Gawronski noted that[4] before the experiment began, the therapists accepted only participants that needed an assistive device or ES to stand and walk. Thirty-one of the 40 participants chosen for the study had experienced a partial SCI, and 9 participants suffered from cerebral impairments. Conducted over a 3-month period, this study involved placement of electrodes to the areas where the patients exhibited the most instability when walking. The therapists then applied the electric stimuli through the electrodes using the 1-channel Unistim, Walkaide, or 4-channel Quadstim stimulating devices. Monitoring and videotaping each patient while walking with and without the aid of ES allowed the therapists to review and examine the patients' gait patterns as therapy progressed. This study included four trials, each trial consisting of a rapid 5-meter walk with and without ES, from which the therapist measured the stride lengths and cycle times of each patient.

Scremin also conducted an experiment in which the participants suffered from spinal cord injuries, but this study measured the change in the muscle mass of unexercised limbs due to ES. Consisting of thirteen men with SCI, the study involved a 3-phase exercise program. The first phase of the program concentrated on strengthening the quadriceps. The second phase focused on achieving a pedaling motion through progressive sequential stimulation via electrodes placed on[5] the quadriceps, hamstrings, and gluteal muscles. The third phase included a 30-minute exercise program in which the therapist applied ES to produce a motion in the legs similar to that in riding a bicycle. Only when patients met the objectives in the previous phase did they progress to the next phase. Throughout each phase, therapists progressively measured the muscle mass of the quadriceps throughout the study.[6]

Unlike Scremin's study, the experiment organized by Bogataj, Gros, Miroljub, Kljajic, Acimovic, and Malezic studied the effect of ES on different neuromuscular disabilities.[7] The study included twenty patients suffering from severe hemiplegia, or partial paralysis of a certain side of the body. Because this experiment compared the effects of conventional therapy and those of ES therapy, participants performed conventional therapy and ES therapy for only three weeks, half the duration of the entire experiment. The patient attended therapy once a day, five days a week, for a full 6 weeks. Before experts accepted patients into the study, the participants needed to meet certain standards of health and wellness. Therapists examined each patient to ensure each had a healthy cardiovascular system, an adequate reflex response, full cognitive ability, and the motor abilities to stand alone or with moderate support. Experimenters then randomly assigned the chosen participants into two groups.[8] Group 1 consisted of five males and five females who began the experiment performing conventional therapies. Group 2 consisted of six males and four females who all began therapy receiving ES therapy and finished the experiment performing conventional therapies.[9] The conventional therapy within the experiment consisted of gait and balance training, strength exercises, and range of motion exercises. When participants received ES, the therapists applied the electrical stimuli to the peroneal nerve and soleus muscle for ankle movement, the hamstring muscles and quadriceps femoris musculature for knee movement, the gluteus maximus muscle for hip extension, and the triceps brachii muscle for arm movement. The therapist applied ES as the patient walked along a 100-meter pathway. To compare later in the study, a stride analyzer measured certain aspects of the patients' gait as they walked. As therapy progressed, the distance walked increased for each patient. Because the ES therapy applied only to gait training with each patient, all results represented the effect of ES in conjunction with conventional therapy.

An experiment by Lewek, Stevens, and Snyder-Mackler studied the effect of ES on a patient with musculoskeletal injuries, while the previous experiments included only patients with neuromuscular injuries. This experiment investigated the effect of ES on a 66-year-old man recovering from a total knee arthroplasty on his left knee. As in previous experiments, the patient performed a conventional therapy program containing range of motion exercises 3 times a week for 6 weeks. The patient continued with his regular rehabilitative therapy including range of motion, bicycle, strength, and resistance exercises, in addition to[10] daily ice and elevation of the injured knee.[11] To determine the needed dose of ES, the patient performed isometric contractions three times. After programming

the Versa-Stim 380 for 10 contractions, the therapist increased the stimulation amplitude to the maximum toleration for each session. To ensure a fast recovery, the patient also performed volitional[12] strengthening exercises with weights.

ES proved effective for several types of injuries by increasing muscle mass, decreasing the duration of therapy, and increasing the muscle strength. Unlike in previous experiments, Bircan, Senocak, Peker, Kaya, Tamci, Gulbahar, et al. investigated the effect of ES on healthy patients. For this study, the experimenters recruited[13] 30 healthy medical students and separated them into three groups of ten. Group A and group B both received varying levels of electrical stimulation, while group C remained the control group receiving no electrical stimulation at all. The supervising therapist applied electric stimulation for 15 minutes a day at the maximum tolerated intensity. Patients received this ES regimen five days a week, for three weeks.

RESULTS

Used in conjunction with traditional therapies, electrical stimulation promotes faster rehabilitation, an increase in the muscle mass of unused limbs, and an increase in the likelihood of a full recovery from injury. The case study completed by Lewek, Stevens, and Snyder-Mackler (2001) proved that ES, when performed in addition to conventional therapies, decreased the time necessary for rehabilitation. A 66-year-old man with a total knee arthroplasty, when treated by both ES and traditional therapies[14] acquired an 86% force gain of the quadriceps femoris muscle, in 18 sessions of therapy[15] (Lewek, et al. 2001).[16] According to Lewek et al., such results exceeded the expectations noted in other studies reported in the medical literature. The study conducted by Lewek et al., however, did not measure the increase in strength due to ES. To answer this question, Bircan et al. (2002) designed an experiment showing the effect of ES on a healthy patient. Data collected before and after the 3-week study showed a significant increase in the isokinetic strength of the quadriceps femoris muscles in the two groups receiving varying degrees of ES (Bircan et al.[17] 2002). The group denied the use of ES in the study organized by Bircan et al. (2002) showed no improvement in isokinetic strength.

Scremin (2000) prepared an experiment that measured not only muscular strength increases but also the increases in the muscle mass of participants' unutilized limbs due to ES. The participants in this experiment suffered from complete SCI, producing total immobility of the lower extremities. The calves and thighs showed signs of significant increase in the muscle to fat ratio, and the muscle mass of the legs and thighs increased by approximately 24% after the ES therapy (Scremin, 2000). Unlike Scremin's study, Bogataj, Gros, Kljajic, Acimovic, and Malezic (1995) created a study in which the participants receive[18] both traditional and ES therapies. After 6 weeks of research, Bogataj et al. concluded that ES therapy is an effective treatment when used in conjunction with conventional treatments. Bogataj et al. noted that ES therapy allowed patients to begin gait rehabilitation at the start of therapy without training or strengthening before beginning,[19] but stressed that ES therapy should not replace conventional therapies.

A study organized by Wieler, Stein, Ladouceur, et al., and reported on by Gawronski (2000), measured the effects of ES on walking ability and gait patterns, but with patients with SCIs and cerebral impairments.[20] After the application of the ES, walking speeds of the participants increased by 0.14 meter per second (m/s) (Gawronski, 2000). After calculations, the mean walking speed of the participants measured at a 45% total increase. Among the participants with SCI, the mean walking speed increased by 55%, while increasing by 19% in the participants with cerebral impairments (Gawronski, 2000). This study showed how different injuries and disabilities respond to ES therapy in varying degrees (Gawronski, 2000).

CONCLUSION

The experiments produced evidence that ES increases the muscle mass and strength of immobile limbs. Data indicated that ES is effective for patients with various types of injuries and that rehabilitation is faster and more effective with the use of ES. As research into the possibilities of ES continues, new uses of ES are uncovered,[21] and researchers have already begun testing the use of ES for speech and breathing impairments, bladder control, and pain relief. Although most of the reports stress that ES therapy is effective only when used as a collaborative method of treatment for all injuries, medical experts need to determine the most effective uses for ES through highly accurate and controlled experiments.

References

Bircan, C., Senocak, O., Peker, O., Kaya, A., Tamci, S. A., Gulbahar, S., et al. (2002). Efficacy of two forms of electrical stimulation in increasing quadriceps strength: A randomized controlled trial [Electronic version]. *Clinical Rehabilitation, 16,* 194–203. Retrieved November 11, 2002, from MEDLINE.

Bogataj, U., Gros, N., Kljajic, M., Acimovic, R., & Malezic, M. (1995). The rehabilitation of gait in patients with hemiplegia: A comparison between conventional therapy and multichannel functional electrical stimulation therapy [Electronic version]. *Physical Therapy, 75,* 40–53. Retrieved November 11, 2002, from Health Reference Center Academic database.

Gawronski, S. (2000). Multicenter evaluation of electrical stimulation systems for walking [Electronic version]. *Physical Therapy, 80,* 198. Retrieved November 11, 2002, from Health Reference Center Academic database.

Lewek, M., Stevens, J., & Snyder-Mackler, L. (2001). The use of electrical stimulation to increase quadriceps femoris muscle force in all [sic] elderly patient following a total knee arthroplasty [Electronic version]. *Physical Therapy, 81,* 1565–1573. Retrieved November 11, 2002, from Health Reference Center Academic database.

Scremin, E. (2000). Increasing muscle mass in spinal cord injured persons with a functional electric stimulation exercise program [Electronic version]. *The Journal of the American Medical Association, 283,* 719. Abstract retrieved November 11, 2002, from Health Reference Center Academic database.

COMMENTS

1. The term "electrical stimulation" needs to be written out before the abbreviation can be used. (Check for this point after revisions in which text is moved.)

2. Now, the abbreviation is not needed here.

3. The commas setting "in combination with traditional therapy" are not needed.

4. A comma is needed here.

5. "applied to"

6. This phrase is awkward.

7. Some of the sentences in the paragraph are rearranged for coherence.

8. This sentence is changed for coherence.

9. These two sentences need to be combined and changed for coherence within the paragraph.

10. This needs to be changed to make it an independent clause.

11. More information needs to be given on where the electrical stimulation was applied.

12. Unnecessary word

13. Incorrect word choice

14. A comma is needed here.

15. Awkward

16. Incorrect citation

17. A comma is needed after the period in this citation.

18. "received"

19. No comma is needed here.

20. Awkward

21. Awkward

Draft #5

Electrical Stimulation Therapy and Its Effects on Muscular Rehabilitation

INTRODUCTION

In rehabilitating patients with immobilizing injuries, maintaining the strength, range of motion, and muscle mass of the injured limb proves difficult, but it is[1] necessary. Loss of these functions increases the time of rehabilitation and decreases the probability of a complete recovery. Applying electrical stimulation (ES) while patients are immobile enables rehabilitation to start immediately after surgical recovery. By decreasing the time the muscles remain inactive, ES increases the likelihood of a full recovery. Muscle weakening and atrophy also remain common problems when treating patients lacking movement in their limbs due to spinal cord injuries (SCIs), stroke, or injuries causing a loss of muscle control and/or a decrease in the use of certain muscles. For patients with partial paralysis or loss of muscle control, regaining normal gait patterns, balance control, and stride length requires a lengthy, strenuous rehabilitation. In recent studies, ES proved effective for increasing the muscle mass, strength, and control of unutilized limbs.

Consisting of a series of programmed electrical stimuli produced by a stimulator and conducted to the nerves and muscles through electrodes attached to the skin, ES produces movement in the initially immobile[2] muscle. The stimuli produce movement in the muscles the injured and disabled patients cannot exercise. Although experts have proved ES effective for use on these unutilized muscles, many therapists do not perform ES therapy at all. Studies show that ES in combination with traditional therapy increases the muscle mass in unutilized limbs, allowing the patient to regain control over gait patterns and balance faster and easier than with conventional therapy alone. It[3] is necessary that therapists review such findings to ensure that patients receive the most efficient care possible.

METHODS

Recently, therapists and medical experts organized and conducted experiments to determine the effects of ES on healthy, injured, and diseased patients. Wieler, Stein, Ladouceur, et al. completed a study measuring[4] the effects of ES on the walking ability of patients with SCIs and cerebral impairments. Gawronski, a certified physical therapist in New York, wrote about this experiment. Gawronski noted that, before the experiment began, the therapists accepted only participants that[5] needed an assistive device or ES to stand and walk. Thirty-one of the 40 participants chosen for the study had experienced a partial SCI, and 9[6] participants suffered from cerebral impairments. Conducted over a 3-month period,[7] this study involved the placement of electrodes to the areas where the patients exhibited the most instability when walking. The therapists then applied the electric stimuli through the electrodes using the 1-channel Unistim, Walkaide, or 4-channel Quadstim stimulation devices. Monitoring and videotaping each patient while walking with and without the aid of ES allowed the therapists to review and examine the patients' gait patterns as therapy progressed. This study included four trials, each trial consisting of a rapid 5-meter walk with and without the application of the ES, during which the therapist measured the stride lengths and cycle times of each patient.

Scremin also conducted an experiment in which the participants had SCIs, but this study measured the change in the muscle mass of unexercised limbs due to ES. Consisting of thirteen[8] men with SCI, the study involved a 3[9]-phase exercise program. The first phase of the program concentrated on strengthening the quadriceps. The second phase focused on achieving a pedaling motion through progressive sequential stimulation via electrodes applied to the quadriceps, hamstrings, and gluteal muscles. The third phase included a 30-minute exercise program in which the therapists applied ES to produce a motion in the legs similar to the motion produced when riding a bicycle.[10] Only when patients met the objectives in the previous phase did they progress to the next phase. Throughout each phase, therapists progressively measured the muscle mass of the quadriceps.

Unlike Scremin's study, the experiment organized by Bogataj, Gros, Miroljub, Kljajic, Acimovic, and Malezic studied the effect of ES on different neuromuscular disabilities. Before experts accepted patients into the study, the participants needed to meet certain standards of health and wellness. Therapists examined each patient to ensure each had a healthy cardiovascular system, and adequate reflex response, full cognitive ability, and the motor abilities to stand alone or with moderate support. The study included twenty[11] patients suffering from severe hemiplegia, or partial paralysis of a certain side of the body. Because this experiment compared the effects of conventional therapy and those of ES therapy, participants performed conventional therapy and ES therapy for only 3 weeks, half the duration of the entire experiment. The patients attended therapy once a day, five[12] days a week, for a full 6 weeks. Within the first session, the therapists randomly assigned the chosen participants into two groups. Consisting of five males and five females, group 1 received the conventional therapies within the first three[13] weeks of the experiment, while group 2 consisted of six males and four females and performed the conventional therapies within the last three[14] weeks of the experiment. The conventional therapy within the experiment consisted of gait and balance training, strength exercises, and range of motion exercises. When participants received ES, the therapists applied the electrical stimuli to the peroneal nerve and soleus muscle for ankle movement, the hamstring muscles and quadriceps femoris musculature for knee movement, the gluteus maximus muscle for hip extension, and the triceps brachii muscle for arm movement. The therapist applied ES as the patient walked along a 100-meter pathway. To compare later in the study,[15] a stride analyzer measured certain aspects of the patients' gait as they walked. As therapy progressed, the distance walked increased for each

patient. Because the ES therapy applied only to gait training with each participant, all results represented the effect of ES in conjunction with conventional therapy.

An experiment by Lewek, Stevens, and Snyder-Mackler studied the effect of ES on a patient with musculoskeletal injuries, while the previous experiments included only patients with neuromuscular injuries.[16] This experiment investigated the effect of ES on a 66-year-old man recovering from a total knee arthroplasty on his left knee. As in previous experiments, the patient performed a conventional therapy program containing range of motion exercises 3[17] times a week for 6 weeks. The patient continued with his regular rehabilitative therapy including range of motion, bicycle, strength, and resistance exercises, and he received daily ice and elevation treatments on the injured knee. Applying 10 minutes of neuromuscular ES every session, the therapist attached the electrodes over the distal vastus medialis and proximal vastus lateralis muscles. To determine the needed dose of ES, the patient performed isometric contractions three times. After programming the Versa-Stim 380 for 10 contractions, the therapist increased the stimulation amplitude to the maximum toleration for each session. To ensure a fast recovery, the patient also performed strengthening exercises with weights.

ES proved effective for rehabilitating several types of injuries by increasing muscle mass, decreasing duration of therapy, and increasing the muscle strength. Unlike in previous experiments, Bircan, Senocak, Peker, Kaya, Tamci, Gulbahar, et al. investigated the effect of ES on healthy patients. For this study, the experimenters accepted 30 healthy men and women and separated them into three groups of ten.[18] Group A and group B both received varying levels of ES, while group C received no ES at all. The supervising therapist applied ES for 15 minutes a day at the maximum tolerated intensity. Patients received this ES regimen five[19] days a week, for three[20] weeks.

RESULTS

Used in conjunction with traditional therapies, ES promotes faster rehabilitation, an increase in the muscle mass of unused limbs, and an increase in the likelihood of a full recovery from injury. The case study completed by Lewek, Stevens, and Snyder-Mackler (2001) proved that ES, when performed in addition to conventional therapies, decreased the time necessary for rehabilitation. A 66-year-old man with a total knee arthroplasty, when treated by both ES and traditional therapies for 18 sessions, acquired an 86% force gain of the quadriceps femoris muscle (Lewek et al., 2001). According to Lewek et al., such results exceeded the expectations noted in other studies reported in the medical literature. The study conducted by Lewek et al., however, did not measure the increase in strength due to ES. To answer this question, Bircan et al. (2002) designed an experiment showing the effect of ES on a healthy patient. Data collected before and after the 3-week study showed a significant increase in the isokinetic strength of the quadriceps femoris muscles in two groups receiving varying degrees of ES (Bircan et al., 2002). The group denied the use of ES in the study organized by Bircan et al. (2002) showed no improvement in isokinetic strength.

Scremin (2000) prepared an experiment that measured not only muscular strength increases but also the increases in muscle mass of participants' unutilized limbs due to ES. The participants in this experiment suffered from complete SCI, which produces total immobility of the lower extremities. The calves and thighs showed signs of significant increase in the muscle to fat ratio and the muscle mass of the legs and thighs increased by approximately 24% after the ES therapy (Scremin, 2000). Unlike Scremin's study, Bogataj, Gros, Kljajic, Acimovic, and Malezic (1995) created a study in which the participants receive both traditional and ES therapies. After 6 weeks of research, Bogataj et al. concluded that ES therapy is an effective treatment when used in conjunction with conventional treatments. Bogataj et al. noted that ES therapy allowed patients to begin gait rehabilitation at the start of therapy without training or strengthening before beginning, but he stressed that ES therapy should not replace conventional therapies.

A study organized by Wieler, Stein, Ladouceur, et al., and reported on[21] by Gawronski (2000), also measured the effects of ES on the walking ability and gait patterns in patients with spinal cord injuries and cerebral impairments. After the application of the ES, walking speeds of the participants increased by 0.14 meter per second (m/s) (Gawronski, 2000). After calculations, the mean walking speed of the participants measured at a 45% total increase. Among the participants with SCI, the mean walking speed increased by 55%, while increasing by 19% in the participants with cerebral impairments (Gawronski, 2000). This study showed how different injuries and disabilities respond to ES therapy in varying degrees (Gawronski, 2000).

CONCLUSIONS

The experiments produced evidence that ES increases the muscle mass and strength of immobile limbs. Data indicated that ES is effective for patients with various types of injuries and that rehabilitation is faster and more effective with the use of ES. As research into the possibilities of ES continues, experts uncover new uses of ES, and researchers have already begun testing the use of ES for speech and breathing impairments, bladder control, and pain relief. Although most of the reports stress that ES therapy is effective only when used as a collaborative method of treatment, medical experts need to determine the most effective use for ES through highly accurate and controlled experiments.

COMMENTS

1. "they are"
2. Awkward word choice
3. Vague word choice
4. Change the phrase to "measured."
5. "who"
6. "nine"
7. "period of 3 months"
8. 13
9. "three"
10. These sentences need some variation.
11. 20
12. 5
13. 3
14. 3
15. This phrase is awkward where it is.
16. Awkward sentence
17. "three"
18. 10
19. "5"
20. "3"
21. Incorrect word choice

Final Draft

Running head:
ELECTRICAL STIMULATION THERAPY

Electrical Stimulation Therapy and Its Effects on Muscular Rehabilitation

INTRODUCTION

In rehabilitating patients with immobilizing injuries, maintaining the strength, range of motion, and muscle mass of the injured limb proves difficult, but they are necessary. Loss of these functions increases the time of rehabilitation and decreases the probability of a complete recovery. Applying electrical stimulation (ES) while patients are immobile enables rehabilitation to start immediately after surgical recovery. By decreasing the time the muscles remain inactive, ES increases the likelihood of a full recovery. Muscle weakening and atrophy also remain common problems when treating patients lacking movement in their limbs due to spinal cord injuries (SCIs), stroke, or injuries causing a loss of muscle control and/or a decrease in the use of certain muscles. For patients with partial paralysis or loss of muscle control, regaining normal gait patterns, balance control, and stride length requires a lengthy, strenuous rehabilitation. In recent studies, ES proved effective for increasing the muscle mass, strength, and control of unutilized limbs.

Consisting of a series of programmed electrical stimuli produced by a stimulator and conducted to the nerves and muscles through electrodes attached to the skin, ES produces movement in the immobile muscle. The stimuli produce movement in the muscles the injured and disabled patients cannot exercise. Although experts have proved ES effective for use on these unutilized muscles, many therapists do not perform ES therapy at all. Studies show that ES in combination with traditional therapy increases the muscle mass in unutilized limbs, allowing the patient to regain control over gait patterns and balance faster and easier than with conventional therapy alone. Therapists need to review such findings to ensure that patients receive the most efficient care possible.

METHODS

Recently, therapists and medical experts organized and conducted experiments to determine the effects of ES on healthy, injured, and diseased patients. Wieler, Stein, Ladouceur, et al. measured the effects of ES on the walking ability of patients with SCIs and cerebral impairments. Gawronski, a certified physical therapist in New York, wrote about this experiment. Gawronski noted that, before the experiment began, the therapists accepted only participants who needed an assistive device or ES to stand and walk. Thirty-one of the 40 participants chosen for the study had experienced a partial SCI, and nine participants suffered from cerebral impairments. Conducted over a period of 3 months, this study involved the placement of electrodes to the areas where the patients exhibited the most instability when walking. The therapists then applied the electric stimuli through the electrodes using the 1-channel Unistim, Walkaide, or 4-channel Quadstim stimulation devices. Monitoring and videotaping each patient while walking with and without the aid of ES allowed the therapists to review and examine the patients' gait patterns as therapy progressed. This study included four trials, each trial consisting of a rapid 5-meter walk with and without the application of the ES, during which the therapist measured the stride lengths and cycle times of each patient.

Scremin also conducted an experiment in which the participants suffered from SCIs, but this study measured the change in the muscle mass of unexercised limbs due to ES. Consisting of 13 men with SCI, the study involved a three-phase exercise program. The first phase of the program concentrated on strengthening the quadriceps. Focusing on achieving a pedaling motion in the second phase, therapists applied electrodes to the quadriceps, hamstrings, and gluteal muscles. Later, in the third phase, therapists applied ES for 30 minutes to produce a motion in the legs similar to that in riding a bicycle. Only when patients met the objectives in the previous phase did they progress to the next phase. Throughout each phase, therapists progressively measured the muscle mass of the quadriceps.

Unlike Scremin's study, the experiment organized by Bogataj, Gros, Miroljub, Kljajic, Acimovic, and Malezic studied the effect of ES on different neuromuscular disabilities. Before experts accepted patients into the study, the participants needed to meet certain standards of health and wellness. Therapists examined each patient to ensure each had a healthy cardiovascular system, and adequate reflex response, full cognitive ability, and the motor abilities to stand alone or with moderate support. The study included 20 patients suffering from severe hemiplegia, or partial paralysis of a certain side of the body. Because this experiment compared the effects of conventional therapy and those of ES therapy, participants performed conventional therapy and ES therapy for only 3 weeks, half the duration of the entire experiment. The patients attended therapy once a day, 5 days a week, for a full 6 weeks. Within the first session, the therapists randomly assigned the chosen participants into two groups. Consisting of five males and five females, group 1 received the conventional therapies within the first 3 weeks of the experiment, while group 2 consisted of six males and four females who received the conventional therapies within the last 4 weeks of the experiment. The conventional therapy within the experiment consisted of gait and balance training, strength exercises, and range of motion exercises. When participants received ES, the therapists applied the electrical stimuli to the peroneal nerve and soleus muscle for ankle movement, the hamstring muscles and quadriceps femoris musculature for knee movement, the gluteus maximus muscle for hip extension, and the triceps brachii muscle for arm movement. The therapist applied this ES as the patient walked along a 100-meter pathway. A stride analyzer measured certain aspects of the patients' gait as they walked, to compare later in the study. As therapy progressed, the maximum distance walked increased for each patient. Because the ES therapy applied only to gait training with each participant, all results represented the effect of ES in conjunction with conventional therapy.

While the previous experiments included only patients with neuromuscular injuries, an experiment by Lewek, Stevens, and Snyder-Mackler studied the effect of ES on a patient with musculoskeletal injuries. This experiment investigated the effect of ES on a 66-year-old man recovering from a total knee arthroplasty on his left knee. As in previous experiments, the patient performed a conventional therapy program containing range of motion exercises three times a week for 6 weeks. The patient continued with his regular rehabilitative therapy including range of motion, bicycle, strength, and resistance exercises, and he received daily ice and elevation treatments on the injured knee.

Applying 10 minutes of neuromuscular ES every session, the therapist attached the electrodes over the distal vastus medialis and proximal vastus lateralis muscles. To determine the needed dose of ES, the patient performed isometric contractions three times. After programming the Versa-Stim 380 for 10 contractions, the therapist increased the stimulation amplitude to the maximum toleration for each session. To ensure a fast recovery, the patient also performed strengthening exercises with weights.

ES proved effective for rehabilitating several types of injuries by increasing muscle mass, decreasing duration of therapy, and increasing the muscle strength. Unlike in previous experiments, Bircan, Senocak, Peker, Kaya, Tamci, Gulbahar, et al. investigated the effect of ES on healthy patients. For this study, the experimenters accepted 30 healthy men and women and separated them into three groups of 10. Group A and group B both received varying levels of ES, while group C received no ES at all. The supervising therapist applied ES for 15 minutes a day at the maximum tolerated intensity. Patients received this ES regimen 5 days a week, for 3 weeks.

RESULTS

Used in conjunction with traditional therapies, ES promotes faster rehabilitation, an increase in the muscle mass of unused limbs, and an increase in the likelihood of a full recovery from injury. The case study completed by Lewek, Stevens, and Snyder-Mackler (2001) proved that ES, when performed in addition to conventional therapies, decreased the time necessary for rehabilitation. A 66-year-old man with a total knee arthroplasty, when treated by both ES and traditional therapies for 18 sessions, acquired an 86% force gain of the quadriceps femoris muscle (Lewek et al., 2001). According to Lewek et al., such results exceeded the expectations noted in other studies reported in the medical literature. The study conducted by Lewek et al., however, did not measure the increase in strength due to ES. To answer this question, Bircan et al. (2002) designed an experiment showing the effect of ES on a healthy patient. Data collected before and after the 3-week study showed a significant increase in the isokinetic strength of the quadriceps femoris muscles in two groups receiving varying degrees of ES (Bircan et al., 2002). The group denied the use of ES in the study organized by Bircan et al. (2002) showed no improvement in isokinetic strength.

Scremin (2000) prepared an experiment that measured not only muscular strength increases but also the increases in muscle mass of participants' unutilized limbs due to ES. The participants in this experiment suffered from complete SCI, which produces total immobility of the lower extremities. The calves and thighs showed signs of significant increase in the muscle to fat ratio and the muscle mass of the legs and thighs increased by approximately 24% after the ES therapy (Scremin, 2000). Unlike in Scremin's study, in the experiment conducted by Bogataj, Gros, Kljajic, Acimovic, and Malezic (1995), the participants received both traditional and ES therapies. After 6 weeks of research, Bogataj et al. concluded that ES therapy is an effective treatment when used in conjunction with conventional treatments. Bogataj et al. noted that ES therapy allowed patients to begin gait rehabilitation at the start of therapy without training or strengthening before beginning, but these investigators stressed that ES therapy should not replace conventional therapies.

A study organized by Wieler, Stein, Ladouceur, et al. and reported on by Gawronski (2000) also measured the effects of ES on the walking ability and gait patterns in patients with spinal cord injuries and cerebral impairments. After the application of the ES, walking speeds of the participants increased by 0.14 meter per second (m/s) (Gawronski, 2000). After calculations, the mean walking speed of the participants measured at a 45% total increase. Among the participants with SCI, the mean walking speed increased by 55%, while increasing by 19% in the participants with cerebral impairments (Gawronski, 2000). This study showed how different injuries and disabilities respond to ES therapy in varying degrees (Gawronski, 2000).

CONCLUSIONS

The experiments produced evidence that ES increases the muscle mass and strength of immobile limbs. Data indicated that ES is effective for patients with various types of injuries and that rehabilitation is faster and more effective with the use of ES. As research into the possibilities of ES continues, experts uncover new uses of ES, and researchers have already begun testing the use of ES for speech and breathing impairments, bladder control, and pain relief. Although most of the reports stress that ES therapy is effective only when used as a collaborative method of treatment, medical experts need to determine the most effective uses for ES through highly accurate and controlled experiments.

References

Bircan, C., Senocak, O., Peker, O., Kaya, A., Tamci, S. A., Gulbahar, S., et al. (2002). Efficacy of two forms of electrical stimulation in increasing quadriceps strength: A randomized controlled trial [Electronic version]. *Clinical Rehabilitation, 16*, 194–203. Retrieved November 11, 2002, from MEDLINE.

Bogataj, U., Gros, N., Kljajic, M., Acimovic, R., & Malezic, M. (1995). The rehabilitation of gait in patients with hemiplegia: A comparison between conventional therapy and multichannel functional electrical stimulation therapy [Electronic version]. *Physical Therapy, 75*, 40–53. Retrieved November 11, 2002, from Health Reference Center Academic database.

Gawronski, S., (2000). Multicenter evaluation of electrical stimulation systems for walking [Electronic version]. *Physical Therapy, 80*, 198. Retrieved November 11, 2002, from Health Reference Center Academic database.

Lewek, M., Stevens, J., & Snyder-Mackler, L. (2001). The use of electrical stimulation to increase quadriceps femoris muscle force in all [sic] elderly patient following a total knee arthroplasty [Electronic version]. *Physical Therapy, 81*, 1565–1573. Retrieved November 11, 2002, from Health Reference Center Academic database.

Scremin, E. (2000). Increasing muscle mass in spinal cord injured persons with a functional electric stimulation exercise program [Electronic version]. *The Journal of the American Medical Association, 283*, 719. Abstract retrieved November 11, 2002, from Health Reference Center Academic database.

Case Study 3
Stages and Strategies

Draft #1
Eliminating Major Grammatical Errors

When patients test positive for the human immunodeficiency virus (HIV), they need to notify their nurses. Arguments exist both for and against the patient's disclosure of HIV-positive serologic status; however, the nurse's knowledge of the diagnosis outweighs the patient's decision not to disclose this information. Several factors hinder this disclosure. By disclosing this information to their nurses, patients believe a violation of their confidentiality has occurred. Patients also express concerns about isolation from other individuals, as well as about lack of care. The thought of preconceived judgments made by nurses also influence[1] the decision of a patient not to disclose this information. Being HIV positive may embarrass patients, and they may wish to keep their disease hidden from other individuals. Validity exists within each of these concerns; however, they are not necessarily true. Disclosing this information simply enhances the overall care of the patient.

Confidentiality plays an important role in the decision of whether or not to disclose a patient's HIV diagnosis. Therefore, the patient decides to whom he or she will disclose this information. However, nurses' cognizance of the patient's HIV-positive diagnosis allows them to aid in the patient's care. Problems arise when nurses do not know of a patient's HIV-positive condition. The patient may begin exhibiting symptoms of HIV infection; consequently, the nurse will begin treating these symptoms. Without proper knowledge of the patient's medical condition, the nurse may treat the ailments incorrectly. If the nurse has no knowledge of the patient's HIV infection, he or she cannot provide the most effective care for the patient. Maintaining confidentiality can exist, however, the nurse's knowledge of the patient's condition remains essential.[2]

Nursing schools stress the importance of not formulating preconceived judgments recently, a case study was conducted to substantiate this point.[3] The study was done in a group of third-year nursing students and dealt with the topic of preconceived judgments and how to effectively deal with them during the education years, so that they do not exist once the nurses start working with actual patients. It is fairly common for people to shy away from caring for someone who is infected with a virus such as HIV. This case study took three different approaches to educating these nurses about HIV and surveyed them on their thoughts of treating the disease, both before and after the education. The results were compared with those from a group of nursing students who did not receive education on the HIV virus.

Many patients feel their nurses hold preconceived judgments when they read in the patient's record that the individual suffers from HIV. Reading in a patient's chart that an individual's diagnosis is HIV positive does not differ from reading that the individual has hepatitis, muscular dystrophy, or any other form of an illness. Unfortunately, preconceived judgments do happen; however, these judgments do not differ from judgments made about gender, age, or ethnicity.

People face embarrassment throughout their lives for a variety of reasons. Many people do not tell their nurse personal facts about themselves because of a fear of embarrassment. However, the nurse can better understand the fears and the concerns of a patient, as well as the patient's physical symptoms, if the nurse knows the patient's history in its entirety. Disclosing the facts of an individual's health to his or her nurse should not lead to embarrassment. If mandating that HIV become known to nurses. Patients can rest assured that nothing will surprise the nurses.[4]

Many patients feel that if nurses learn of their HIV status, then solitary confinement within the hospital will take place. To the patients, this act of isolation means that everyone will realize they have HIV, and the opportunity to interact with other patients will no longer exist. HIV patients do receive their own rooms. However, that does not segregate them within the hospital, to alert other patients to their HIV-positive status. Several factors influence who receives a single room within a hospital.

Initially, reasons exist that make a nurse's knowledge of a patient's positive test for HIV unimportant. However, after a closer investigation, one can see the importance of telling a nurse that a patient has HIV. This disclosure does nothing more than enhance the overall care of the patient. No negative repercussions follow.

COMMENTS

1. The first major error is a subject-verb disagreement. Subjects and verbs must match in their forms. For example, a plural verb requires the plural form of the verb. Many subject-verb disagreement problems arise when prepositional phrases follow the subject but precede the verb. In this case, "The thought," singular, influences the decision; thus, the verb should end with an *s*.

   REVISION: The thought of preconceived judgments made by the nurses influences . . .

2. The comma splice is the second major error. In a comma splice, a writer uses only a comma to join two or more independent clauses. Each section on either side of the comma is an independent clause, a complete thought with a subject and verb. To correct a comma splice, a writer may insert a period between the two clauses, a semicolon between the clauses, or a conjunction such as "and" after the comma. In this example, the clauses before and after the however are both independent clauses. Therefore, the sentence requires a semicolon before "however."

   REVISION: Maintaining confidentiality can exist; however, the nurse's knowledge of the patient's condition remains essential.

3. Run-on sentences are a third major error. Writers create run-on sentences when they join two independent clauses without any form of punctuation or conjunction. A writer can correct a run-on sentence in the same manner as correction of a comma splice. This sample sentence requires the addition of a period, with a capital letter to begin the new sentence.

   REVISION: Nursing schools stress the importance of not formulating preconceived judgments. Recently, a case study was done to substantiate this point.

4. The final major error made by writers is the sentence fragment. A sentence fragment is an incomplete thought punctuated as a complete sentence. Dependent clauses cannot be punctuated as a complete sentence, or independent clauses. Writers must include a dependent clause in the same sentence as that containing the independent clause to which it refers. In this sample sentence, the "If" indicates a dependent clause, so this fragment must be included with the following sentence.

   REVISION: If mandating that HIV become known to nurses, patients can rest assured that nothing will surprise the nurses.

Draft #2
Implementing a Verb–Based Writing Style

When patients *test* positive for the human immunodeficiency virus (HIV), they *need to notify* their nurses. Arguments *exist* both for and against the patient's disclosure of HIV-positive serologic status; however, the nurse's knowledge of the diagnosis *outweighs* the patient's decision not to disclose this information. Several factors *hinder* this disclosure. By disclosing this information to their nurses, patients *believe* a violation of their confidentiality has occurred. Patients also *express* concerns about isolation from other individuals, as well as about lack of care. The thought of preconceived judgments made by nurses also *influences* the decision of a patient not to disclose this information. Being HIV positive may *embarrass* patients, and they may *wish* to keep their disease hidden from other individuals. Validity *exists* within each of these concerns; however, they *are* not necessary. Disclosing this information simply *enhances* the overall care of the patient.

Confidentiality *plays*[1] an important role in the decision of whether or not to disclose a patient's HIV diagnosis. Therefore, the patient *decides* to whom he or she will disclose this information. However, nurses' cognizance of the patient's positive HIV diagnosis *allows* them to aid in the patient's care. Problems *arise* when nurses do not know of a patient's HIV-positive condition. The patient may *begin exhibiting* symptoms of HIV infection; consequently, the nurse *will begin treating* these symptoms. Without proper knowledge of the patient's medical condition, the nurse may *treat* the ailments incorrectly. If the nurse *has* no knowledge of the patient's HIV infection, he or she cannot *provide* the most effective care for the patient. Maintaining confidentiality can *exist*; however, the nurse's knowledge of the patient's condition *remains* essential.

Nursing schools *stress*[2] the importance of not formulating preconceived judgments. Recently, a case study *was conducted* to substantiate this point. The study *was done*[3] on a group of third-year nursing students and dealt with the topic of preconceived judgments and how to effectively deal with them during the education years, so that they do not exist once the nurses start working with actual patients. *It is*[4] fairly common for people to shy away from caring for someone who is infected with a virus such as HIV. This case study *took*[5] three different approaches to educating these nurses about HIV and *surveyed* them on their thoughts of treating the disease, both before and after the education. The results *were compared* with those from a group of nursing students who did not receive education on the HIV virus.

Many patients *feel* their nurses hold preconceived judgments when they read in the patient's record that the individual suffers from HIV. Reading in a patient's chart that an individual's diagnosis *is*[6] HIV positive does not *differ* from reading that the individual *has* hepatitis, muscular dystrophy, or any other form of an illness. Unfortunately, preconceived judgments *do happen*; however, these judgments *do not differ* from judgments made about gender, age, or ethnicity.

People *face*[7] embarrassment throughout their lives for a variety of reasons. Many people do not *tell*[8]

their nurse personal facts about themselves because of a fear of embarrassment. However, the nurse can better *understand* the fears and the concerns of a patient, as well as the patient's physical symptoms, if the nurse *knows* the patient's history in its entirety. Disclosing the facts of an individual's health to his or her nurse should not *lead to*[9] embarrassment. If mandating that HIV become known to nurses, patients can *rest assured*[10] that nothing will surprise the nurses.

Many patients *feel* that if nurses learn of their HIV status, then solitary confinement, within the hospital, *will take place*.[11] To the patients, this act of isolation *means* that everyone will realize they have HIV, and the opportunity to interact with other patients will no longer exist. HIV patients do *receive* their own rooms. However, that does not *segregate* them within the hospital, to alert other patients to their HIV-positive status. Several factors *influence* who receives a single room within a hospital.

Initially, reasons *exist* that make a nurse's knowledge of a patient's positive test for HIV unimportant. However, after a closer investigation, one can *see*[12] the importance of telling a nurse that a patient has HIV. This disclosure does nothing more than *enhance* the overall care of the patient. No negative repercussions *follow*.

COMMENTS

For each essay, the writer should create a draft that focuses strictly on verb-based writing techniques. In any writing piece, strong verbs create a more professional tone and a greater sense of formality. In addition, stronger verbs can be more effective in portraying the writer's ideas. When a writer employs verb-based writing strategies, the reader appreciates the effort the writer has invested into writing the piece. Writers often insert the "to be" verb and its conjugations, lessening the strength of the essay. Oftentimes, the writer can replace the "to be" verb and many subsequent verbs with a much stronger verb. In this particular essay, the writer uses many strong verbs (verbs are italicized). However, some verbs—indicated with underscores—require further adjustment to enhance the overall quality of the paper.

1. Oftentimes, writers choose a verb that they would choose when in conversation with another individual. Writers should avoid conversational language whenever possible. The chosen verbs should reflect the writer's true intentions and should not provide ambiguity. The verb "play" in this sentence is not appropriate. Confidentiality, an intangible noun, cannot "play." To improve the sentence, the noun that performs an action in the sentence can be rearranged to the front of the sentence.

   REVISION: When deciding whether or not to disclose an HIV diagnosis, a patient considers confidentiality an important factor.

2. In this sentence, a stronger verb choice would be "emphasize." "Emphasize" has a more direct meaning than "stress," which normally functions as a noun.

   REVISION: Nursing schools emphasize the importance . . .

3. The use of the "to be" verb (helping verb) in addition to a main verb often represents a case in which a stronger, more effective verb can be used. Also, in this sentence, "was done on" is a poor verb choice in discussing an experiment.

   REVISION: The study was conducted with . . .

4. Again, the "to be" verb does not represent a strong verb choice. In addition, the "it" functioning as the noun does not refer to anything in the previous sentence. Therefore, the writer must eliminate both.

   REVISION: Nurses commonly shy away from . . .

5. Using literal meanings, "took" is inappropriate in this sentence because the study did not "take" anything.

   REVISION: This case study used . . .

6. Obviously, the use of the "to be" verb weakens the overall quality of the sentence. Also, note that the *patient* is HIV positive, not the diagnosis.

   REVISION: . . . that a patient is HIV positive . . .

7. Using the verb "face," the writer includes conversational language. Everyone does not "face" embarrassment.

   REVISION: People experience embarrassment . . .

8. Although correct in this situation, "tell" exemplifies the use of weak verbs. The writer should substitute a stronger verb.

   REVISION: Many people do not inform . . .

9. When read literally, "lead to" becomes inappropriate in this sentence. The weak verb choice demonstrates use of conversational language. Simply by choosing a stronger verb, the writer improves the quality of the sentence.

   REVISION: . . . his or her nurse should not result in . . .

10. In this case, "rest assured" demonstrates the use of purely conversational language; it is a phrase that has no definite meaning. In addition, the entire sentence does not contribute to the paragraph. The writer must reevaluate his or her thoughts and create another sentence.

11. Again, "take place" is wordy, and the writer can replace the two-word verb with a single, strong verb.

    REVISION: . . . within the hospital, will result.

12. The use of " to see" exemplifies the use of conversational language because no one literally "sees" or visualizes the importance.

    REVISION: . . . one can acknowledge . . .

Draft #3
Finding the Precise Words: Word Choice and Diction

When patients test positive for the human immunodeficiency virus (HIV), they need to notify their nurses. Arguments exist both for and against the patient's disclosure[1] of HIV-positive serologic status; however, the nurse's knowledge of the diagnosis outweighs the patient's decision not to disclose[1] this information. Several factors hinder this disclosure[1]. By disclosing[1] this information to their nurses, patients believe a violation of their confidentiality has occurred. Patients also express concerns about isolation from other individuals, as well as about lack of care. The thought of preconceived judgments made by nurses also influences the decision of a patient not to disclose[1] this information. Being HIV positive may embarrass patients, and they may wish to keep their disease hidden from other individuals. Validity exists within each of these concerns; however, they are not necessary. Disclosing[1] this information simply enhances the overall care of the patient.

When deciding whether or not to disclose an HIV diagnosis, a patient considers confidentiality an important factor. Therefore, the patient decides to whom he or she will disclose this information. However, nurses' cognizance of the patient's HIV-positive diagnosis allows them to aid[2] in the patient's care. Problems arise when nurses do not know of a patient's HIV-positive condition. The patient may begin exhibiting symptoms of HIV infection; consequently, the nurse will begin treating these symptoms. Without proper knowledge of the patient's medical condition, the nurses may treat the ailments incorrectly. If the nurse has no knowledge of the patient's HIV infection, he or she cannot provide the most effective care for the patient. Maintaining confidentiality can exist;[3] however, the nurse's knowledge of the patient's condition remains essential.

Nursing schools emphasize the importance of not formulating[4] preconceived judgments. Recently, a case study was conducted to substantiate this point. The study was conducted with a group of third-year nursing students and dealt with[5] the topic of preconceived judgments and how to effectively deal with[5] them during the education years, so that they do not exist once the nurses start working with actual patients. Nurses commonly shy away from[6] caring for someone who is infected with a virus such as HIV. This case study used three different approaches to educating these nurses about HIV and surveyed them on their thoughts of treating the disease, both before and after the education. The results were compared with those in a group of nursing students who did not receive education on the HIV virus.

Many patients feel their nurses hold preconceived judgments when they read in the patient's record that the individual suffers from HIV. Reading in a patient's chart that the person suffers from HIV does not differ from reading that a patient has hepatitis, muscular dystrophy, or any other form of an illness. Unfortunately, preconceived judgments do happen;[7] however, these judgments do not differ from judgments made about gender, age, or ethnicity.

People experience embarrassment throughout their lives for a variety of reasons. Many people do not inform their nurse of personal facts about themselves because of a fear of embarrassment. However, the nurse can better understand the fears and the concerns of a patient, as well as the patient's physical symptoms, if the nurse knows the patient's history in its entirety. Disclosing the facts of an individual's health to his or her nurse should not result in embarrassment. If mandating that HIV become known to nurses, patients can rest assured[8] that nothing will surprise the nurses.

Many patients feel[9] that if nurses learn of their HIV status, then solitary confinement, within the hospital, will result. To the patients, this act of isolation means that everyone will realize they have[10] HIV, and the opportunity to interact with other patients will no longer exist. HIV patients do receive their own rooms. However, that does not segregate them within the hospital, to alert other patients to their HIV-positive status. Several factors influence who receives a single room within a hospital.

Initially, reasons exist that make a nurse's knowledge of a patient's positive test for HIV unimportant. However, after a closer investigation, one can acknowledge the importance of telling a nurse that a patient has HIV. This disclosure does nothing more than enhance the overall care of the patient. No negative repercussions follow.

COMMENTS

1. In the introduction, the writer uses the word *disclose* and other derivations of the word too frequently. Substitution of other words could eliminate the redundancy.

   REVISION: . . . patient's decision not to reveal . . .

2. The choice of the verb *to aid* does not express the writer's intended meaning for the sentence. The knowledge of the diagnosis only enhances the nurse's ability to care

for the patient. However, the use of the word "aid" creates the idea that the nurse cannot treat the patient without that knowledge. Therefore, the writer should eliminate the verb and recast the sentence.

> REVISION: . . . positive HIV diagnosis enhances the nurse's ability to treat the patient . . .

3. The wording and verb tenses chosen create a sentence that does not make sense. In the sentence, "maintaining" acts as the noun. However, "maintaining" cannot exist. Therefore, the sentence and verb tenses require alteration.

> REVISION: Confidentiality can be maintained . . . or Maintaining confidentiality is possible . . .

4. In this case, simple verb substitution can simplify the use of *not* in combination with another verb. Generally, one verb exists as the "opposite" of another.

> REVISION: . . . emphasize the importance of avoiding . . .

5. The use of the phrase "deal with" demonstrates the use of conversational language. If the phrase were spoken in such a context, the listener would understand the idea the speaker wished to convey. However, writers must eliminate the use of such conversational language, to avoid misinterpretation by the reader.

> REVISION: . . . involved the topic . . . and . . . to effectively eliminate them . . .

6. Again, the use of conversational language decreases the professional format of the essay.

> REVISION: . . . avoid caring for . . .

7. Judgments do not happen; they exist.

> REVISION: . . . judgments do exist.

8. In addition to poor word choice, this sentence does not make sense. The sentence does not adequately summarize the preceding paragraphs or refer to the thesis. Therefore, the writer should eliminate the entire sentence.

9. The idea expressed in the sentence refers to a fear held by many patients. Therefore, the writer could replace the verb "feel."

> REVISION: Many patients fear . . .

10. The patients do not "have" HIV but have tested positive for or have been diagnosed with the disease. The use of the verb "have" is not the best word choice when describing organisms that cause diseases.

> REVISION: . . . realize they are HIV positive

Draft #4
Building Coherence throughout the Document

When patients test positive for the human immunodeficiency virus (HIV), they need to notify their nurses. Arguments exist both for and against the patient's disclosure of HIV-positive serologic status; however, the nurse's knowledge of the diagnosis outweighs the patient's decision not to reveal this information. Several factors hinder this disclosure. By disclosing this information to their nurses, patients believe a violation of their confidentiality has occurred. Patients also express concerns about isolation from other individuals, as well as about lack of care.[1] The thought of preconceived judgments made by nurses also influences the decision of a patient not to reveal this information. Being HIV positive may embarrass patients, and they may wish to keep their disease hidden from other individuals. Validity exists within each of these concerns; however, they are not necessary. Disclosing this information simply enhances the overall care of the patient.

When deciding whether or not to disclose an HIV diagnosis, a patient considers confidentiality an important factor.[2] Therefore,[3] the patient decides to whom he or she will disclose this information. However, nurses' cognizance of the patient's HIV-positive diagnosis enhances the nurse's ability to treat the patient.[4] Problems arise when nurses do not know of a patient's HIV-positive condition. The patient may begin exhibiting symptoms of the HIV infection; consequently, the nurse will begin treating these symptoms. Without proper knowledge of the patient's medical condition, the nurse may treat the ailments incorrectly. If the nurse has no knowledge of the patient's HIV infection, he or she cannot provide the most effective care for the patient. Confidentiality can be maintained; however, the nurse's knowledge of the patient's condition remains essential.

Nursing schools emphasize the importance of avoiding preconceived judgments.[5] Recently, a case study was conducted to substantiate this point. The study was conducted with a group of third-year nursing students and involved the topic of preconceived judgments and how to effectively eliminate them during the education years, so that they do not exist once the nurses start working with actual patients. Nurses commonly avoid caring for someone who is infected with a virus such as HIV. This case study used three different approaches to educating these nurses about HIV and surveyed them on their thoughts of treating the disease, both before and after the education. The results were compared with those from a group of nursing students who did not receive education on the HIV virus.

Many patients feel their nurses hold preconceived judgments when they read in the patient's record that the individual suffers from HIV.[6] Reading on a patient's chart that the person suffers from HIV does not differ from reading that a patient has hepatitis, muscular dystrophy, or any other form of an illness. Unfortunately, preconceived judgments do exist; however, these judgments do not differ from judgments made about gender, age, or ethnicity.[7]

People experience embarrassment throughout their lives for a variety of reasons.[8] Many people do not inform their nurse of personal facts about themselves because of a fear of embarrassment. However, the nurse can better understand the fears and the concerns of a patient, as well as the patient's physical symptoms, if the nurse knows the patient's history in its entirety. Disclosing the facts of an individual's health to his or her nurse should not result in embarrassment.

Many patients fear that if nurses learn of their HIV status, then solitary confinement, within the hospital, will result. To the patients, this act of isolation means that everyone will realize they are HIV positive, and the opportunity to interact with other patients will no longer exist. HIV patients do receive their own rooms. However, that does not segregate them within the hospital, to alert other patients to their HIV-positive status. Several factors influence who receives a single room within a hospital.

Initially, reasons exist that make a nurse's knowledge of a patient's positive test for HIV unimportant.[7] However, after a closer investigation, one can acknowledge the importance of telling a nurse that a patient has HIV. This disclosure does nothing more than enhance the overall care of the patient. No negative repercussions follow.

COMMENTS

1. Within this one sentence, two isolated ideas are expressed as one. Attaching one idea directly after another creates a sense of insignificance of the second idea. To avoid this problem, the writer must develop two separate sentences, each of which adequately addresses the individual point that will be discussed in the body of the paper.

2. This introductory statement does not pertain to the information included in the remainder of the paragraph. After reading the first sentence, the reader expects a paragraph discussing the confidentiality issues involved in the disclosure of HIV status. However, the paragraph states the problems that arise when nurses care for patients that choose not to disclose their HIV status. The writer must formulate a statement that correctly introduces the information that will be discussed in the following paragraph.

3. The use of the word "therefore" is inappropriate in this situation. When used properly, "therefore" provides a transition between two ideas in which the latter statement describes the result of the prior. In this case, the writer has not established any point before the use of the transition word, thus creating an incorrect attempt at a transition statement.

4. As with the the previous error, the writer has used a transition word incorrectly. "However" provides a transition between two contrasting ideas. This requirement has not been fulfilled prior to the use of the transition word, again creating a transitioning error.

5. The second body paragraph addresses the instruction provided to nurses in nursing school regarding the treatment of patients with diseases such as HIV. This information is a shift from the previous paragraph regarding care by practicing nurses. To increase effectiveness, the paragraph discussing training of nurses should precede the paragraph about nurses in practice. Ordering the paragraphs in such a realistic sequential order provides easier transitioning for the reader.

6. As with every other body paragraph, this paragraph begins with a subject verb combination in a simple sentence. This format becomes redundant and the reader may lose interest. Sentence variation, which is discussed in the next draft, must be employed to create a more professional essay.

7. In this essay, the writer intends to persuade the reader that patients should disclose a HIV-positive status to their nurses and physicians. With this statement, the writer contradicts the positive points that had been previously established and creates a coherence break. In a persuasive essay, a writer may introduce the arguments presented by the opposition, but he or she must refute that opposition. In this case, the writer introduces this contradictory statement without any refutation, thereby weakening his or her argument.

8. Again, a simple sentence creates a sense of redundancy. In addition, the introductory sentence for this paragraph does not adequately prepare the reader for the paragraph to follow. When this sentence is read, the reader can easily become confused about what point the writer is trying to establish. Therefore, the writer must create a connection between previous body paragraphs and the ones to follow. Otherwise, the essay seems choppy and unprofessional.

Overall, this essay is choppy. The writer moves from one point to another without any use of transitions. A simple transition word or statement can ease the switch even between seemingly unconnected ideas. Without transitions, the essay lacks coherence, and the reader may become confused and uninterested. Also, the final sentence of each body paragraph should reconnect the paragraph to the thesis statement. In doing this, the writer ensures that the reader is constantly reminded of the overall purpose of the essay.

Draft #5
Sentence Variation

When patients test positive for the human immunodeficiency virus (HIV), they need to notify their nurses. *(complex)*[1] Arguments exist both for and against the patient's disclosure of HIV-positive serologic status; *(simple)*[2] however, the nurse's knowledge of the diagnosis outweighs the patient's decision not to reveal this information. *(simple)*[3] Several factors hinder this disclosure. *(simple)*[4] By disclosing this information to their nurses, patients believe a violation of their confidentiality has occurred. *(complex)*[5] Patients fear inadequate care as a result of their condition. *(simple)*[6] Also, patients express concerns about isolation from other individuals. *(simple)*[7] The thought of preconceived judgments made by nurses also influences the decision of a patient not to reveal this information. *(simple)*[8] Being HIV positive may embarrass patients, and they may wish to keep their disease hidden from other individuals. *(compound)*[9] Validity exists within each of these concerns; *(simple)*[10] however, they are not necessary. *(simple)*[11] Disclosing this information simply enhances *(gerund)* the overall care of the patient. *(simple)*[12]

Nursing schools emphasize the importance of avoiding preconceived judgments. Recently, a case study was conducted to substantiate this point. The study was conducted with a group of third-year nursing students and involved the topic of preconceived judgments and how to effectively eliminate them during the education years, so that they do not exist once the nurses start working with actual patients. Nurses commonly avoid caring for someone who is infected with a virus such as HIV. This case study used three different approaches to educating these nurses about HIV and surveyed them on their thoughts of treating the disease, both before and after the education. The results were compared with those from a group of nursing students who did not receive education on the HIV virus.

When deciding whether or not to disclose an HIV diagnosis, a patient considers confidentiality an important factor. *(complex)*[1] In addition, patients should contemplate the effects of disclosure or nondisclosure on the nurses' ability to provide adequate care. *(simple)*[2] Nurses' cognizance of the patient's HIV-positive diagnosis enhances their ability to treat the patient. *(simple)*[3] Problems arise when nurses do not know of a patient's HIV-positive condition. *(simple)*[4] The patient may begin exhibiting symptoms of HIV infection; *(simple)*[5] consequently, the nurse will begin treating these symptoms. *(simple)*[6] Without proper knowledge of the patient's medical condition, *(prepositional)* the nurse may treat the ailments incorrectly. *(simple)*[7] If the nurse has no knowledge of the patient's HIV infection, he or she cannot provide the most effective care for the patient. *(complex)*[8] Confidentiality can be maintained; *(simple)*[9] however, the nurse's knowledge of the patient's condition remains essential. *(simple)*[10]

Many patients feel their nurses hold preconceived judgments when they read in the patient's record that the individual suffers from HIV. Reading on a patient's chart that the person suffers from HIV does not differ from reading that a patient has hepatitis, muscular dystrophy, or any other form of an illness. Unfortunately, preconceived judgments do exist; however, these judgments do not differ from judgments made about gender, age, or ethnicity.

In addition to the fear of preconceived judgments on the part of the medical staff, many patients do not inform their nurse of personal facts about themselves because of a fear of embarrassment. However, the nurse can better understand the fears and the concerns of a patient, as well as the patient's physical symptoms, if the nurse knows the patient's history in its entirety. Disclosing the facts of an individual's health to his or her nurse should not result in embarrassment.

Many patients fear that if nurses learn of their HIV status, then solitary confinement, within the hospital, will result. To the patients, this act of isolation means that everyone will realize they are HIV positive, and the opportunity to interact with other patients will no longer exist. HIV patients do receive their own rooms. However, that does not segregate them within the hospital, to alert other patients to their HIV-positive status. Several factors influence who receives a single room within a hospital.

While a patient may have initial hesitations about revealing a positive diagnosis of HIV, a closer investigation allows him/her to acknowledge the importance of informing a nurse that he suffers from HIV. This disclosure does nothing more than enhance the overall care of the patient. No negative repercussions follow.

COMMENTS

Paragraph 1 (sentences 1 to 12): In this introductory paragraph, the writer uses three types of sentences: simple, complex, and compound. However, the use of simple sentences becomes redundant in this paragraph. Following the first complex sentence, the writer creates three simple sentences with the same subject-verb-object format. When reading such sentences, the reader may lose interest in the essay.

The second and third sentences can be combined to form a complex sentence.

REVISION: While arguments exist both for and against the patient's disclosure of HIV, the benefit of the nurse's knowledge of the virus outweighs the patient's decision not to reveal this information.

Combining sentences 6 and 7 creates a compound-complex sentence.

REVISION: When deciding whether or not to reveal their diagnosis, patients fear inadequate care as a result of their condition, and they express concerns about isolation from other individuals.

By combining sentences 10 and 11, another complex sentence is created.

REVISION: Although validity exists within each of these concerns, they are not necessary.

Also in the introductory paragraph, the writer uses only two gerund phrases. To avoid redundancy in a paper, writers should incorporate all five types of phrases. In this introductory paragraph, the writer has used gerunds in sentences 9 and 12. By rearranging the wording in sentence 9, the writer can create a participial phrase.

REVISION: Fearing embarrassment, patients may wish to keep their disease hidden from other individuals.

Paragraph 3 (sentences 1 to 10): Again, the writer focuses on redundant simple sentences rather than on more interesting sentence types. The constant subject-verb-object format may bore the reader and makes the essay appear unprofessional.

Combining sentences 5 and 6 creates a compound sentence.

REVISION: The patient may begin exhibiting symptoms of the HIV virus, and the nurse will begin treating these symptoms.

Sentence 3 can be reworded to include another type of phrase. Phrases can also help decrease the monotony of simple sentences.

REVISION: To enhance the nurse's ability to treat the patient, the patient should inform the nurse of his or her HIV-positive diagnosis.

The final type of phrase, the appositive, can be created to provide the reader with nonessential information without disturbing the intended message of the sentence.

Exercises

EDITING, REVISING, AND PROOFREADING

■ Editing

Directions: Revise the following passage by demonstrating your knowledge of professional/academic writing skills. You may consider reorganizing and rewriting the entire passage to make it a coherent whole.

The new director of physical therapy has submitted a report which he has outlined several problems that he feels is responsible for the department's failure to receive compensation for treatments. The first problem he identifies is when therapists are not clear in stating their rationale for treatment, additionally, he cites poor writing skills as the main reason for the following: There are often significant differences between therapists writing but he says that most students cannot organize his/her thoughts clear. Which is a major problem. Although many students are taking writing classes. After taking such writing classes, the documents are often plagued with other problems such as: sentence fragments, run on sentences and the therapists constantly write comma splices. Another problem is not describing the medical necessity of procedures. But this is getting better because students are being taught to define medical necessity in their documentation. Documentation should say the appropriateness of treatment too; as this demonstrates that the Therapists work is of the quality of meeting general medical standards. It is also found that documentation is needed to educate payors and patients as well. All therapists must be able to educate others or the profession will suffer. And this brings us to statement five, we need to get reimbursed for your services which are rendered. It is also a problem that writers/therapists' don't know how to use commas, or other marks of punctuation accurately. Writers/therapists also don't use good sentence variety. They have several short sentences that are choppy. They sho uld have sentences that show the four types of sentences and the five types of phrases. They use verbs that are weak and passive too. Sentence combination skills are required by many educated people to provide this. Because subordination and coordination of an idea is good for readers. Proofreading and editing skills are needed and therapists should always remember what is needed for documentation that is effective.

■ Revision

Directions: Employing the strategies of writing and revising that you have learned, rewrite the following essay.

The new manager of Buffalo Allied Health has submitted a report in which she has outlined several problems that she feels are responsible for the low production that has been plaguing her facility. The first problem that she identifies is that employees and therapists are working with equipment that they have not been specifically trained to use. There are often significant differences that she has identified between the preparation workers have and the actual tasks that they are expected to perform. She feels that this is the primary reason for poor productivity. Her report also indicates that absenteeism in the Therapy Clinic is 15% higher that that which is experienced by the surrounding clinics and hospital facilities. It is also noted in her report that she can find no reason for the higher absenteeism. She is willing to speculate that there is a relationship between poor training and low morale. This can cause employees to be absent from work. The third problem in the clinic noted in her report is that because the Clinic operates some of the company's oldest equipment, down time and a lack of spare parts leave many workers idle for what she calls "extended periods." The manager speculates that these three problems could be the causes for low productivity. She adds that until the Clinic has newer equipment and better training for its personnel, productivity will continue to be a problem.

■ Editing and Proofreading an Evaluation

Directions: Find and fix all the problems with this evaluation.

Upon treating Jane Smith for the past four months, she has gained movement, sensation, and balance back on her left side after having a stroke last March. Mrs. Smith is able to perform some of her daily functional activities. She has been discharged two weeks ago. I would appreciate a reimbursement for the services rendered.

Dr. Thomas referred Jane to physical therapy. She desires to ambulate a normal distance in order to do her daily activities. Jane, a 55-year-old female that lives with her husband in an apartment. She was a healthy person with no medical history prior to the stroke. She has been working as a library clerk for 20 years. Jane's goal is to go back to work after physical therapy. She suffered a mild stroke. The most important exercises for Mrs. Smith at this time is maintaining her balance and coordination. Mrs. Smith did not have any physical therapy prior to her visit to the clinic. Upon evaluation, the patient has shown capability to stand and ambulate with one physical therapist assisting her. Transferring from chair to bed also needs to be worked on. The patient's left arm and leg requires strengthening exercises. To test the patient's strength and ability, I went through some active and passive ROM. I wanted to evaluate how severely the stroke effected her.

■ Editing and Proofreading a Reimbursement Narrative

Directions: Find and fix the errors in all facets of the writing process.

Mr. James recently arrived in the hospital emergency room with a very serious heart condition. James happens to be covered under your insurance policy for up to $5000 for an emergency room visit. In closely evaluating this policy, with reference to Mr. James' specific case, I am fully aware that reimbursement for services rendered will only be satisfied when the payor deems the patient's treatment "medically necessary." Therefore, I intend to validate the options of treatment that I administered to James and prove their crucial necessity.

Mr. James, referred to us by Dr. Carlton, possesses a history of ventricular fibrillation which previously resulted in two cardiac arrests. In addition, he suffered from a double by-pass surgery whereby he emerged with the presence of a minimal functional strength deficit in both his lower extremities. A systematic evaluation of his electrocardiogram records over the past five years, beginning with his first cardiac arrest, illustrates a gradual increase in the severity of his ventricular fibrillation. Before his recent visit to the emergency room the fibrillation discomfort and general strength deficit have persisted as his only complaints.

James arrived by ambulance in full cardiac arrest. Responding to the seriousness of the situation, he underwent resuscitation. With no response, I immediately defibrillated him to initiate a steady heart rhythm.

■ Editing and Proofreading: Sentences and Passages

Directions: Find and correct all the errors in the following sentences and passages.

The therapists in this department are going to work with the patient to get his ROM and strength back to where it needs to be to function properly.

It is important to have early motion because it decreases effusion, pain, and inhibits fear. Weights should also be used early, but in small amounts and little by little.

It is essential for her to attend physical therapy to repair her ROM of the petellofemoral joint and strength of the quadriceps and hamstring muscles.

She was able to handle 25 lbs. of weights.

The onset began when she fell.

The left biceps and triceps had 5 out of 5.

The patient received treatment for her right shoulder. The treatment consists of electrical stimulation, ultrasound, joint mobilization, and exercises from active assisted and active free ROM to active resisted. The exercises included using pulleys, and pedulum. The exercises were used to strengthen the patients' strength, and ROM.

Patient's ability to perform daily activities should show a little improvement.

She has problems going from wheelchair to shower. The use of crutches is a must.

On the other hand, she will receive treatment.

No specific action was recalled by the patient.

The patient was requested to participate in exercises and attending therapy.

Edna fractured her right radius on 3/3/00. She injured her radius by slipping on ice.

The patient is not allowed to put weight on leg, no coordination can be measured.

The pain can be intense at time, on a scale of 1-10, she says it can vary.

The stairs will be slow going, however she will have a ramp to help these things.

She may lean to far and end up hurting herself.

Patient should have been able to increase movement back to it's original status. Although the therapy proved unsuccessful because the patient still experiences problems.

In evaluating the information obtained during the exam, they can be organized and interpreted in the following way.

Patient demonstrates normal ROM, and this is where we will concentrate our efforts.

He will be encouraged to continue those exercises when he is not in the clinic and he will also be given additional exercises for home.

Good posture is essential for him because it will help with his aerobic capacity for sports, and it will benefit treatment because posture affects joint integrity which is what we are trying to get the most out of.

Dr. Meyers diagnosed the patient on 9/8/00 and on 9/15/00 reconstructive surgery was performed.

The treatment that Mr. Smith receives on a regular basis would improve his ROM, and strengthen his muscles gradually.

The patient being an avid basketball star has experienced many problems.

The patient will attend 5 sessions three or four times per week.

Some of the injuries are listed below,
  1. Torn ACL
  2. Dislocated knee
  3. Sprain to knee

The patient engages in strenuous exercises such as; running, jumping, and swimming.

2

Writing for Academic Purposes

The following chapters examine the various types of writing assignments that students will encounter in an academic setting. Most people thinking about their academic career can remember a few papers that they wrote; however, only a few of those people can recall the organizational principles that guided those assignments. This section of the text serves to reinforce the strategies for organizing and presenting information. It covers the rhetorical devices, such as definition, cause and effect, and process analysis. It also expands on the principles of logic and reasoning required for argumentation. Finally, it delineates the processes of research writing and writing the thesis. The final chapter on writing for publication is relevant both to this section and to the next and final section, "Writing for Administrative Purposes."

TYPES OF ACADEMIC WRITING

In Section 1, we established that in academic or professional writing, you usually will write in either of two arenas: to inform or to persuade. In either case, knowledge and understanding of the organizational principles that guide such writing are essential.

Expository (Informative) Writing

Expository writing (sometimes called *informative writing*) provides the reader with information, or it helps to explain a set of circumstances. It is most often used in the medical profession to set forth the findings in a study. This type of writing requires the writer to back up or support his or her claims with hard facts or data. Informative writing assignments never take on a subjective slant; they are written with an objective eye for accuracy and clarity, but they do, in some ways, attempt to guide the thinking of the reader. All writing in academic circles does so. Consider what you read in journals or textbooks as classic examples of expository writing; these forms of writing educate the reader. Educational material should not be slanted, but it should inform and guide the reader, and the results should be verifiable by anyone interested in contesting the information presented. Conversely, some people think that newspaper and magazine articles are written in this mode. This is not always the case, as some authors carefully conceal their biases and ultimately seek to persuade the reader. Such writing is not expository or informative writing. Expository writing uses conventions of organization to plan out the approach to explaining a set of circumstances. These conventions include methods such as definition, cause and effect, and comparison and contrast.

Argument

Argumentative writing (often called *persuasive writing*) attempts to reinforce an already existing opinion or sway a reader to change opinions. Some writing instructors teach the persuasive essay as a mechanism of argument because the essay presents a side to an argument and then reinforces it with evidence. Indeed, the persuasive essay is an argument. However, the effective argument is well supported with convincing evidence. Most persuasive essays are written in the health professions through professional forums, such as newspapers or journals, or through administrative writing to convince administrators or others in the field to shift their stance or support a claim on a debatable issue.

Many beginning writers fail to comprehend the purpose of this type of assignment or this form of writing because they believe that since they have an opinion about a subject, they have an argument. This is not the case, because everyone's opinion is not truly valid, for academic or professional purposes, until it is supported with some verifiable evidence or experience. Using personal experience is often considered a weak form of evidence because it may not be easily reproducible. Consequently, as a writer, you are saddled with the responsibility of supporting your ideas with facts and hard evidence.

The important element to remember in writing a persuasive essay is that everyone has an opinion, and some or most of your readers may disagree with your stance on the issue that is being debated. Tact and understanding should be applied liberally. Your goal here is not to offend those who disagree but to present information in such a way that those who disagree might change their opinion. Meeting this challenge requires understanding your audience and using the correct tone in the words you choose.

KNOWING YOUR AUDIENCE

Although the main goal of an essay is to inform, persuade, or argue a particular side, knowing the audience is the key to success. Using appropriate language, or language written on the same intellectual and emotional level as the audience's, helps align you with the audience, dissenters and all. You are neither writing to clear your head of ideas nor to verify that you can think. You are writing essays and argumentative documents to convince others to believe what you believe, or at least to believe that you have provided a rational argument with reasonable claims. If you fail to realize that you are writing for others, you will never be a successful writer.

Also, successful writers tailor their messages, or the content, to the needs and values of the audience. To do so, writers must analyze the needs and values of the audience before writing. An audience analysis includes observing or identifying the target audience and grasping fully who they are in order to develop the message that will meet their needs. Defining the audience helps writers set communication goals.

The most obvious approach to determining the profile of the audience is to examine demographic figures: age, gender, class (socioeconomic group), group affiliations (medical societies, and church, civic, or social groups), ethnicity, and education. However important these may seem, they may not always develop a full picture of the audience's needs. Demographic analysis can be helpful, but it may not provide a means to determine how an audience thinks. A psychographic analysis asks writers to consider the audience's world views, to assess how and why they believe what they believe, to understand what concerns them, to determine how they make decisions (based on political, social, economic, moral, or ethical standards), and to identify which of these factors motivates them to act.

Abraham Maslow determined that people are motivated to act according to certain needs, which he categorized in a hierarchy. Others such as Rokeach and also Osborn and Osborn identified needs and values to supplement Maslow's work. Still others—Gronbeck, McKerrow, Ehninger, and Monroe—devised systems to explain human motivation based on appeals. Much of this research is based on advertising or reaching an audience in an academic setting, but the principles are the same for writing for the health professions: The more we know about the audience, the better we can influence the ability of all of its members to react and make decisions.

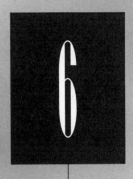

Expository

Writing

Key Terms

Bidirectional A cause-and-effect organizational pattern in which either an event may be explained by its causes or the effects of that event on the future may be explained

Bullets Typographical symbols used to indicate elements for which a specific order is not necessary

Categorical approach In comparing/contrasting, analysis of both subjects through a predetermined set of categories

Classification Organizes large bodies of information into categories

Directional process analysis Explains how to accomplish a goal, for example, a recipe of giving directions to someone who is lost

Division Classifies the parts of the whole

Expanded definition Redefining terms or concepts through logic

Expository writing Writing that provides information, using patterns of organization to create well-reasoned text

First person Using "I" in subjective case and "me" in the objective

Heading A signpost indicating to the reader that information is compartmentalized for convenience

Informational process analysis Explains how a process works

Narration Chronological sequencing of events; telling the story

Negation Defining an object or a concept by what it is not

Numbers Used to indicate order

Objective description Clear statement of facts as they occur

One-to-one correspondence Relationship between cause and effect in which only one factor is the cause of an event or a condition, with other factors discounted as causes

Second person Using "you" in subjective and objective case

Simple definition The dictionary definition of a word, term, or concept

Subjective description Interpretation of the facts or events

Third person Telling the story using *he*, *she*, or *they* or using the passive voice

Topical approach In comparing/contrasting, discussion of one subject first in its entirety and then another subject in its entirety

chapter objectives

On completion of this chapter, the reader should be able to

1. Organize ideas and communicate through patterns of reasoning and logic.
2. Understand the needs of an audience and choose an appropriate mode.
3. Employ descriptive language to suit the scene.
4. Organize information by means of standard use of headings, numbers, and bullets

For **expository writing** in any context, we present and organize information to meet the demands or expectations of our audience. Such patterns of organization help our readers gather the information we intend to communicate in a manner that is logical. Depending on the nature of the topic, different patterns of organization can be applied. Certain patterns fit certain purposes better than others.

NARRATION

The most recognizable pattern of organization is the narrative. We have all told stories, and **narration** is the storytelling mode that uses an orderly time sequence to divulge the facts in an order determined by the writer. When a writer seeks to *explain* a topic, narration is the mode of choice.

The narrative process is used most readily to explain how to perform a task or a series of tasks: treatment modality, office protocol, or filling out paperwork. Additionally, the chronological sequencing of events can be applied to other patterns of organization. For example, if explaining the causes of an issue in a cause-and-effect essay, you may be required to provide a sketch of the events leading up to the issue. A good writer uses many organizational patterns, which are interdependent.

Narration is the pattern of organization that writers use to tell a story. For example, when patients explain how an injury occurs, they usually follow a sequence of events arranged in chronological order. A writer in the medical professions will choose the narrative mode when the situation dictates it, such as to chronicle the events that lead to a patient's illness or injury or to describe a series of events in which the writer was a participant or observer. The most recognizable pattern of organization, narration fits the storytelling mode, but many inexperienced writers feel that it is too informal to be used in the profession. This is not true. This chapter dictates when the narrative mode is acceptable in professional writing environments.

Understanding Reader Expectations

With the telling of any story, readers develop expectations. They want to know who was involved, what happened, where it happened, when it happened, why it happened, and how it happened. Although all of these elements may not be necessary when chronicling the events leading up to a patient's injury or ailment, a thorough investigator will record the necessary facts and reinvent them in a strategy that will be useful to others who read the document. Likewise, creating a simple list of events will not be sufficient. Readers will want to be placed into the scene to experience the events. Consequently, developing a strategy for writing the narrative is important to the medical writer.

When chronicling the events told by another person, a writer must be aware of shifts in setting or circumstance that may mislead the reader or divert attention away from the main point. Consequently, the writer must be judicious when eliminating information that a patient presents. Sometimes, what may seem to be inconsequential may actually prove to be key; likewise, you will not want to overburden your reader with extraneous or trivial bits of information, especially if they detract from the continuity and flow of the writing. Additionally, managing information in this form requires the use of strong transitional words and phrases that signal changes. A reader will become bored or confused with the repetition of the word *next* as a sentence opener. A strong writer will use subordination and coordination strategies to emphasize the main points of the passage and to create appropriate transitions between events of importance.

Determining Purpose

When introductory writing instructors assign narration in their classrooms, they want their student writers to develop the schemes to tie events together, but, more important, they want their writers to develop an understanding of the thesis or the overall purpose of the sequence of events. In other words, when someone tells a story, he or she should have an ultimate purpose in mind. For example, a student wrote an essay about the first time he scaled an icy mountain in which he described the event in great detail; however, by the end of the essay, I as a reader did not understand why he was telling this story. In the essay, he described how he suffered a variety of difficulties on his journey and how he feared for his life. These events were described, but the ultimate message or purpose of the essay was not clear. In other words, he had no thesis to direct the events. When he added a thesis about the first time he ever faced death and related the body paragraphs to that topic, his essay became unified.

Lack of a thesis is a common problem with narration. Many writers become engrossed in the process of storytelling, but they fail to direct the reader's attention to the overall purpose for telling the story.

Determining Point of View

When writing in the narrative mode, writers choose a perspective from which to tell the story. For example, in an essay about my work with developing writers, the appropriate form would be the **first person**. The first person is the mode using *I:*

> *I* studied the effects of computer-enhanced learning on a group.
> *I* divided the sample into two groups.
> *I* gathered the results.
> *I* concluded that computer-enhanced learning is an effective strategy to teach writing.

The first person form signifies to the reader that the events are the result of direct experience.

Writers face a dilemma, however, with the first person form. As the preceding example indicates, the use of *I* becomes boring and repetitive and even borders on egotistical. Many writers attempt to avoid the use of *I* by employing the passive voice. Instead of claiming responsibility for the action, however, the sentence now focuses on the action instead of the actor.

EXAMPLE

> I divided the sample into two groups.
> The sample was divided into two groups.

This is an acceptable practice for many research writers. The actors in the project have

been identified. The repetition of the word *I* is needless, and the focus can now be shifted to the action.

The **third person** perspective is appropriate for telling the story of others. Writers in the health professions use this form when discussing the work of others from a research perspective or when chronicling events that are discussed by a patient. In this form, the pronouns *he, she,* and *they* are used (or *him, his, her, their, them*).

The third person point of view is used most often in academic writing and writing in the professions because it sends a message of objectivity. The writer has processed the events and is delivering them to the reader through an editorial filter. For example, when a patient discusses the events that led to an injury, the practitioner will decide what information is appropriate and necessary for other readers. When discussing the published work of other researchers, the writer will pull from the original research the passages or events that influence the purpose of the paper being written. Ultimately, the writer controls how the reader absorbs information that is provided by others.

The **second person** form is used when a writer directly addresses the reader, as I have done in this text. Using the pronoun *you,* I have sought to engage the readers of this text by making them active participants.

> **EXAMPLE:** When you use passive voice, know when it is acceptable and when it is not.

Such direct address will indicate to the readers that their participation is necessary.

Many writers, when instructing others, fail to recognize that use of the second person voice is an effective strategy. They feel that the use of the second person may be overbearing, and they attempt to write "around" the pronoun, creating awkward constructions:

> **EXAMPLE:** When finished with the floor cleaning, sweep the steps.

The use of *you,* however, also has its difficulties. Many writers will attempt to include the reader and mistakenly add the reader to a group. This is a simple problem of reading for accuracy:

EXAMPLE: When you enter junior high school, you must adjust to changing rooms for different classes.

The problem here is that I, the reader, am not entering junior high school. This writer has failed to recognize that the intended audience may be outside the preconceived limits.

EXAMPLE: When you quantify the active range of motion, you must write your measurements in degrees.

This writer assumes that I, the reader, am a therapist, which I am not. Again, I have been placed into a group of which I am not a part. This mistake creates confusion for the reader or distances the reader from the ultimate purpose by excluding him or her from the audience.

Choosing Language Appropriate to the Scene

To fully communicate the experience of the narrative, a writer must be aware of readers' expectations. All readers need to be engaged, and this can be accomplished by using language that is strong and action oriented. The section on verb-based writing strategies in Chapter 3 reinforces this point, but the point is worth repeating here. Readers need a clear picture of the events or the players in the events. The language the writer chooses determines the effectiveness of the passage.

In many cases, writers simply choose the language that comes to mind quickly when describing events. Descriptive terms, especially strong verbs, can help a reader *see* and *feel* the events.

Consider the different effect each of the following sentences has on you:

WEAK: The passage from Dr. White's article deals with the subject of bulimia.

BETTER: Dr. White discusses bulimia in her article.

In the "weak" example, the subject, *the passage*, is not significant. Furthermore, the verb *deals with* does not convey a specific meaning. In the "better" example, the focus of the sentence shifts to a *conversation* that Dr. White has with the reader. This promotes the idea to readers that they are exchanging information with the experts.

Although the preceding example indicates that objective, descriptive terms must be used to communicate clearly, in some cases, the opposite is true. When patients describe symptoms or events, for example, they often use language that is appropriate to their experience. This should not be ignored. Use direct quotes to indicate terms from the dialogue.

EXAMPLE: The patient complained of pain radiating down his arm, like "a thousand knives stabbing" him.

This example provides some necessary information in that the pain is not dull but shooting, and the term *stabbing* may indicate that the pain is periodic instead of chronic.

Sample Student Essay
NARRATION

After Benjamin Christopher Lewis tore his anterior cruciate ligament (ACL) while skiing at the Peak'n Peek Ski Resort on December 17, 2001, he underwent ACL reconstructive surgery by Dr. Phillip C. Carnes at St. Vincent's Hospital in Erie, Pennsylvania. Following his surgery, Mr. Lewis implemented a home rehabilitation treatment program, which not only hindered his recovery time owing to his lack of motivation in the program but also resulted in the formation of excess scar tissue within the knee joint capsule. At this time, Dr. Timothy N. Banks performed surgery to remove the scar tissue and referred him to Erie Rehabilitation. On January 8, 2002, I admitted Mr. Lewis into my care.

Most patients who have undergone ACL reconstruction demonstrate full extension and a flexion of 140° at the 3-week post-ACL surgery period; however, Mr. Lewis displayed only a 170° extension and a 140° flexion during his first visit. These impediments resulted from both the unsuccessful home treatment program and his second surgery to remove scar tissue. Despite these initial shortcomings, Mr. Lewis displayed full flexion and extension by the end of his 6-month treatment, and consequently, I am discharging Mr. Lewis at this time.

At the beginning of each therapy visit, I applied a moist hot pack to Mr. Lewis's knee for approximately 20 minutes prior to his exercise program and ended with 15 minutes of icing. During the first week, the patient concentrated on regaining some of his lost flexion by performing three sets of heel, shuttle, and wall slides for 15 repetitions each. To aid in his full extension efforts, Mr. Lewis completed the same amount of heel props, prone hangs, and towel stretches during this first week. At the end of his first week with me, Mr. Lewis made significant progress and increased his flexion to 124°. At the start of the second week of treatment, I established a plan to help Mr. Lewis regain patellar tendon strength to better support his knee joint, which was done by adding step-down exercises, leg presses, and knee extensions. Mr. Lewis executed three sets of 12 repetitions for each of these exercises. By the end of the third week, Mr. Lewis had reached full extension and a flexion of 135°. After almost a month of treatment, the patient not only enhanced his strength and conditioning by utilizing the Stairmaster and bicycle for 20 minutes each day but also increased his sport-specific agility by adding forward and backward running, lateral slides, and jumping rope. At this point in his recovery, I reduced his weekly visits to the clinic from the original four or five times a week to only twice a week. In addition to the exercises that Mr. Lewis performed within our clinic, he also completed several in-home exercises to help regain strength in his quadricep and calf muscles by performing three sets of 10 repetitions of both partial squats on the involved leg and calf raises to better stabilize his knee.

At this time, which is 6 months from the first time I met with Mr. Lewis, he has achieved a full recovery. Even though Mr. Lewis underwent a full functional progression back to activity to include near-normal strength, decreased swelling, full motion, excellent stability, and complete running program, I still urge him to continue his strengthening exercises while returning to his normal activities at home. In addition, I also created a specific knee-strengthening program for Mr. Lewis to decrease the possibility of further knee injuries. The patient will stand on one leg, bending the other leg behind his body, concentrating on a single stance one-third knee bend. Continuing the exercise at a steady rate for 3 minutes, working up to 5 minutes on each leg, Mr. Lewis will complete a series of flexions and extensions from approximately 30° to 80°. I also recommended to Mr. Lewis that he add specific hamstring and side-to-side exercises as a preseason and intraseason workout. This 20-minute-a-day program, concentrating on the knee musculature, will improve performance, increase strength, and diminish injuries for Mr. Lewis during ski season.

As a result of Mr. Lewis's full recovery of strength following his ACL tear, I am discharging him from my care at Erie Rehabilitation. He may return to all of his normal activities, including skiing, and wear his sports brace when participating in activities, if needed.

DESCRIPTION

When writers describe a subject or topic, they develop in their readers' minds a sense of place, the scene, a person or group, and time. Obviously, much writing for the health professions depends on this pattern, as professionals are often required to describe an incident, injury, or events leading to an injury, as in writing a report.

As established in the previous chapter, a reader wants to *see* and *feel* the scene, in order to gather the full meaning of the event or the nature or characteristics of the person, and descriptive language helps achieve this goal. However, description does not exist on its own. Rarely would a medical practitioner simply describe a person or an event. The writer must have a purpose for describing, and often, that purpose is achieved if descriptive elements are combined with other patterns of exposition.

Consider the example from the foregoing sample student essay illustrating narration. The essay tells the story of the therapist's work on a particular patient; however, the story cannot be told without describing the details of the event that caused injury or the events that took place in therapy. Consequently, the second paragraph of the text turns to a general description of therapy and the advances made. Additionally, the writer, using both narration and description, comes back to the ultimate purpose for telling the story and describing the events. In other words, the thesis statement controls the reasons for explaining such information. Examine the passage again as it is reproduced here:

After Benjamin Christopher Lewis tore his anterior cruciate ligament (ACL) while skiing at the Peak'n Peek Ski Resort on December 17, 2001, he underwent ACL reconstructive surgery by Dr. Phillip C. Carnes at St. Vincent's Hospital in Erie, Pennsylvania. Following his surgery, Mr. Lewis implemented a home rehabilitation treatment program, which not only hindered his recovery time owing to his lack of motivation in the program but also resulted in the formation of excess scar tissue within the knee joint capsule. At this time, Dr. Timothy N. Banks performed surgery to remove the scar tissue and referred him to Erie Rehabilitation. On January 8, 2002, I admitted Mr. Lewis into my care.

Most patients who have undergone ACL reconstruction demonstrate full extension and a flexion of 140° at the 3-week post-ACL surgery period; however, Mr. Lewis displayed only a 170° extension and a 140° flexion during his first visit. These impediments resulted from both the unsuccessful home treatment program and his second surgery to remove scar tissue. Despite these initial shortcomings, Mr. Lewis displayed full flexion and extension by the end of his 6-month treatment, and consequently, I am discharging Mr. Lewis at this time.

People use description as a mode of communication in everyday discussions, but medical professionals rely on it for success in their profession. Many practitioners will ask patients to tell the events that lead up to an injury (narration), but the description of the pain, the location, the sounds, and the feelings associated with it help practitioners qualify the injury. Most important, the patient's description helps practitioners clarify the specific details of the injury or illness. These feelings need to be recorded with precision. Consequently, the language used should be clear, exact, and precise in order to prevent any misunderstanding between the caregivers or between the patient and the caregivers.

The purpose for describing, however, is sometimes lost when writers communicate in the workplace. Often, a practitioner, when charting a patient's condition, will provide both objective and subjective responses to the patient's words. These need careful consideration because they can affect the purpose of the document.

Objective description reports the information without interpretation. The writer simply reproduces in words the feelings or other observable traits of the patient. Additionally, writers can also objectively describe the activities in a research project, keeping in mind that the activities must be verifiable. **Subjective description** reports the information but does so through an interpretive lens. The writer imposes his or her feelings or impressions on the event or behavior being described, and this interpretive process is often done in response to the writer's values or belief system.

For example, consider the patient who comes into the emergency department complaining of back pain. She sits comfortably on the examination table and, during the examination, describes classic symptoms of lower back pain but then asks for a specific type of drug, a narcotic, used to treat extreme pain. In the objective sense of description, the practitioner would simply record these events. In the subjective sense, the practitioner may be skeptical of the patient's condition because she sat comfortably on the table. Furthermore, the patient asks for a specific type of drug, a narcotic. These circumstances may indicate that the patient is a drug seeker and is looking for a way to find those drugs and have the insurance company pay for them. Although the objective recording of this event cannot make this assessment, the subjective description can. The practitioner can impose his or her experiences on the subject or react to a patient history. In either case, the purpose of writing is determined by the mode.

Ultimately, writers must choose the language that best represents the observations they can make, but the passages of description must serve a purpose. Remember that the reason for describing rests in making a case. Bring your reader back to that case frequently to reinforce the thesis.

Sample Student Essay
OBJECTIVE AND SUBJECTIVE DESCRIPTION

Directions: Examine the different modes of description employed in the following student essay. The ultimate purpose of the essay is to provide a critical analysis of the character's condition. Be sure that the modes contribute to the purpose. Note the narrator's position and the writer's response as well as the practitioner's response.

In the short story "The Yellow Wallpaper," by Charlotte Perkins Gilman (1899), Gilman depicts the life of a mentally ill woman. The story centers on a woman's descent into madness, which is escalated by medical influence that was supposed to have helped her. This woman's life story, from her point of view, portrays to the reader the digression of her mental illness as she struggles to become an independent individual.

Gilman describes a hysterical woman suffering from nervous depression. Her loving husband, John, who is a medical doctor, overprotects her. He took her to a summer home, away from society, for rest therapy. The narrator is placed into a room alone, and she "forbidden to work until she is well again" (Gilman, 1899, p. 1). She is encouraged to rest; she is not even allowed to write. John's dislike of the narrator's writing is demonstrated when she says, "Here comes John, and I must put this away,—he hates to have me write" (Gilman, 1899, p. 3). He believes that writing will create more stress for her. This demonstrates the structure of John's life and the control that he possesses over her. Her feelings regarding her writing are the opposite of John's. She states, "I think sometimes that if I were only well enough to write a little it would relieve the press of ideas and rest me" (Gilman, 1899, p. 4). Writing is her way of relieving stress in her life and expressing herself. She tries to rest, and to do as she is told but she continues to suffer because John does not feel that she is ill. Since he does not listen to her concerns, she feels inferior and unsure of her own sanity. John enforces the inactivity that pushes her deeper into madness and in effect causes her to rebel.

John forces her into a secluded room with no escape. This room has bars on the windows and a stationary bed nailed to the floor. She sees images of women stooping down and creeping behind the wallpaper; she cannot help but fixate on them. "The wallpaper has a kind of sub pattern in a different shade, a particularly irritating one, for you can only see it in certain lights . . . " (Gilman, 1899, p. 5). "At night in any kind of light, in twilight, candlelight, and worst of all by moonlight, it [the image] becomes bars! The outside pattern I mean, and the woman behind it is as plain as can be. By daylight she is subdued, quiet . . . " (Gilman, 1899, p. 9). This quote supports the idea that the room is increasing her insanity and forcing her to see things that are not really there. There is visibility during the daylight; therefore, she creeps around by night, and when she cannot sleep, it is more "interesting to watch the developments" (Gilman, 1899, p. 10). While she is in the room, her developing insanity is a form of rebellion and a way for her to gain her own independence.

Later in the story, she locks herself in her room, and notices a "very funny mark on the wall, . . . near the mopboard" (Gilman, 1899, p. 11). She rapidly crawls around the room on her hands and knees following the streak. This action she performs shows that she has taken the images and marks on the wallpaper to a deeper level of insanity, and it is mentally disturbing her. She sees the same woman creeping in the paper during the daytime. She can relate to daylight creeping because she does the same thing so that John does not get suspicious, and this is also why her door is locked at night. She acts out wildly, " . . . I wasn't alone a bit! As soon as it was moonlight and that poor thing began to crawl and shake the pattern, I got up and ran to help her. I pulled and she shook, I shook and she pulled, and before morning we had peeled off yards of that paper" (Gilman, 1899, p. 13). This amplifies the violent anger that accompanies the narrator's fight to free herself both from her husband and her room. She believes the wallpaper is strangling her, restraining her from freedom.

She creeps and crawls around her room. In the final scene, John is shocked by the woman's actions and he faints. The narrator creeps over him, saying, "I've got out at last . . . in spite of you and Jane. And I've pulled off most of the paper, so you can't put me back" (Gilman, 1899, p. 15). This comment illustrates her attainment of complete insanity. She does not appear to be concerned that she has crawled over her husband, and achieved her independence from her submission to John.

Gilman demonstrates the woman's digression into insanity throughout the story. The story begins with long descriptive paragraphs in which the narrator was disturbed about losing her baby and not being able to write. By the end, the paragraphs and thoughts become shorter because the mentally ill woman is unable to speak coherently. The rest cure, involving the removal of stimulation and socialization from her life, with time, becomes unbearable for her. She was incapable of coping with the environment in which she was living; therefore, she rebelled.

The woman found the loss of her baby and the strict ways of her husband to be too overpowering. Once she was put into the room, her mental state only became worse, as the actions she demonstrated were signs of her regression. The yellow wallpaper and the images the narrator sees in the paper maddened her. Once she rips down the paper, she achieves her independence; nobody could control her, and she was not dependent on others for survival. The narrator gains her independence, but in return, she trades her sanity.

PROCESS ANALYSIS

If you have ever explained how to assemble a toy or machine or if you ever explained to someone how something works, you have engaged in a *process analysis*. A process analysis can be the simple writing of directions, like a recipe, or it can be a series of explanations that demonstrate the complexities of an operation, such as the description of how to solve mathematical equations or the explanation of cell respiration. In each of these instances, the writer is aware of the audience's need for structure. For every process analysis, the structure is sequential: The process is a series of steps that takes the reader to an expected goal or outcome. Process analyses have two forms: directional and informational.

The **directional process analysis**, like a recipe, explains to the reader how to perform a series of tasks or an activity. In this form, the sequence of events is vital to the success of the instructions and the document. If the reader fails to follow the set procedure, the goal will not be achieved. For example, if you explain the process of brushing your teeth, you cannot instruct the reader to insert the toothbrush into the mouth if he or she has not filled the brush with toothpaste. At the professional level, the writing of directional processes is often vital to the functioning of the office or the performance of the appropriate treatments. In the office, certain procedures and protocol must be followed for charting information, filling out paperwork, or even caring for equipment. These processes are not always evident to employees, and a simple directional process document can save time and money. Likewise, the performance of a certain treatment modality follows a certain procedure. For example, for suturing a wound, you cleanse, prepare, and drape the area in sterile fashion; inject the wound site with anesthetic; close the wound site with six vertical sutures; and apply antibiotic cream and dressing. You cannot begin suturing without preparing the area or anesthetizing; the procedures follow a sequence that must be met for reasons of safety and consistency of practice.

The **informational process analysis** provides information that explains how something works or how certain functions are accomplished. Unlike the directional form, which asks readers to follow instructions, the informational form asks readers to examine the reasons underlying the process to promote their understanding of the process, often with practical applications. For example, patients in rehabilitative medicine often complain of radicular symptoms, or nerve-related problems, such as numbness, weakness, or tingling electric pain. Rehabilitation specialists who treat such problems want the patient to understand the process that produces the pain. For instance, the patient may be suffering from a disk herniation. In this event, a disk compresses one of the large spinal nerves, which causes irritation and inflammation of that nerve. That large nerve branches into smaller nerves that feed the patient's extremities. The pain at the larger nerve extends to the smaller nerves at the periphery, such as lower extremities, or legs and feet. Thus, the damage to the large nerve at the spine affects the nerves at the periphery and manifests itself as the tingling pain about which the patient complains. With appropriate information, the patient will understand that the treatment procedure to follow is not one that directly treats the legs and feet, where the pain occurs. Instead, the practitioner's treatment will focus on the back.

Organizing the Steps

In writing directional process analyses, the sequence of the steps is essential to the success of the activity. Consequently, the steps should be carefully presented to clearly dictate that order. To help organize information, writers often use typographical conventions to indicate this pattern: **numbers** and **bullets** to form lists and **headings** to separate tasks within the procedure. Not only do these conventions help the reader organize the steps in sequence, but the separation of this information from the "wall of words" in the explanatory sections draws attention to them and gives them importance. Listing information vertically, instead of horizontally, creates space around the lists and headings, which ultimately serves as a sign of significance.

Numbers are used to indicate order. If the process depends on the exact sequence of events, such as directions, your reader should be alerted to this demand. Such order is signified with the use of numbers. Think about the sets of directions you receive with new products that require assembly. Each element of assembly is divided into a sequence that must be followed. These are listed as numbers, not letters. Additionally, the style manual of the APA and other style manuals dictate specific formats to be followed. Most, however, follow a standard format:

1. Indent five spaces or one strike of the tab key.
2. Type the numeral.
3. Skip two spaces, and then begin typing.

Note: If the words in the list create full sentences, then use a period at the end of each. If the words are fragments or single words, use no terminal mark of punctuation. Also, if the sentence leading to the list is a complete sentence, use a colon to introduce the list. If the words preceding the list do not compose a sentence, use no mark of punctuation before the list (or at the end of the lead). If the words in the list complete the sentence that was started, use a period after the last element in the list to end the sentence.

If the process requires no order, use bullets. For example, instructions often specify materials to be used, and these may be presented to the reader in list form. If use of the items requires no specific sequence or order, use bullets—for example:

Go to the hardware store and purchase
- one hammer
- two circular saws
- two boxes of nails.

The order in which these are purchased is inconsequential to the procedure. Therefore, bullets are used instead of numbers. The rules of sentence creation and punctuation apply here as well.

Finally, many writers compartmentalize information by using headings. The APA style manual provides specific instructions for developing headings, as most manuals do, but some common sense can be applied here to create your own system if one is not provided.

Headings not only divide information but also indicate importance. Primary headings are usually centered, with all the letters of every word capitalized. Secondary headings may be centered, but usually only the first word and all important words are capitalized. Tertiary headings are usually aligned on the left margin and capitalized according to sentence-style form, meaning that only the first word and any proper nouns are capitalized. Other headings that follow will most likely be indented five spaces and underlined, also with sentence-style format. These are standard heading formats used in a variety of writing environments because they help readers identify major sections of the text or changes to the sequence of an order. Headings that are centered and/or capitalized are more important to the organizational structure than are headings positioned on the left margin.

Although most people use headings as signposts, they often fail to recognize that readers will expect consistency in their use. For example, headings should not appear at the bottom of the page unless at least two lines of text accompany the heading. Also, there should be at least two headings of any specific level—for example, a paper that has one secondary heading should also include at least one other secondary heading. This assures the reader that the organizational structure is developed with some depth.

When creating headings, be sure that each heading is accompanied by text. No heading should exist stacked on top of another. If this happens, the organizational structure should be revised. Finally, if a single-word heading is used, do not start the first sentence of the text with the word *This*. Headings are markers, not part of the text. Your reader will scan the page for information, but the writer should not assume that the reader will recognize that the pronoun's antecedent is the heading.

Finally, in constructing headings or lists, the elements of each entry must be parallel in structure to those like it. When explaining the order without the use of headings and lists, or within the text, indicate shifts or new procedures or tasks by providing transitional words and phrases.

Sample Student Essay
PROCESS ANALYSIS

Directions: Not all essays are entirely written in one mode. Examine the progress report below and highlight the passages that use the process analysis technique. Notice also the student's use of a list and a table to manage information.

Michael Geigger was seen 3 days a week as recommended by the physical therapist. He attended physical therapy from March 22, 2000, to April 17, 2000, for a total of 12 sessions, and he missed zero appointments. His consistent attendance assisted in the exceptional rehabilitation of his left shoulder. The girth measurement of the patient's shoulder at the time of initial evaluation was 46 centimeters, and his present girth measurement is 49 centimeters. The skilled care provided by the physical therapist influenced the increase in the patient's girth measurement; the strengthening exercises increased the muscle capacity of the patient's shoulder. The strengthening of the patient's shoulder diminished the acute aching that he sensed in his shoulder. In the initial evaluation, the patient sensed acute pain when he reached back, up above his shoulder, or to the right and left side with weight over 15 pounds; currently, he can reach above his head with a maximum of 20 pounds without pain. The continuation of skilled care will persist to reduce the acute pain and increase the girth measurement in his left shoulder.

The controlled exercises assigned by the therapist facilitated improvements in the patient's posture and resulted in an increase in the range of motion (ROM) of his left shoulder. On March 22, 2000, the physical therapist recorded the ROM of the patient in the supine position:

Measurements of patient's left shoulder	Measurements at the March 22, 2000, session	Measurements at the April 17, 2000, session
Flexion, active	116°	150°
Flexion, passive	130°	160°
Abduction, active	70°	71°
Abduction, passive	72°	78°
Internal rotation	45°	48°
External rotation	20°	26°

The patient reports that he continues to sense a dull pain in his deltoid muscle, resulting in an inability to complete the exercises assigned by the physical therapist. The patient's active and passive ROM have not improved as stated in the goals established in the initial evaluation; therefore, the continuation of physical therapy in a controlled setting is necessary to assist in complete rehabilitation of the left shoulder.

The patient demonstrates functional strength within his available range. The strengthening of his muscles also assisted in the improvement of his ROM. The therapist instructed the patient to use the upper body exercise machine (UBE) for 10 slow repetitions, to perform 25 repetitions of pulleys, to complete 10 repetitions of wall ladders, and to complete upper body rows for 10 minutes. Initially, the patient received a 2 out of a possible 5 on the strength examination because of his inability to move actively through his full range of motion; currently, he receives a 4/5. Previously, he was unable to lift a 4-pound weight, recording the level of pain as a 2/5. The patient demonstrates the ability to lift 15 pounds with his left shoulder; the pain level is a 1/5. The increase in motion range and the ability to lift an increasing amount of weight, when compared with findings on the initial evaluation, enables him to perform his necessary activities of daily living (ADL). With the professional assistance from a physical therapist, the patient will continue to regain his ROM, strength, and functional use.

The mobility and strength of the patient has increased; therefore, he is able to return to work lifting objects with a maximum weight of 15 pounds above his waist no more than 40 times a day. The continuation of skilled care will enable the patient to remain at work and continue to increase the amount of weight he is capable of lifting. The persistence of skilled care will improve the functional abilities, the ROM, the level of pain, and the strength of the patient's left shoulder. With continued treatment provided by the physical therapist, the patient will gain up to 95% of his initial ROM and 100% of his functional use. In a controlled setting, the skilled physical therapist supervises the activities performed by the patient to ensure that the strengthening and training are completed properly and to assist him when necessary. Such supervised training also provides instruction that aids the patient in the performance of exercises at home.

The physical therapist performs the following actions to aid in the rehabilitation of the patient's left shoulder. I apply moist heat and phonophoresis for 10 minutes at 0.4 watt per square centimeter; these modalities relax the deltoid muscle, resulting in a reduction of pain and an increase of the ROM. The patient proceeds in the plan of treatment by making use of clinical equipment to strengthen the upper body. The patient utilizes overhead pulleys to strengthen and increase the functional use of his left shoulder. The supervision of skilled care during this plan of treatment ensures that the tasks are properly acted out, which will reduce the risk of further injury.

The current problems of the patient, which have affected his life at home and at work, are the same as stated in the initial evaluation but less severe. The following are the patient's problems that continue to require attention:

- decreased mobility in the left shoulder
- decreased strength of left shoulder
- decreased functional use of left shoulder.

Controlled care, three times per week, will aid the patient increasing mobility, strength, and functional use. The sessions must continue for 2 additional weeks to ensure complete recovery from his accident. The patient must repeat the sessions, which the physical therapist instructs, three times per week to ensure proper healing. The physical therapist supervises the assigned exercises to guarantee that tasks are done correctly and to the patient's fullest potential. Thorough supervision by the therapist and dedication by the patient ensure proper healing in the shortest possible time period.

With the previous standard for care established by the physical therapist, I have developed a plan for future treatment. After intensive therapy in the controlled facility, the physical therapist will instruct the patient to perform arm lifts at home, initially with no weight and gradually increasing the weight to 10 pounds. The patient will perform small arm lifts, gradually increasing the range, until he has the ability to lift his arm parallel to the floor. The patient will complete the second exer-

cise, arm circles, as for the arm lifts, increasing the weights and the size of the circles gradually. The physical therapist will encourage the patient to visit a local gym and/or aquatic facility to receive the maximum benefit from rehabilitation. The explicit instructions as stated will increase the patient's ROM and strength of the left shoulder.

The patient's improved functional use depends upon the continuation of skilled care to assist in the strengthening of the left shoulder. The therapist instructs the patient, as well as the family of the patient, to perform the instructed exercises, which continuously strengthen the left shoulder and prevent future injury.

The short-term goals of the patient, as stated in the initial evaluation, were to improve his mobility by at least 10° in his ROM; this goal was met on April 7, 2000. The new goal is to improve his ROM by an additional 15° by April 30, 2000. The pain in his shoulder has been reduced by 75% with the 2-week time period. Consequently, with this progress, the patient's functional mobility will return to the minimum of 160° of flexion and abduction, allowing the patient to reach over his head with no pain by May 15, 2000, instead of the original goal of June 1, 2000. The patient has the potential to regain 95% of his original range of motion after the completion of the three remaining physical therapy sessions. He will return to work by May 1, 2000, with no restrictions, and perform everyday tasks such as dressing himself and brushing his teeth without pain. His rehabilitation potential is exceptional.

CLASSIFICATION AND DIVISION

Scientists and health professionals often use systems of classification and division to help them make sense of their complicated worlds. **Classification** allows a writer to organize information into convenient categories, while **division** identifies the parts of the whole subject and defines how each part contributes to the function of the whole.

Classification, as a pattern of exposition, sorts complex information into manageable forms. For example, all scientists are familiar with the taxonomic system of classification for all living things. Scientists use several types of phyla to define the different groups in the animal kingdom. The system of classification becomes more specific as we analyze order, genus, and species. Many health care providers will use classification in patient education literature such as manuals about ways to improve cardiovascular health, ways to maintain flexibility, kinds of arthritis, or types of food to eat for a healthy diet. Although classification in these examples is a means to manage complex or overwhelming amounts of information, classification also can be used to define and sort as few as two types in the same system. Consider the use of classification in the following student essay.

Sample Student Essay
CLASSIFICATION

Types of Hip Replacement Methods

In the past 10 years, total hip arthroplasty has become more common. As techniques and technology improve, doctors can provide more patients with better prostheses to accommodate their active lifestyles. Also, new components used for re-creating the hip joint are more effective, allowing younger, active people to return to their active lifestyles. In response to some of these advancements, researchers have begun to study the two types of prostheses—cemented acetabular and cementless acetabular fixation—used in replacing the hip joint, to determine the advantages of using the cementless method.

In the past, the dominant prosthesis technique used was cemented acetabular fixation, but this method reduced the range of motion in the joint after surgery and prevented patients from performing many of the tasks they executed before surgery. In the cemented method, the joint is fused together, causing stiffness and rigidity and inhibiting motion in the limb; however, the cementless method allows the joint to be free moving, and the only fixed position is in the acetabulum of the pelvis, which provides patients with a larger range of motion than would be provided with the cemented prosthesis.

Unlike classification, which categorizes various entities into manageable groups, division breaks down one entity and discusses the relationship of the parts to the whole. For example, when we discuss the writing process, we break up the complex process into its component

parts: prewriting, writing, revising, rewriting, editing, and proofreading. The success of the final product depends on how well each of these components works within the system, which is the result of the writer's commitment to engaging each of the phases in a deliberate manner. The process of using division as pattern of organization depends on your need to examine the component parts of a particular subject.

In the sample student essay used to demonstrate classification, the student discussed two types of hip replacement procedures. In the following example, she divides one of the categories into a discussion of its component parts to demonstrate its effectiveness:

Sample Student Essay
DIVISION

In almost all of the research conducted, scientists compared the use of cemented and cementless acetabular components and concluded that the cementless component supplied patients with the greatest amount of relief. In any hip replacement procedure, three components determine its success: bone growth, reduced amount of aseptic loosening, and reduction of pain. The cementless procedure provides all three components.

In studies conducted by Whaley, Berry, and Harmsen (2001), the cementless procedure supplied patients with the greatest amount of bone ingrowth. One of the advantageous qualities of the cementless procedure is the ability for the vital bone in the patient's femur to grow into the prosthesis. Researchers found that the ability of the bone to grow into the component provides further fixation; therefore, patients experience less aseptic loosening, which ultimately results in no need to cement the acetabular component into the femur and hipbone. With any invasive procedure, patients can experience varying degrees of postoperative pain; however, total hip replacement surgery can cause patients pain for years following the surgery and has left some bedridden. Grubl and colleagues (2002) examined 123 patients after surgery and for 10 years following. They reported no hip pain from 106 patients of the cementless component implementation, and only 4 complained of moderate pain. Consequently, the cementless procedure allows for bone growth and reduced aseptic loosening and reduces pain.

To differentiate between classification and division, use the following rule: You will use classification to indicate *types*; you will use division to indicate *components*. Your purpose in writing will dictate the system of organization you use.

COMPARISON AND CONTRAST

By bringing together two subjects, we can explore their similarities and differences to better understand them. For example, a patient presents a variety of symptoms. To rule out one diagnosis over another, the practitioner may need to demonstrate how the symptoms may appear to be due to one disorder but in reality may reflect an entirely different disorder that requires a different approach to treatment.

Writers often compare and contrast subjects to determine ways in which they are different or similar. Such a technique helps a reader in two ways: In one approach, a comparison/contrast essay may help a reader solidify definitions of the subjects. For example, some people may not understand the difference between chiropractors and physical therapists. Consequently, a comparison/contrast of the two professions will help define the scope of practice of each. In another approach, a comparison/contrast essay allows demonstration of the merits of one subject relative to another, to help a reader make a choice or decision between the two. For example, a comparison/contrast essay may be used to highlight advantages of one type of therapy over another, as was the case in the previous essay about the cemented and cementless approaches to hip replacement. The example was used to explain a definition organizational strategy, but the ultimate purpose of the essay was to determine that cementless replacements are more effective than cemented replacements.

Ultimately, a comparison/contrast pattern of writing helps readers distinguish between two subjects for identification purposes, or it is used to show that one subject is preferable to another.

Be sure that your reader knows your purpose when you begin the essay.

When analyzing the subjects, approach them in one of two strategies to provide a clear organizational structure to the essay: topical or categorical. In the **topical approach**, write about one subject in its entirety first; then discuss the same principles as they appear in the other. In short analyses or papers, this works best. For example, if you are considering the choice between one type of stapler to buy for the office versus another, you can highlight the strengths and weaknesses in short paragraphs because staplers do not have complex sets of features to compare. In the **categorical approach**, divide the essay into the categories of analysis first; then compare both subjects within the framework of each category. For example, if you are comparing political candidates, you may want to itemize the issues that interest you, such as character, commitment to health care issues, and economic principles. With these category sets, address each political candidate's position on the issues, and develop your paragraphs around these topics.

Sample Student Essay
COMPARISON AND CONTRAST

During the past four years, the American Physical Therapy Association (APTA) and the American Chiropractic Association (ACA) have fought in court to determine who can manually manipulate a patient's spine to repair a subluxation, a partial separation of the articular surface of a joint. Physical therapists use manual manipulations, and insurance companies reimburse them for their services. Chiropractors argue that insurance companies unjustly repay therapists for this service because manipulation is not a legal service that physical therapists can provide, as stated in the law. The scope of practice of each profession needs clarification to determine the principles of this issue.

According to the Social Security Amendment in 1972, Medicare providers included chiropractic services as a physician's service (McAndrews, 2000). This document also included provisions requiring chiropractors to earn a state license, setting standards for practicing physicians, and establishing rules for treating patients by means of manual manipulation only (McAndrews, 2000).

The amendment states that physical therapists may utilize manipulation techniques if they use a nonspecific force and no momentum to redirect the vertebrae into the center of the patient's anatomy (McAndrews, 2000). The nonspecific force terminology means that therapists cannot direct the vertebrae into a specific position, but they can manipulate the tissues surrounding the bone for realignment. Therapists cannot use any type of momentum when manipulating a patient because forceful manipulation is a chiropractic service.

By definition, subluxations interfere with the transmission of nerve impulses, which create pain and contribute to weakened states of health (Bruno, 1999). Manual manipulation is a method to correct the problem. Chiropractors believe that realignment of the vertebrae in the spine contributes to the health and wellness of the patient. Physical therapists use manipulation to alleviate pain, but they do not believe that the spine controls the body and allows the body to naturally heal itself.

The APTA uses the argument that physical therapists are authorized, under their licensure, to manipulate the spine and that Medicare did not interpret the statute correctly because the definition of a subluxation is unclear. The position taken by the APTA is that therapists can provide manual manipulation of the spine to repair a subluxation because they believe that manual manipulation and manipulations of the spine are synonymous. However, chiropractic professionals believe that therapists charge for a service they cannot legally provide. Supporters of the ACA agree that the laws in place sufficiently state the difference between chiropractic manipulation and physical therapy manipulations. The applied technique and the desired outcome determine the difference. Additionally, chiropractors can refer patients to other medical professionals for additional testing and x-rays. Therapists may suggest to their patients that they seek other treatment, but they do not possess the independence of the chiropractor when outsourcing patient treatments.

The difference in their practices is determined by their education. Therapists, although educated in treating the spine, are educated in treating the soft tissue and joint manipulation techniques, not the manipulation of the vertebrae. Chiropractors are trained to manipulate the vertebrae of the spine for overall health and wellness.

Although chiropractors and physical therapists manipulate patients and receive reimbursement for their services in different ways, laws prohibit manual manipulation by the use of force by thera-pists to correct a subluxation of the spine. All states restrict therapists from repairing the spine and authorize manual manipulation treatment for licensed chiropractors.

References

Bruno, L. (1999). *Chiropractic.* Gale Encyclopedia of Medicine (1st ed.). Retrieved April 3, 2002, from Health Reference Center Academic Database.

McAndrews, G. P. (2000). Opposition to APTA's motion. Retrieved March 1, 2002, from *American Chiropractic Association Today Online:* www.acatoday.com

CAUSE AND EFFECT

Scientists spend their careers asking why certain things happen. For example, when a patient presents a list of symptoms, the practitioner asks, "Why does this happen?" and seeks the answer to this question. The answer, obviously, is the reason for the occurrence of the symptoms. When practitioners of any kind seek the reasons to explain a set of events, they are searching for *causes*. Causes explain the occurrence of effects. For example, if a patient complains of pain in her knee (the effect), a health care professional seeks to know if the patient has experienced trauma to the area or if the pain has developed chronically. When the patient responds, the causes are evident and the health care professional can now treat the causes to eliminate the effect.

Consider another example concerning behavior. In the college experience, some first-year students cannot leave their dorm room without making it neat and orderly, whereas at home, they are sloppy and their rooms are always a mess. Why does this happen? Some theories of human behavior explain that people who feel a sense of disorder in their lives will attempt to impose an order by organizing their possessions. This theory of human behavior explains the effect by describing causes.

Issues of causation are written about frequently in the medical and allied health professions. Often, a practitioner will discuss a current problem and attempt to articulate what has caused it. In other words, this pattern focuses on why an event happened. For example, a patient who develops a sore joint over time may look back to several events or circumstances that may have contributed to the problem. Conversely, the effect can be seen in the future as a writer examines present issues and determines that changes will be effected in the future. For example, if physical therapists are afforded reimbursement for patients who seek treatment from them without a referral (direct access), the future of the profession will be altered dramatically.

Ultimately, the cause-and-effect organizational pattern can work in various directions or be **bidirectional**. A writer may find an event and explain the causes of the event, or a writer may find an event and discuss the effects of that event on the future. For example, gambling is a topic of much scientific research. In a cause-and-effect essay, a writer could establish gambling as the effect and then explain the causes of gambling. If explaining the consequence of an event, a writer uses an "if . . . , then . . . " development scheme. However, gambling as a topic does not have to be the effect; it can also be the cause. For example, a writer could explore the effects of gambling addiction on family, finances, education, or personal relationships. In this pattern, the writer is predicting the future by relying on probability. Often, a word or phrase from the following list accompanies this pattern:

arises from	may	probable
stems from	might	possible
is produced by		

Other Cause-and-Effect Devices

In the previous examples, the focus of the essay is purposely reduced to an answerable question. Writers should do the same when gathering information and developing the essay. However, using questions in your final draft is not appropriate in the formal writing environment. For example, many writers may be inclined, in error, to use the question as a means to deliver the thesis statement, as in the following example:

With the development of casinos across New York State and with the popularity of the state lottery system, many people have reported problems with gambling, and treatment centers for addictions have reported a double-digit rise in gambling cases at their facilities. Gambling is a topic of much scientific research, but why does it occur? What leads a person to mismanage money to support a game?

In this example, the focus of the essay rests on a question. The purpose of any essay should be to answer questions, not impose them. Consider also that a question should elicit a response. Expecting your reader to answer out loud or write the answer in the margin is thoughtless. Some writers, however, defend the act of asking questions by posing them as rhetorical questions. If the question has an obvious answer, the writer should, most likely, not ask it, or the writer should mold the question into a simple statement. Ultimately, asking questions in professional writing is sophomoric and detracts from the purpose of the essay: to give answers.

Another Way of Looking at the Cause-and-Effect Essay: Problem Solving/Solution Seeking

Practitioners' jobs often include problem solving and solution seeking. They identify and clarify the problem and then propose and implement various solutions. For example, patients may complain that they are not receiving the appropriate feedback from the practitioner; the practitioner attempts to find a way to open the communication path. Also, patients are often in need of basic physical fitness. The practitioner can explain to them how to meet that need by setting up a plan.

Errors in Reasoning in the Cause-and-Effect Essay

Writers of cause and effect can fall into problems in reasoning that may skew the results of the information provided in a document. Obviously, we can never be sure that a **one-to-one correspondence** is at work in our discussion.

For example, we may conclude that gambling is caused by displaced feelings of inadequacy. Several cases may indicate that people with gambling problems have low self-esteem, but these cases cannot possibly indicate that low self-esteem is the *only* cause of gambling. Many other factors can influence a person's behavior. Low self-esteem may be one of several causes, and this issue must be made clear to the reader.

In addition to ignoring multiple causes, a writer may also fail to reason accurately by confusing the results of chronological events. For example, in a recently published article about the effects of prayer on healing, the author pointed to several cases in which the patients recovered after a group of people engaged in thoughtful prayer for the patients' recovery. However, simply because people recover from illnesses after others have prayed on their behalf does not mean that the prayer was the deciding factor in their wellness. Determining that the chronology of events signals the causes is a mistake in reasoning. Indeed, prayer may be the cause for their recovery, but if prayer does cause healing, it cannot be proved. Consider the following sample student essays:

Sample Student Essay
UNVEILING THE FALLACY OF CHRONOLOGY IN CAUSE AND EFFECT

The mind is a strong element used in the road to recovery after an illness or physical problem. Even though the mind is an amazing tool used during healing, it is not the cure-all answer to all the problems in the human body. In addition to other medical rehabilitation and treatments, alternative medicine forms such as prayer, meditation, herbal treatments, and massage therapy may aid in the restoration of one's well-being, but these alternative medicine forms, on their own, cannot completely heal medical problems. Instead, the mind works with the body to heal.

Intercessory prayer is a technique in which an outside person prays for the health and well-being of another who is ill. The effectiveness of this alternative medicine form is questionable. In Randolph C. Byrd's 1988 study, the control group "required ventilatory assistance, antibiotics, and diuretics more frequently than patients in the IP [intercessory prayer] group," and therefore, Byrd concluded that intercessory prayer is a beneficial technique that should be used in the curative process (Murphy, 2001). Murphy countered these findings stating that Byrd's study was not complete and questioned, "How does one interpret the fact that many people in the IP groups didn't show any improvement at all?" (Murphy, 2001). In other words, if intercessory prayer is reportedly beneficial, then everyone should experience improved health, which is not the case in Byrd's study. Murphy states, "Personal prayer can be a healthful activity," but it should not be the only form of treatment that should be administered to a patient (Murphy, 2001). Murphy references the 1965 study by C. R. B. Joyce and R. M. C. Welldone, who discovered no real clear pattern between the hospitalized patients who were prayed for and those who were not. However, even though intercessory prayer has not been proved to be 100% effective in recovery efforts, it should not be eliminated entirely in the improvement process. Instead, intercessory prayer should be used hand in hand with other medical techniques. Because prayer is an extremely powerful device, it is also involved in the placebo effect. If a patient knows that others are praying for him to get well, he will have a firm faith that God will come through for him and aid in his recovery. With this thought, the patient becomes more positive in his outlook, and his condition may even start to improve, allowing the patient to believe that his recovery is the direct result of the prayers.

Both massage therapy and meditation are two other forms of alternative medicine. Meditation, for example, is a calming mental exercise that is proved to help reduce stress, tension, panic, and anxiety. Besides these soothing effects, meditation is also a scientifically verified way to relieve chronic pain and reduce high blood pressure and may even be helpful for both headaches and respiratory problems, including asthma. Like meditation, massage therapy also provides relief from the symptoms of anxiety, stress, insomnia, depression, and tension as well as headaches, muscle pain, and back pain, but is not capable of curing any serious or life-threatening medical disorders. Just as prayer allegedly does, meditation and massage both help to alleviate some of the other factors that are related to the illness but do not eliminate the underlying cause. Once these factors or symptoms are eliminated by the alternative medicine mind-relaxation techniques, the patient, his body, and medical practitioners can all work together to cure the primary root of the problem.

Because the mind and body work so closely together, both forms of treatment are more effective if practiced together.

Herbal remedies, which have become quite popular in the last decade, are one final form of alternative medicine that act on the placebo effect and do not necessarily give promising results. In fact, British alternative medicine researcher Dr. Edzard Ernst conducted a study in which he tested *Gingko biloba*, St. John's wort, *Echinacea*, ginseng, and several other herbs that constitute over $590 million in sales annually in the United States alone (Bouchez, 2002). After carrying out 16 well-conducted clinical trials, Ernst found no support that ginseng is an effective way to treat any condition (Bouchez, 2002). In actuality, his research indicated many potential side effects including insomnia, severe headaches, hypertension, nausea, and diarrhea. Despite these findings, people still continue to utilize these herbs. These sustained actions have to do with the placebo effect. People who take herbs are convinced that these herbs, such as ginseng, have life-altering effects that can help promote a healthy lifestyle. Believing what the labels and advertisements say, their minds believe it to be true and trick their body into thinking the same. Like the other forms of alternative medicines, however, these herbs do not remove the underlying cause of a person's illness.

In times of illness or physical distress, the mind tends to take over and makes the body believe something that may not actually be true. For this, the mind is truly a magnificent instrument used on the road to wellness. However, the emphasis that the mind is the main healing factor is false. While it is true that practices such as prayer and herbs improve the mind and relieve other symptoms of an illness, they do not make a bone mend any faster or make rheumatoid arthritis disappear. Instead, medical intervention is needed to yield successful recoveries in these examples. If both the mind and medical involvement are intertwined, however, the healing process will occur at a more rapid pace.

References

Bouchez, C. (2002, January 4). Some herbs don't deliver on promises. Retrieved January 23, 2002, from http://dailynews.yahoo.com/h/hsn/20020104/hl/some_herbo_don_t_deliver_on_promises_1.html

Murphy, C. (2001). Intercessory prayer. Retrieved January 23, 2002, from www.theatlantic.com

Sample Student Essay
CAUSE AND EFFECT

INTRODUCTION

Medical records reveal that, throughout history, as many as 300 million people worldwide suffered from the disease known as lymphedema (Wozniewski, Jasinski, Pilch, & Dabrowska, 2001). Nonstandardized care for lymphedema results in a variety of treatment options: manual lymphatic drainage (MLD), skin care, exercises, compression pump, multilayer bandaging, compression garments, pneumatic compression, elevation, laser treatment, pharmacological management, psychosocial support, and surgical treatment. Caregivers alter the treatment based on the individual's needs and personal preferences, but most therapy programs include MLD, exercise, and compression produced by bandages, garments, or sleeves. Physical therapists all over the world employ these same treatments, which, supported with adequate research, should become standard protocol.

The lymphatic system, a network of lymphatic vessels, lymph, lymphoid tissues, and lymphoid organs, functions to maintain normal blood volume by transporting lymph from peripheral tissues to the circulatory system (Silverthorn, 2001). A patient may experience improper reabsorption of lymph from the tissues, which causes a dysfunction in capillary-lymph exchange, leading to edema (Silverthorn, 2001). The presence of parasites or cancer, the growth of fibrotic tissue, or the removal of lymph nodes, often a result of cancer treatment, leads to a decrease in the flow of lymph, which may also cause edema (Silverthorn, 2001).

The medical community arranged lymphedema into two classes: primary and secondary (Gillham, 1994). A person diagnosed with primary lymphedema, a result of a genetic abnormality, may lack sufficient valves in the lymphatic vessels or may possess vessels either too large or small for the existing valves (Gillham, 1994; Reynolds, 1996). Unlike primary lymphedema, secondary lymphedema derives from the removal of lymph nodes and vessels, infection, paralysis or immobilization, scars or burns from surgery, or other diseases (Buren & Linton, 2000; Reynolds, 1996).

To determine the effectiveness of complex decongestive therapy, which includes MLD, bandaging or garments, exercises, and a compression pump, Lydia Gillham completed a case study titled "Lymphoedema and physiotherapists: Control not cure." Physicians diagnosed Mrs. Smith, a 51-year-old woman, with primary lymphedema of both legs and mild secondary lymphedema of the arm. Using a weighted measuring tape and a pre-programmed computer, Gillhan plotted a graph of clinical measurements, and she estimated retention of 11 pints of excess fluid in Smith's legs. Smith's treatments consisted of massage, multilayered graduated compression bandaging left on for 24 hours, exercises, compression pump applied for 2 hours every visit, and skin care. After 2 weeks of this intense treatment regimen, a graph of new measurements revealed a loss of 3½ pints of fluid from Smith's left leg and 4½ pints from her right leg.

Weiss conducted a study titled "Treatment of leg edema and wounds in a patient with musculoskeletal injuries." Following an injury and several surgical procedures, the patient developed edema of the lower limb and two sores and required physical therapy. The patient participated in a therapy program consisting of MLD, compressive bandages, exercise, and skin care. Throughout the 7 weeks of therapy, 89% of the patient's wounds healed, and the edema in the leg decreased by 74%.

Determining the efficiency of the complex physical therapy method in treating patients with lymphedema of the extremities, Wozniewski et al. (2001) conducted a study titled "Complex physical therapy for lymphedema of the limbs." Complex physical therapy consists of intermittent pneumatic compression, exercises, and MLD. The study comprised 208 women between the ages of 17 and 83 years of age; 188 had lymphedema of the upper limb and 20 had lymphedema of the lower limb. Completing calculations both before and after complex physical therapy allowed Wozniewski et al. to determine the decrease in lymph volume in the limbs of the affected individuals. Lymphedema resolved completely in the upper extremity of 32 patients, in the lower extremity of 4 patients with primary lymphedema, and in the lower extremity of 4 patients with secondary lymphedema. Wozniewski et al. calculated an average decrease of 43% in patients with slight edema, 33% in those with moderate edema, and 19% in individuals with severe edema.

No surgical or conservative methods currently available possess the capability of curing lymphedema. Health care professionals caring for patients with lymphedema must accept the inability to treat the disease and instead try to control the effects of lymphedema (Gillham, 1994). In the

past, medical professions refused to treat lymphedema, but now the debilitating disease gains more attention than ever from physical therapists (Reynolds, 1996). The unavailability of continuing education programs encompassing lymphedema prohibited interested physical therapists from attaining the necessary information for deliverance of treatment (Reynolds, 1996). Leading them to seek out new treatment options, physical therapists found that traditional methods produced unsatisfactory results (Reynolds, 1996). Abandoning these traditional techniques, such as the compression pump and elevation, therapists develop new treatment programs that often include MLD, exercise, and compression (Reynolds, 1996).

The decline in skin elasticity, range of motion, and overall mobility resulting from edema necessitates the inclusion of exercise in the treatment plan (Reynolds, 1996). In the treatment of lymphedema, the use of exercise assists patients by producing enhanced lymph movement, muscle contraction, and deep breathing (Gillham, 1994). Activating the venous and lymphatic pumps, muscle activity contributes to the drainage of excess fluid from the tissues (Gillham, 1994). Exercising patients require careful supervision because an increase in vasodilation, heart rate, and temperature, due to excessive exercise, escalates lymph production (Buren & Linton, 2000).

Use of compression bandages, garments, and sleeves during the exercise period maintains the progress made during the program period (Gillham, 1994). Patients wear compression garments and sleeves, as in intermittent pneumatic compression, to prevent the return of fluid to the limb (Gillham, 1994). Low-stretch bandages, applied with padding, create low pressure during rest, which provides comfort, and high pressure during activity, which improves the function of deep vessels.

To maintain the effects of the various treatments such as MLD, physical therapists fit patients with compression garments. Applied in conjunction with other techniques, MLD, a type of gentle massage, directs lymphatic fluid away from damaged vessels and into healthy axilla (Gillham, 1994). The massage creates an augmentation in the uptake of lymph in superficial lymphatic vessels (Gillham, 1994).

Apart from the care provided by physical therapists and other health care professionals, physical therapists advise lymphedema sufferers on the importance of proper skin care. Patients dealing with lymphedema may experience transformations in the skin and underlying tissues due to the abundance of protein found in lymph fluid (Gillham, 1994). To reduce the threat of infection, affected persons must adequately care for their skin. Physicians may recommend the use of nonallergenic soaps and moisturizers (Gillham, 1994). Daily moisturizing and wearing protective clothing, such as gloves, help to prevent sores and cracking, both of which open up the body to infection (Gillham, 1994). Lymphedema also necessitates the evasion of trauma to the affected limb, as further injury could cause an increase in swelling and eventually scarring, which causes additional damage to the superficial lymphatic vessels (Gillham, 1994).

Although no standard treatment for lymphedema currently exists, most physical therapists create treatment plans including most if not all of the aforementioned techniques. The studies performed by Gillham, Weiss, and Wozniewski et al. all involved MLD, a form of compression, and exercise. The techniques employed produced desired outcomes in all of the studies mentioned above. To prove the methods effective, medical personnel must conduct additional research and, provided a positive outcome, MLD, compression, exercises, and skin care should become the standard practice for lymphedema.

Jacobs believes that "[t]o bring lymphedema treatment into the 21st century, the health care community must focus their attention on this condition and work as a team to develop better prevention and treatment options" (Reynolds, 1996). Despite the lack of research and standard procedures, the combination of MLD, compression, and exercise proves effective. This combination, as well as skin care precautions, should become the protocol for treating patients with lymphedema.

References

Buren, J. M., & Linton, C. (2000). The role of exercise in treating lymphedema. *Rehab Management: The Interdisciplinary Journal of Rehabilitation, 13,* 26–31.

Gillham, L. (1994). Lymphoedema and physiotherapists: Control not cure. *Physiotherapy, 80,* 835–842.

Reynolds, J. P. (Ed.). (1996). Lymphedema: An "orphan" disease. *PT Magazine, 4,* 54–63.

Silverthorn, D. U. (2001). Blood flow and the control of blood pressure. In *Human physiology: An integrated approach* (pp. 461–462). Upper Saddle River, NJ: Prentice-Hall.

Weiss, J. M. (1998). Treatment of leg edema and wounds in a patient with severe musculoskeletal injuries. *Physical Therapy, 78,* 1104–1113.

Wozniewski, M., Jasinski, R., Pilch, U., & Dabrowska, G. (2001). Complex physical therapy for lymphoedema of the limbs. *Physiotherapy, 87,* 252–255.

DEFINITION

In most cases, people are familiar with definitions because they help explain the meaning of a word with which they may not be familiar. This form is the **simple definition** and is the one found in the dictionary. The use of definition as an organizational pattern for expository writing does not follow this simple formula. Instead, definition used in academic or professional writing usually attempts to expand the reader's understanding of a term or to clarify an abstract concept. This is called an **expanded definition**.

In the health professions, practitioners will often need to define the malady they are treating. For example, in the following sample student essay, the writer defines amyotrophic lateral sclerosis, or Lou Gehrig's disease, to determine if physical therapy is a viable treatment option for someone with this degenerative disease. The student defines the disease by characteristics; then she approaches the characteristics through the scope of practice of the physical therapist. Ultimately, she concludes that physical therapy is a viable treatment protocol for this degenerative disease because therapists treat these symptoms regularly. She has expanded the definition of *scope of practice*.

Ultimately, the writer, when defining the subject, must consider, as this student does, several forms of reasoning that help a reader define the term or event. The most likely support mechanism for defining an event or issue is the example. Additionally, writers often will define the history of the event to demonstrate how the condition or event came about in its present form. Using a more creative approach, writers can define their subjects by describing what they are *not*—that is, by **negation**. In other words, a writer can compare one event or item with another and determine for the reader that they are similar and deserve the same definition or that one is different from the other and therefore deserves a separate definition.

Sample Student Essay
DEFINITION — EXAMPLE 1

Treatment of Amyotrophic Lateral Sclerosis

Amyotrophic lateral sclerosis (ALS), more commonly known as Lou Gehrig's disease, advances quickly and attacks and deteriorates the voluntary motor system, including the upper motor neuron (UMN) and the lower motor neuron (LMN) (Galinski-Malaguti, Malaguti, Andres, Munsat, 1996; Peruzzi & Potts, 1996). The distinctive properties of ALS include skeletal muscle atrophy, spasticity, skeletal muscle weakness, and function loss due to denervation of the skeletal muscles, along with spontaneous contractions known as fasciculations (Galinski-Malaguti et al., 1996; Thibodeau & Andres, 1987).

Causes of ALS remain unclear, but some theories state that a genetic link may predispose some people to develop it, as 5% to 10% of those people with a family history of the disease become afflicted with the disease (Galinski-Malaguti et al., 1996). According to Galinski-Malaguti et al., some environmental factors include exposure to lead and viral infections. Roughly 1 in 100,000 people annually develop ALS, with the average onset of ALS occurring between 50 and 70 years of age (Galinski-Malaguti et al., Thibodeau & Andres, 1987).

Exerting themselves physically may cause ALS (Peruzzi & Potts, 1996). Lou Gehrig, the first and most famous person diagnosed with ALS, played first base for the Yankees in the 1920s and 1930s. He played a then-record 2,630 consecutive games, ending the streak in 1939, as a result of a sudden lack of coordination, just before his diagnosis of ALS. He never played baseball again.

Typical manifestations of ALS consist of fasciculations; muscle atrophy (wasting away); clumsiness; dysphagia (painful swallowing); muscle cramps; shortness of breath; weight loss; fatigue; and hyperflexia (excessive movement), followed by loss of reflexes and paralysis (Galinski-Malaguti et al., 1996; Thibodeau & Andres, 1987). ALS deteriorates the motor system in a linear and parallel fashion, usually beginning with the hands and progressing up the upper extremities and down the rest of the body, ending in the death of the patient due to respiratory failure (Galinski-Malaguti et al., 1996; Thibodeau & Andres, 1987). Death often occurs within 3 years after diagnosis, but some patients live as long as 10 years (Galinski-Malaguti et al., 1996; Peruzzi & Potts, 1996).

ALS spares all involuntary systems, such as cardiac and smooth muscle, sensation, sphincter control, and mental processes (Thibodeau & Andres, 1987). With mental operations preserved, patients feel depressed because of their recognition of their deteriorating body and the burden they place on their loved ones (Thibodeau & Andres, 1987). To counteract these emotions, according to Thibodeau & Andres (1987), the primary care physician may refer the patient to a psychiatrist or psychologist for help in dealing with such emotions in a healthy way. If the physician fails to take notice of the patient's unbalanced emotional state, progression to deep depression is possible, with subsequent suicide attempts in an effort to end the patient's suffering. Family members may need emotional support of their own, and support groups may help them cope with the turmoil they feel regarding their afflicted loved one (Thibodeau & Andres, 1987).

Despite the unavailability of a cure, treatment options exist to help patients live more comfortable lives, and physical therapy (PT) plays a large role in the treatment of ALS (Galinski-Malaguti et al., 1996; Peruzzi & Potts, 1996; Thibodeau & Andres, 1987). Tailoring a specific strengthening program to each individual helps to maintain range of motion (ROM) and prevent contractures (i.e., shortening of muscles) (Thibodeau & Andres, 1987). Physical therapists should teach their patient energy preservation methods as well (Peruzzi & Potts, 1996; Thibodeau & Andres, 1987).

"Physical therapy intervention for persons with amyotrophic lateral sclerosis," by Anna C. Peruzzi and Ann F. Potts, defines and describes the physiology of ALS. The article also illustrates a detailed example of the type of program that physical therapists should implement for their ALS patients based on the five most common problems that PT can help, including special equipment needed.

In "Amyotrophic lateral sclerosis; A comprehensive review," Dana Galinski-Malaguti, Raymond Malaguti, Patricia Andres, and Theodore Munsat discuss the physiology of ALS along with the epidemiology. This review demonstrates the evaluation and diagnosis processes and overall treatment of ALS beyond the scope of physical therapy including education, psychotherapy, respiratory therapy, drug therapy, and surgery options.

Linda M. Thibodeau and Patricia L. Andres, in "Physical therapy management of patients with ALS," outline ALS and discuss the importance of a PT program and what that program should entail. Along with the psychological issues that may arise, it also explains the different types of equipment that the disease necessitates.

Richard W. Bohannon describes the strengthening program of a 56-year-old woman with ALS in "Results of resistance exercise on a patient with amyotrophic lateral sclerosis: A case report." The article gives background information on previous studies, and it explains the patient's initial condition, including specific measurements, the specific exercise program prescribed for her, and her condition after the study ended.

The general concerns that PT addresses involve muscle weakness and fatigue, pain, respiratory dysfunction, changes in passive range of motion (ROM), and problems with activities of daily living (ADL) (Peruzzi & Potts, 1996). Mild resistive exercises can strengthen those muscles unaffected thus far by ALS (Thibodeau & Andres, 1987). In doing so, the increased strength in unaltered muscles can compensate for the loss of strength in other muscles and expand the patient's functional abilities (Peruzzi & Potts, 1996).

Multiple studies show that a strengthening program consisting of resistance exercises can augment strength in a patient with ALS (Bohannon, 1983; Peruzzi & Potts, 1996). One such study conducted in a 56-year-old woman involved training her arms with proprioceptive neuromuscular facilitation and slow reversals (Bohannon, 1983). Her exercises included different patterns and combinations of abduction and adduction, flexion and extension, and internal and external rotation performed against manual resistance (Bohannon, 1983). She performed the movements 6 days a week for 75 days (Bohannon, 1983). The results showed no regular trend, but static strength increased in 14 muscle groups and decreased in 4 other muscle groups (1983). The patient reported that she developed the ability to pivot her wheelchair on a carpeted surface because of the training course.

Other suitable exercises, besides a strengthening program, include swimming, walking, and riding a bicycle, and other low-impact aerobic activities (Thibodeau & Andres, 1987). All symptoms amplify with fatigue, so an avoidance of exhaustion should occur in an effort to maintain optimal performance (Thibodeau & Andres, 1987).

Patients complain of pain caused by hypersensitivity to touch, muscle aches, and cramping (Peruzzi & Potts, 1996). Decreased ROM, caused by an inability to move due to a decrease in strength, causes cramping. Mobilization of the joints and soft tissues, along with ROM exercises, can relieve that pain (Peruzzi & Potts, 1996; Thibodeau & Andres, 1987). Rest, stretch, massage, moist heat, and transcutaneous electrical nerve stimulation help to ease the pain as well. To compensate for hypersensitivity, the caregiver should use modified handling techniques, massage, and limb elevation (Peruzzi & Potts, 1996).

The respiratory dysfunction caused by upper airway blockage, secondary to impairment of inspiration and expiration muscles, is not reversible (Peruzzi & Potts, 1996; Thibodeau & Andres, 1987). Passive trunk mobilizations and deep breathing exercises help increase chest expansion to prevent atelectasis (incomplete expansion of a lung) (Peruzzi & Potts, 1996; Thibodeau & Andres, 1987). Minimizing bed rest, incentive spirometry, and deep breathing and coughing techniques are essential (Peruzzi & Potts, 1996; Thibodeau & Andres, 1987). Toward the end of the clinical course in ALS, breathing can occur only with mechanical ventilation, which family members should discuss with their loved one ahead of time, as it raises ethical questions (Peruzzi & Potts, 1996).

As strength declines in individuals with ALS, joint ROM decreases, which can lead to contractures or deformities (Peruzzi & Potts, 1996). Gentle heating, along with joint mobilization and stretching, aids in maintaining and increasing ROM (Peruzzi & Potts, 1996). Active assisted or passive ROM exercises, depending on the patient's level of weakness, prevent reductions in passive ROM (Peruzzi & Potts, 1996).

To aid in performance of ADL, the patient uses assistive devices and equipment (Peruzzi & Potts, 1996; Thibodeau & Andres, 1987). ALS patients often have difficulty ambulating as a result of "foot drop"; thus, the use of an ankle orthotic enables safe ambulation by preventing tripping (Thibodeau & Andres, 1987). Walkers and crutches also help the patient move about; however, the patient will require a wheelchair in the final stages of the disease, and the physical therapist should plan for this eventuality (Thibodeau & Andres, 1987). Bathroom equipment and strategically placed bars along walls assist the patient with ADL as well (Thibodeau & Andres, 1987).

When the disease advances to the final stages, the emphasis of PT shifts from therapeutic care to palliative care and education of loved ones and caregivers (Thibodeau & Andres, 1987). To improve the quality of life, proper neutral positioning and passive ROM become increasingly important (Thibodeau & Andres, 1987). In end-stage disease, the extensive motor neuron loss causes the patient to depend on others for all aspects of care (Thibodeau & Andres, 1987). The physical therapist must teach the caregivers how to properly assist the patient using correct body mechanics to avoid injuring themselves (Thibodeau & Andres, 1987).

The best treatments for ALS incorporate a multidisciplinary approach (Galinski-Malaguti et al., 1996). The treatment for ALS should involve, along with PT, psychotherapy, occupational therapy (OT), speech therapy (ST), respiratory therapy, and drug therapy (Galinski-Malaguti et al., 1996). OT provides assistive devices, which help with ADL, and ST helps manage dysphagia (Galinski-Malaguti et al., 1996).

Prescribed drug therapy includes riluzole, amitriptyline HCl, diazepam, quinine, and antibiotic therapy (Galinski-Malaguti et al., 1996). Riluzole, recently approved by the Food and Drug Administration, slows the progression of the symptoms of ALS according to a European study (Galinski-Malaguti et al., 1996). Multiple studies in the United States continue to try to confirm the results of the European study (Galinski-Malaguti et al., 1996). Amitriptyline HCl reduces emotional stress by reestablishing and maintaining normal sleeping patterns (Galinski-Malaguti et al., 1996). Diazepam, baleen, and quinine sulfate reduce muscle cramping, and antibiotic therapy helps infections (Galinski-Malaguti et al., 1996).

With continued research projects, a new theory has been developed about the cause of ALS. This hypothesis states that an excess of glutamate, an essential central nervous system neurotransmitter, causes ALS (Galinski-Malaguti et al., 1996). This conjecture drives most research today (Galinski-Malaguti et al., 1996).

While researchers continue to look for a cure for ALS, physical therapists will continue to treat ALS with the most effective treatments available. PT helps ALS patients live comfortable and functional lives for their remaining years.

References

Bohannon, R. W. (1983). Results of resistance exercise on a patient with amyotrophic lateral sclerosis: A case report. *Physical Therapy, 63*(6), 965–968.

Galinsky-Malaguti, D., Malaguti, R., Andres, P., & Munsat, T. (1996). Amyotrophic lateral sclerosis; A comprehensive review. *Physician Assistant, 20*(8), 65–76.

Peruzzi, A. C., & Potts, A. F. (1996). Physical therapy intervention for persons with amyotrophic lateral sclerosis. *Physiotherapy Canada, 48*(2), 119–126.

Thibodeau, L. M., & Andres, P. L. (1987). Physical therapy management of patients with ALS. *Clinical Management in Physical Therapy, 7*(4), 6–8.

Sample Student Essay
DEFINITION—EXAMPLE 2

Multiple studies are being conducted to determine the effectiveness of alternative methods of medicine. One of these alternative methods is intercessory prayer.

Intercessory prayer is defined as prayer by one person for the health of another. Dr. Herbert Benson, the founder of the Harvard-affiliated Mind/Body Institute, studies the effects of both relaxation and prayer on healing. His studies validate that a reduction in mental stress will lead to positive physical changes, which is referred to as the "relaxation response." His newest studies focus on the benefits, if any, of intercessory prayer. Some studies show that a patient participating in prayer, or a patient's knowledge that another person is praying for him or her, may have a positive effect on the health of this patient. The state of well-being that is produced in some patients after they practice meditation or prayer is believed to be due to the placebo effect and the connection between mind and body. No research can prove that prayer actually has any effect on a patient when the patient is unaware that he or she is being prayed for.

There is no way to prove whether this type of intercessory prayer is actually beneficial to the patient or not. The studies done seem to be conducted as an effort to prove whether or not there is a God or higher power that has an effect on the well-being of humans, and no clear proof can be given either way.

In the nineteenth century, Sir Francis Galton conducted a study on the effectiveness of intercessory prayer. The study compares the life span of royalty, who are assumed to receive the most prayer from others, with the life span of commoners. His studies show that royalty, excluding those who were killed or died accidentally, had the shortest life span overall. In a further study conducted by C. R. B. Joyce and R. M. C. Welldon at the London Hospital Medical College, patients diagnosed with a "stationary or progressively deteriorating psychological or rheumatic disease" were assigned to one of two groups. Teams were set up to provide prayer for one of these groups, while the other group received no organized prayer. No clear pattern of an improved state of well-being for those who received prayer from the organized groups is presented by this study.

Further studies, completed in 1988 and 1999, indicate that intercessory prayer is a factor in healing. The Council for Secular Humanism and the Committee for the Scientific Investigation of Claims of the Paranormal believe that intercessory prayer has absolutely nothing to do with improved health in patients. These organizations believe that the studies are invalid because the researchers did not eliminate all outside factors. The patients not receiving intercessory prayer from a set group of intercessors may be receiving it in other ways from family or friends. The presence of factors such as outside prayer makes it impossible to prove that intercessory prayer is the one factor affecting the health of the patients. Prayer and meditation by the individual may cause improvements in his/her health through the placebo effect, but it cannot be concluded with any certainty that intercessory prayer can improve the health of an individual. There are far too many factors to validate any conclusion made from these studies.

Many alternative techniques for healing, such as meditation, acupuncture, and chiropractics, all prove to be beneficial practices for the individuals involved. Intercessory prayer, however, cannot possibly be proved effective.

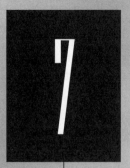

CHAPTER

7

Writing the

Argument

Key Terms

Argument Objectively stating claims, defending positions, and refuting opposition

Authoritative Work that represents good science and can be verified

Categorical argument Attempts to prove that an entity (a term, object, person, and so on) fits into the parameters of an established design or mechanism

Causal argument Reasoning based on a chain of events that explain the problem or issue in reasonable and rational terms

Circular reasoning Evidence used to support the claim is essentially the claim itself

Classical argument structure A logical sequence to argument; strategy for outlining

Deduction The principle has categories; if an object fits a category, it fits the principle

Definitional argument Reasoning based on an expanded definition

Hasty generalization A claim made with insufficient evidence

Implicit argument Writing that defends a position although the language and support is objective

Induction If several show the same principle, the principle applies to all

Primary evidence Data, such as results of experiments, that can be verified

Red herring Misdirecting the reader to support other causes, not the original claim

Secondary evidence Data from studies conducted by others that are used by a writer

chapter objectives

On completion of this chapter, the reader should be able to

1. Recognize that all writing is a form of argument.

2. Choose appropriate language to persuade the audience and not inflame dissenters.

3. Avoid basing arguments on subjective categories (emotional, religious, or political assumptions) and choose objective categories.

4. Read about a subject and derive questions or concerns through critical analysis that helps develop an argument.

5. Develop an argumentative essay through the classical argument structure.

6. Recognize patterns of reasoning and their weaknesses to formulate a logical argument.

7. Read his or her own work as both a supporter and a dissenter to create a rational and logical argument.

8. Understand fallacies and guard against them in argument essays.

*M*uch of our writing in an academic setting is persuasive in nature. Even the most fact-based research paper convinces the audience to understand and accept a principle that is based in opinion. For example, a research paper may contend that physical therapy benefits patients who suffer from degenerative neuromuscular diseases. No one will argue that muscle and joint manipulation or stimulation will not provide benefit for a patient, but the element of contention rests in the fact that the effects of degenerative diseases will not subside with muscle or joint manipulation or stimulation. The treatment affects only the symptoms, not the cause of the disease. In effect, the research paper devoted to factual evidence asks the reader to accept a side to a preexisting argument.

FORMULATING THE ARGUMENT

In the **argument** essay, the writer simply presents a controversial issue and then chooses a side to defend. Support for that position depends on evidence, reasons, and examples. As another element of the essay, the writer may present and attempt to refute opposing viewpoints on the topic. Ultimately, the central purpose of the essay is to defend one side of a controversial issue, not to "straddle the fence" or find equal weight on both sides. The support of the argument essay, then, seeks to find answers to questions and to persuade others to view the topic from the writer's perspective.

Formulating an argument is standard practice for writers. Most if not all writing involves some aspect of argument. An argument, by definition, states a controversy and supports a position about the debatable topic. Some arguments are explicit, meaning that a controversial issue is clearly presented and the writer takes a position on the issue as a thesis statement or controlling idea. Other arguments are implicit. In an **implicit argument**, the writer may not blatantly present the topic of controversy and attempt to persuade the reader, but the elements of controversy and of soliciting support exist because the position of the writer (and results of studies, if applicable) can be argued. The writer, in any document, comes to the paper with "baggage." Writers and researchers may be grounded in politics, social conditions, economics, theories, or even emotions, that influence their reasoning. For example, in a sample student essay presented in earlier chapters, a student presents a claim that physical therapy is a worthwhile treatment of patients suffering from Parkinson's disease. Although the subject seems objective and clearly without outside influence, it is not. The writer has essentially formulated an argument against the standard practice. Currently, health insurers will not reimburse therapists for treatment of degenerative diseases beyond a set number of visits. The reasoning behind this set limit is that the disease is degenerative, and consequently, the patient will never recover fully from the effects of the disease no matter how many times he or she visits a therapist. No treatment of the musculature will solve the patient's problems, since the debilitating effects of the disease derive from issues of neurology. Consequently, payment for services rendered is limited. However, the writer argues that the degenerative effects of the disease can be managed more effectively through therapy because therapeutic exercise can offset the muscle rigidity of the disease and provide a better quality of life for the patient. Therefore, the writer argues, implicitly, that the payment for services rendered should be extended to meet the needs of palliative care.

Such a position is influenced by the writer's philosophical baggage: the writer believes that the insurer should pay for services that influence a patient's quality of life. This type of reasoning, although in the best interest of the patient, is not in the best interest of the business of the insurer. Research conducted by the insurer would produce much different results. The insurer would examine the costs of covering all patients' quality-of-life issues and then would determine that such a move would drain the system and draw money away from the insurer's ability to pay for direct treatments that cure other diseases or illnesses.

The influences that determine any writer's position in any field are many and varied. As a result, the field develops a scholarly dialogue in which ideas are exchanged and debated. Everything published can be scrutinized, and the ideas presented can be challenged. This process of scrutiny and challenge constitutes the academic experience. We are not certain that we can discover a "right" or absolute answer, but we can examine an issue thoroughly and provide workable solutions through the exchange of ideas.

Considering Audience

Defending a position is a difficult process because not everyone agrees with your opinion. A majority may not agree with you. The thrust of argumentative writing is to take on the dissenters and argue persuasively for your side. Arguing for the purpose of convincing others requires the ability to think critically and to analyze all of the possible refutations to your position. Arguing your side is easy; refuting the opposition is difficult and requires that you see the issue from all angles, especially those with which you do not agree.

To write an effective argumentative essay, the words you choose must not inflame readers with an opposing view. You are targeting them as an audience. Choose words and phrases carefully, and attempt to "sell" your position objectively. Many people fail to convince others to swing to their side because they are not objective in their tone or in their argument or evidence. Not considering their argument or planning well, they toss out evidence that does not convince but instead simply reinforces their position. Many writers, when faced with this task in lower-level college courses, choose the easiest form of argument to support their position. Take, for example, the argument that rages between abortion rights activists and abortion protestors. The argument for or against abortion usually derives from a person's deep convictions based on religious or moral thinking. Convincing a Catholic to convert to Protestantism, or vice versa, is nearly an impossible task—for no other reason than the fact that

people's identities are rooted in their religious, cultural, or ethical value systems. Changing people's beliefs is like trying to change their entire state of being. Consider the wisdom of what Linus says in *It's the Great Pumpkin, Charlie Brown*: "You should never discuss in public religion, politics, or the Great Pumpkin." These subjects are avoided in argument not simply out of courtesy but because no one will win. Our belief systems are deeply and firmly rooted.

Consequently, we can learn a lesson from this dilemma. Avoid basing your arguments on emotional, religious, or political assumptions. These are not objective in nature and will damage your argument.

Reasoning and arguing are the cornerstones of much of the progress that we make in our world and in all professions. As professionals, we will be expected to broadcast our ideas in writing (journal articles) and in speech (conference presentations), and we will expect to be challenged. You should feel obligated to challenge assumptions and to argue your position no matter how obtuse you think it is. Developing these skills will help you formulate your philosophical stance on issues as well and help build consistency in your thinking.

CHOOSING A TOPIC

Your genuine interest in your profession may often encourage you to think critically about a subject that is influencing you or your profession. When new information is presented, you may be required to speak or even write about it in an intelligent fashion. For many people, the best way to clarify their ideas and, consequently, to articulate their position is to write them out and analyze them. This exercise in thinking is much like drafting a paper, except that you are writing a short reaction that expresses your views and opinions about new or explosive issues or articles in publications affecting your profession. This writing exercise is often done to help you and others clarify your philosophy of medicine.

Approach the essay by simply responding to the elements of the issue or the publication that directly affect you, your thinking, or the direction such issues or changes can take your profession. You may focus on a central question that has been raised or a problem that has been presented. You may want to criticize certain conclusions or methods of gathering information. However you approach the subject, be sure to use evidence from the text to support your claims. (In doing so, follow the guidelines set forth by the APA for borrowing information from sources.)

When approaching the subject, ask questions to help develop your opinion. In the following exercise, consider the broad scope of topics covered by each question listed.

Exercise

FORMULATING ARGUMENTS

Directions: Read an article and write a short reaction to it to be used later as the foundation to your argument essay. For example, read anything about pain management. Pain management is addressed by several different groups, each claiming effective strategies for treatment. How do you, as a medical or allied health professional, react to this article and the approaches that several million people are taking to ease their pain? As you consider your answer to this question, look at the following list of questions that are also raised in reaction to such information provided in the article. Think of more, and focus your argument on one specific subject.

1. What are the strategies that medical and allied health professionals use for pain management, and how do alternative strategies compare with these?

2. How do you respond to over-the-counter products and self-medication processes?

3. What is your professional opinion about alternative medicines? nutritional supplements?

4. How do you react to the claim that many of these "drugs" have ineffective amounts of ingredients? How should quality be controlled with the distribution of any drug? Does the placebo effect apply here?

5. How do you respond to drug therapy? Is a pill always the answer? Look at products and advertisements, and assess what people want and do.

6. How do chiropractors, massage therapists, accupuncturists, and alternative practitioners compare with professionals in your own health care field? What are the philosophical and practical differences?

7. What does the term *natural* mean?

8. How do you react to the amount of money people are spending on pain management procedures?

9. Ultimately, what is your philosophy of medicine?

Many writers struggle with this type of writing if they are not guided to think about particular issues. Too many arguments exist, and to choose one is an overwhelming task. The following assignments may help you to think about subjects in terms of arguable issues.

A unique way to approach this problem of topic development is through the opposition's eyes. For example, in law school during moot court sessions, students are often asked to argue in support of the side they think is wrong or to defend the guilty party to better understand how the opposition may formulate its case. This intellectual exercise forces the writer to consider all the evidence and to be objective.

For example, in college I was assigned to present a persuasive speech, and I took this tack. I was overwhelmed with signs, posters, and fliers that encouraged environmental awareness (this was the early '80s), the most gripping being the ones exciting us to "Save the baby seals." The posters covered the walls in most buildings, and they appealed to many people's emotions because the posters pictured cute, cuddly, wet-nosed, white baby seals pushing their way helplessly across the ice in the Arctic. It hit me then that the group sponsoring this argument based its claims on the cuteness of the seals. In other words, I felt compelled to save these seals simply because they were cute and cuddly.

In reaction, I gave my persuasive speech on the following topic: "We need to kill more baby seals." It was unpopular at first, but because the case could be made for warm hats and gloves as well as for environmental management of the seal population, or *objective* causes, the emotional appeal faded, and many in the audience were convinced. The opposition was refuted by reminding those in the audience that their opinions would change if the animal was not so cute. Pigs, chickens, and cows are slaughtered daily, and few people make posters on their behalf. This argument is not watertight, but the message is clear: Base your argument on clear, objective evidence and not emotion.

Organizing the Argument

The following formula is a simplified version of the **classical argument structure**, but it can serve as a foundation from which you can begin. Feel free to adjust the order or add sections to this outline to suit your needs.

Introduction: A. Establish that an argument exists by discussing background and explaining the position of the opposing sides.

B. Take a position (thesis).

Body: A. Create evidence paragraph(s) to defend your position.

B. Create evidence paragraph(s) to refute the opposition.

Conclusion: Restate your position in terms of the argument defended and/or refuted.

In standard form, the argument essay fits the classical pattern of presenting a claim, supporting the claim, and reasoning that the evidence provided supports the claim.

EVIDENCE AND PATTERNS OF REASONING IN THE ARGUMENT

To support the claims you make, you must defend your claim with evidence. Various types of evidence exist, but only a few can stand up to the scrutiny of logic: **primary evidence** and **secondary evidence**. If you conduct experiments yourself and then provide proof that your experiments can be reproduced and the results are verifiable, then you are the primary investigator, and the evidence you provide is primary evidence. The experiments that are conducted by others with results written by others constitute secondary evidence. Therefore, when you identify relevant research findings of others and supply that information in your text, as in a research paper, you are conducting secondary research. If you conduct the experiment yourself, such as a thesis project, and report the results in the thesis, your work is primary in nature.

Some textbooks will argue that other forms of support are useful such as personal experience. Although personal experience may seem like primary research, it is often not reproducible, nor may it be researchable. It could simply be a set of events that happened to you.

When using researchable material, either primary or secondary, remember that you are attempting to prove to your audience that your work is **authoritative**. Send the message to your reader that you have scrutinized the evidence and have provided the information that is necessary and accurate. Also, keep in mind the types of reasoning you impose on your audience. Understanding these terms and how they can lead to faulty conclusions will help you develop a logical essay.

Inductive Reasoning

Induction is the form of reasoning that takes several pieces of evidence and then concludes that since these several bits show the same principles, the principle applies to all. For example, we use induction in our primary research. We establish that in a survey of 100 people on campus, a sample population, 90 of them felt that the college does not provide enough parking for students. Consequently, since 90 out of 100 people in the sample agreed on the same subject, then 90% of the college has the same opinion.

Inductive reasoning also applies to our secondary research. When we read and study the work of others in published forums such as journals, we find that, in all the examples we read, all of them produced verifiable evidence. Consequently, we conclude that everything that is published in a journal is verifiable and therefore authoritative.

In reaction to these examples, you should recognize the inherent weaknesses in this type of reasoning. For instance, thinking that all information published in journals is verifiable and therefore authoritative is not safe. Obviously, an article published somewhere in some journal is not verifiable and therefore not authoritative. This, of course, also depends on the definition of the term *publish*.

Deductive Reasoning

In **deduction**, the process of reasoning is reversed from induction. In deduction, you start with a generally accepted truth and then apply pieces of evidence to show that they fit the mold. For instance, you can begin with a generally accepted truth:

> All animals that meow are cats.
> Brutus is an animal that meows.
> Consequently, Brutus is a cat.

In the medical profession, this form of reasoning is used often. For instance:

> December is the start of cold season.
> Patients A, B, and C complain of "runny noses," low fever, coughing, and sneezing.
> Therefore, patients A, B, and C have colds.

Understanding the inherent weaknesses in this form of reasoning is essential to good writing and to creating a solid argument. For example, just because patients exhibit some symptoms does not mean that they have colds. Likewise,

many medical professionals have argued that if we move to a system of socialized medicine, where all people have medical coverage and doctors' wages are paid by the federal government, medical professionals will lose their competitive edge. Since salaries will be controlled, the medical profession will not attract the best and brightest people to work in the medical industry because the salaries are limited. This type of reasoning takes the argument to a logical extreme. Taking the argument to an extreme is an effective means to defeat the opposing position or argument. Know the limitations of this type of reasoning before you employ it.

Patterns of Reasoning

To effectively argue a position, you should recognize the type of support you are using to help you build your case into one that is rational and logical. Additionally, how you organize that information is vitally important. In medical writing, the three dominant patterns of organization are categorical, definitional, and causal. Understanding the patterns of reasoning will help you organize your ideas and then challenge your ideas and your supporting evidence using principles of logic.

Categorical Arguments

In the **categorical argument**, the writer attempts to prove that an entity (a term, object, person, etc.) fits into the parameters of an established design or mechanism. Doing so helps the reader understand an extended definition of a term or see a condition in a new way. In this pattern, the writer operates under the assumption that the audience and the writer agree upon a standard definition of the design or mechanism. For example, in the following sample student essay, the student attempts to prove that chiropractic medicine and physical therapy differ in that physical therapy is a practice grounded in the medical model. The established design or mechanism that the author and audience agree on is the term *medical model*. The writer then attempts to fit physical therapy into the design and to show how chiropractic does not fit into the design. In essence, the writer shows that physical therapy fits into the category and chiropractic does not, to support the practice of physical therapy in the case of patient choice. Notice also the organizational strategy for proving the argument.

Sample Student Essay
CATEGORICAL ARGUMENT

The end of World War I brought the need for rehabilitation aids to help veterans injured in the war. Since that time, the field of rehabilitation care has progressed and evolved into physical therapy. In the latter half of the twentieth century, physical therapy grew rapidly, so rapidly that similar professions began to compete for services. The closest competitors to physical therapy in today's professional market include chiropractors and massage therapists. Recently, the chiropractic community supported legislation that would make spinal manipulation by physical therapists illegal. This effort proved unsuccessful, largely owing to the lobbying efforts of the American Physical Therapy Association (APTA). The topic remains controversial despite the recent ruling.

Although chiropractors focus on the spine and the resulting effects of spinal manipulation, chiropractors are not trained in the medical model. They are a contingent of the healing arts or alternative medicine. Physical therapists receive extensive training in the medical model in bone, muscle, skin, nervous system, and joint care, with an educational background including courses in spinal manipulation. Patients should understand the differences in treatment options before making decisions about their health because the medical model is the standard practice of treatment in today's health care system, and patients choosing to step outside of the medical model are putting their health at risk.

Although the two practices appear similar, they in fact are different in theoretical practice and in administering care. Physical therapists follow a model of education similar to that of a doctor. The science-based education focuses on evaluation and treatment of the heart, lungs, muscles, bones, and nervous system, with clinical experiences to apply and solidify classroom material. Also, physical therapists must meet the standards of practice set by the APTA, which belongs to the American Medical Association. Before being allowed to practice, therapists need to pass the state-licensing examination. In whole health or in the healing arts, chiropractors follow an alternative model of education. Their training places emphasis on alternative medicine principles, techniques, and natural healing. Science courses at a chiropractic college, although similar to those of physical therapy curriculum, do not stress the medical aspects or cover as many subjects and areas of health care. The major point of emphasis relates all education and treatments to the spine. Additionally, chiropractic schools receive accreditation from the Council on Chiropractic Education, but states do not require a comprehensive examination before beginning to practice chiropractic healing. The fact that individual states do not require a comprehensive examination raises questions about the importance of chiropractic practice in the view of the government, the medical community, and even society in general. As a patient, I want health professionals to accommodate and answer to a higher authority than their peers.

The differences in the models of education for each field create inherent differences in their models of practice. A licensed physical therapist evaluates a patient's condition and then plans and administers treatments to promote optimal health. Therapists seek to relieve pain, improve the body's movement and function, maintain cardiopulmonary function, and limit disabilities resulting from injuries or disease. Before a therapist can administer treatment, the patient needs a referral from his or her physician, dentist, nurse practitioner, physician assistant, or podiatrist. Therapists can perform evaluations at any time. With a referral, the therapist will evaluate the patient's condition, discuss the evaluation with the patient, and then formulate a personalized plan of care with the patient's individual goals in mind. Treatments include the following: therapeutic use of hands, exercise, application of therapeutic techniques such as ultrasound and electric stimulation, training in daily living activities, and patient education. Educating patients about their injury and what preventive measures will decrease the risk of reinjury or having a reoccurrence of the condition. Chiropractic is limited in its focus because it attempts to link all maladies to the patient's spine. Although chiropractors may be effective in treating problems associated with the spine, not all patient conditions stem from the spine. Furthermore, since chiropractic is not part of the medical model, moving patients into an appropriate venue for care may be difficult for them. Instead of referring a patient to a medical professional, the chiropractor is more inclined to use other methods of chiropractic treatment or other chiropractors. This may not be in the best interest of the patient, especially if the condition calls for treatment outside chiropractors' scope of practice and knowledge.

Ultimately, the authority in health care is founded in the medical model, and physical therapy is an arm of medicine. Chiropractic, although successful in some arenas of treatment of the spine and pain management, is not part of the medical model, and therefore, patients are limited in their treatment options. Furthermore, because of licensing informalities, chiropractic seems unsupervised. An educated patient will choose the medical model over the healing arts to ensure effective care.

Problems with Categorical Arguments

Like all arguments, categorical arguments have weaknesses, and every writer should be aware of these weaknesses to guard against them. Two methods of challenging the categorical argument are the following:

Disprove the example: To damage the categorical argument, prove that the example does not fit into the categorical design or mechanism. In the sample student essay, you could argue that physical therapy is part of the medical model, but chiropractic also has become part of the medical model. This would dissolve the ultimate claim of the essay.

Disprove the category: In another approach to attacking the categorical claim, focus on the category and prove that it does not have a standard meaning that both the author and audience can agree upon. In the sample, for instance, prove that the medical model is flawed and is no longer the standard for health care practice. Attacking the category will ask the writer to reevaluate the entire claim because the design for reasoning has changed.

Definitional Arguments

Most people, when they think about definitions, think about dictionary definitions, because such definitions are an important part of any written document. For example, a student submitted a paper arguing as follows:

Asynchronous electronic environments are best for the teaching of writing.

Her paper required her to define the term *asynchronous* because, without it, the reader would be lost. She was also required to differentiate between asynchronous and synchronous electronic environments for

clarification in her definition. Her argument could not move forward until she established the working definition of terms. Additionally, her argument hinged not on the definition but on the employment of a certain type of teaching technique. The term itself, however, was not disputed.

In a **definitional argument**, the focus is on definitions of terms that *can* be disputed. In the foregoing example, the terms are not disputed, but the technique may be. However, consider an example in which certain terms may be disputed:

Young people who are 18 years of age are adults and should be allowed to purchase and consume alcohol.

The term *adult* is the disputable term. At what point in people's lives do they become adults? Is this a category that can be defined by age? What is an adult? Does being an adult mean being mature? How is *mature* defined? Does someone have to be mature to drink alcohol?

Notice the types of questions asked and the responses they elicit. Some of the questions seek a formal definition of terms: *What is an adult? How is mature defined?* In addition to defining the terms, consider also how other questions seek to fit the elements of the argument into the definitions: *At what point in people's lives do they become adults? Is this a category that can be defined by age? Does being an adult mean being mature? Does someone have to be mature to drink alcohol?*

In responses to the two different types of questions that can be asked in relation to the subject, the foundation of the argumentative essay can be seen. Any argument based on definition must address two concerns: a definition that exerts some type of meaning on the terms and the molding of circumstances to meet those definitions.

Consider the two concerns of definition in the following example:

Is cloning socially and morally irresponsible?

In response to this question, defining the terms *social responsibility* and *moral responsibility* can be elusive, but the writer is challenged to prove that cloning fits the definition. Consequently, the writer is charged with two tasks: (1) Establish a definition for *social and moral responsibility*, and (2) determine for the reader that *cloning* fits into that definition. The result is a new perspective on the benefits of human cloning.

The following sample student essay attempts to follow this pattern of organization.

Sample Student Essay
DEFINITION

Cloning: The Socially and Morally Responsible Science

In February 1997, a mature ewe gave birth to Dolly, the first mammal cloned from an adult sheep. This announcement from the scientists at the Roslin Institute in Edinburgh, Scotland, attracted massive press interest, creating the theoretical possibility of cloning humans. Following this scientific advance, opponents of human cloning voiced ethical concerns issuing the process as both a moral and a social problem. These opponents claim that human cloning not only deprives humans of their uniqueness but also interferes with the natural process of human development. By interfering with the natural process, opponents argue that scientists tamper with nature. Despite these oppositions to human cloning, however, proponents present stronger evidence why scientists should implement human cloning. Using cloning, scientists will discover breakthroughs affecting the study of genetics, cell development, human growth, and obstetrics. Human cloning not only provides benefits to infertile couples but also allows scientists to clone only certain replacement organs for transplants. Because of all of the advancements that cloning creates for the scientific world, the technological benefits of cloning outweigh the possible social consequences.

Because cloning provides " . . . potential[s] for developing new medical therapies to treat life-threatening diseases and advancing biomedical knowledge . . . " (Larkin, 2001, p. 453), geneticists foresee a number of practical applications for human cloning. For instance, infertile couples who do not wish to adopt may use cloning to produce a biologically related child. In addition, genetic engineers may also employ cloning to produce an offspring free of genetic diseases. For example, flawed genes originating in mitochondria, the

energy-producing structures within the cytoplasm of a cell, produce a variety of disorders affecting the brain, eyes, and muscles of a newborn. If a woman carries a gene for one of these disorders, a geneticist could extract the nucleus of one of her cells, insert new DNA from a healthy donor oocyte into the cell, and implant the resulting embryo into the womb (Larkin, 2001). As a result, the woman would bear a healthy child free of the genetic defect. Furthermore, scientists may also reprogram cells using cloning to treat existing diseases. For example, a genetic engineer could reprogram insulin-producing cells from the pancreas with the genetic material from skin cells of a diabetic. The geneticist would replace the defective material of the pancreatic cells with new DNA from the skin cells and then infuse the new cells back into the pancreas to produce insulin; consequently, the diabetic patient would overcome the disease.

For infertile couples, human cloning also replaces in vitro fertilization or artificial insemination. In in vitro fertilization, the doctor implants many fertilized ova into a woman's uterus, anticipating that one of the eggs will result in pregnancy. Some women, however, can only supply one egg, which limits pregnancy chances (Ridley, 2001). Using cloning, the geneticist divides a single egg into eight different zygotes for implantation creating increased chances for pregnancy. Other women prefer to give birth only once or do not wish to disrupt their career; cloning also allows these women to give birth to a set of identical twins instead of having two different pregnancies.

Today, an organ shortage exists; because of this shortage, thousands of patients die each year before a replacement organ becomes available for transplantation. As a possible solution to this shortage, scientists employ the process of xenotransplantation, transplanting organs from one species to another (Frankish, 2002). Because human cells exhibit different protein coats on their surfaces than donor organisms, this transplantion technique often results in rejection of the transplanted organ (Frankish, 2002). Through cloning advances, however, scientists announced in January 2002 that they successfully cloned pigs that " . . . lack one copy of a gene that prompts the human immune system to reject transplanted pig organs" (Frankish, 2002, p. 137). This problematic gene produces sugar molecules that attach to antibodies in the human body after transplantation causing rejection of the organ (Frankish, 2002). By removing this gene from the surface of the pig cells, scientists not only reduced the chance of organ rejection but also overcame the aggressive response of the human body's immune system to foreign tissue (Frankish, 2002). Therefore, as stated by Robert Lanza, the vice president of medical and scientific development of Advanced Cell Technology, this advancement " . . . sets the stage for human therapeutic cloning as a potentially limitless source of immune-compatible cells for tissue engineering and transplantation medicine . . . " (McCarthy, 2001, p. 1877).

In addition to the recent success of xenotransplantation, human cloning also allows scientists to clone certain organs outside the body to use as replacements for a transplant. Geneticists could clone a fertilized ovum from an individual into several zygotes, implanting one and freezing the others for future use (Ridley, 2001). If the individual required a transplant, the geneticist would implant one of these frozen zygotes and mature it to replace the diseased organ. Because the body would be less likely to reject the organ after a transplant, scientists expect this transplantation procedure to produce a higher success rate than other transplantation techniques such as xeno-transplantation.

In opposition, many people do not support human cloning. Deeming cloning an unnatural process, opponents of human cloning contend that scientists tamper with nature during cloning by genetically manipulating the human embryo before development begins. Numerous religious organizations, including antiabortion groups, that contest cloning contend that cloning is morally wrong because God intended a man and a woman to conceive a child naturally through sexual intercourse (McCarthy, 2001). However, these opponents to cloning do not know God personally, and therefore, they do not know what He intended. Because not everyone believes in God, not all people can support the argument that cloning interferes with God's intentions for how man should reproduce. Also, since infertile couples cannot conceive children naturally, doctors often use in vitro fertilization and fertility drugs to assist these couples in conceiving children. Doctors aid in conception using in vitro fertilization, an unnatural process similar to cloning. In order to demonstrate consistency in their thinking, people who reject cloning should also reject in vitro fertilization since both techniques do not abide by the intentions of God that humans should be reproduced by sexual means without outside human intervention; however, many do not accept both techniques, making their argument invalid.

Because some adversaries believe in genetic determinism, the view that genes determine everything about a human making environmental factors insignificant, they also believe that cloning produces an exact duplicate of another human, depriving the individual of uniqueness. Cloning, however, does not construct an exact replica; instead, cloning yields a genetically identical twin several years younger than the person who donated the cell. For example, even though naturally conceived identical twins represent an exact genetic duplication, two separate individuals result (Larkin, 2001); they differ biologically, psychologically, morally, and legally but not genetically. In fact, their appearances, values, academic achievements, and occupations all can differ based on personal preferences. Therefore, these differences in identical twins result from complex interactions between their genes, environments, and experiences, not by genes alone making each individual unique (Larkin, 2001).

Despite the hopes of some scientists to clone humans, many other scientists object to such plans believing that any attempt to clone a human would result in the death of many embryos before achieving success, just as in the case of Dolly (Larkin, 2001). In fact, scientists fused 277 other oocytes before successfully cloning Dolly in 1997 (Biological uncertainties . . . , 2001). To support the claim that many deaths will occur before attaining success, Irving L. Weissman, professor of pathology, cancer biology, and developmental biology at Stanford University, reports that "[d]ata on the reproductive cloning of animals demonstrates that only a small percentage of attempts are successful, many of the clones die during all stages of gestation, newborn clones often are abnormal or die, and the procedures may carry serious risks for the mother" (Larkin, 2001, p. 453). Therefore, adversaries fear that the same results may occur with human cloning. Since scientists have not yet tested cloning on humans, the possibility of mutation or other biological damage always exists; however, trial and error dominates the scientific world. Using the scientific method for cloning, scientists make advancements; they determine which techniques create successful results and which techniques they can disregard for future use. In fact, by using the trial and error method, researchers have achieved success in producing 8 live embryos for every 10 calf-cloning attempts, producing an 80% success rate (Biological uncertainties . . . , 2001). This research development not only demonstrates a decline in embryo loss but also produces an increase in advances for lifesaving therapies for a wide range of conditions. Therefore, even if geneticists take years to successfully clone another human, the benefits obtained from the procedure will far surpass the hardships and difficulties encountered during the discovery process. If geneticists have to sacrifice 10 embryos in order to save millions of people in the future through organ transplantation or other medical procedures, then scientists should implement cloning immediately to create a better quality of life for many individuals.

Because societal attitudes change and unexpected developments occur, many people make false initial predictions about new medical techniques. Cloning objections parallel those similar to objections raised against previous scientific achievements; for example, society initially rejected heart transplants and test tube babies, but both procedures later became widely accepted. Cloning not only offers many important medical opportunities but also produces many improvements in transplantation and fertility techniques. Through the use of cloning, transplantation processes will become more successful, and more infertile couples will have the opportunity to conceive children. Because cloning helps to improve the overall quality of life of many individuals, the benefits of human cloning far outweigh the negative oppositions.

References

Biological uncertainties about reproductive cloning. (2001). *Lancet, 358*(9281), 519 [Database]. Ebsco Host: MasterFILE Premier.

Frankish, H. (2002). Pig organ transplantation brought one step closer. *Lancet, 359*(9301), 137 [Database]. Ebsco Host: MasterFILE Premier.

Larkin, M. (2001). Click of the week. *Lancet, 359*(9304), 453 [Database]. Ebsco Host: MasterFILE Premier.

McCarthy, M. (2001). US researchers create cloned human embryos. *Lancet, 358*(9296), 1877 [Database]. Ebsco Host: MasterFILE Premier.

Ridley, M. (2001). Sex, errors, and the genome. *Natural History, 110*(5), 43–51 [Database]. Ebsco Host: MasterFILE Premier.

Examining the Weaknesses of the Definitional Argument

In reviewing the argumentative essay based on definition, consider the inherent weaknesses in the process of reasoning. The two areas of weakness are the definition's new or extended meaning and the molding of the circumstances to meet that new or extended meaning.

Consider the areas of weakness that can expose the following argument to criticism: Young people who are 18 years of age are adults and should be allowed to purchase and consume alcohol.

The term *adult*, as we noted earlier, is the disputable term. The term *adult* varies for different people, but most will agree that different people become adults at different ages. Consequently, the argument that all 18-year-olds deserve the right to drink is weakened by the debatable nature of the term *adult*, since most people define it in terms of maturity. Likewise, if the counterargument rests on the issue of maturity, a secondary argument can be made concerning the definition of that term. What, exactly, makes a person mature? How do we know when a person is mature?

The second point of weakness in the definitional essay is the molding of the circumstances to the term. The circumstances may not be an exact fit for the definition because they are too narrow or inaccurate. In the preceding example, this strategy can be applied. If adults can drink because they are mature, then all adults are assumed to be mature. We all know adults who are not mature. Consequently, being 18 does not guarantee that the person will handle drinking as a responsible adult. Furthermore, the counterargument can attack the general principle of the argument. If the age of 18 is arbitrary, then why not lower the age to 16, or why impose an age limit of any kind? Some European countries do not impose age restrictions on drinking, and they have fewer problems with alcohol.

The extent of the counterargument depends on the reach of the definition and the molding of the circumstances to meet that definition. No argument is impenetrable or irrefutable. Your job as a writer is to provide evidence that supports your argument by thinking through the possible counterarguments and guarding against them.

Sample Student Essay
CATEGORICAL AND DEFINITIONAL PATTERNS: FROM OUTLINE TO ARGUMENT

Argument Essay: Is Health Care a Right or a Privilege?

OUTLINE

Health care is a privilege, not a right.

- privilege—private→insurance provided as benefit of a job
- right—government controlled, so that everyone gets equal treatment

Support "privilege" paragraph:

1. system based on private today
   a. receive insurance provided as benefit of a job
2. incentive to work hard→better economy
   a. handouts—incentives no longer there; people will not contribute to society
3. survival of the fittest
   a. make more money→become healthier
   b. why should we support the poor if they do not contribute anything
   c. taxes from upper class would be paying for everyone—the few should not have to support the many
   d. work hard and provide for yourselves
   e. smartest people make the most $— increase quality of care

Refute "right" paragraph:

1. right—health care controlled by government; no one has to pay
2. creates a better quality of life→healthier/ more productive, contributes to the economy→stronger society
   a. why should some people have more access than others?
   b. refute: not enough time to treat everyone equally (waiting lists)
      i. quality of care diminished
      ii. hospital system will be overrun—not enough manpower to back it up
3. everyone deserves an equal chance to get health care
   a. refute: equality will never exist; wealthy will be treated better (wave money so do not have to wait in line)
      i. should not have to pay for cosmetic surgeries

4. government-regulated salaries for doctors (equal pay):
   a. refute: cannot make more; what is the incentive to work or to be more?

Introduction:

1. U.S. health care model exists today as a privilege, not a right, to citizens
2. through this model, individuals receive insurance from job benefits
3. because all individuals do not have equal chances to receive health care, many people contend that this model creates inequality in the health care system
   a. these challengers wish to amend the issue of health care from a privilege to a right in order to create a better quality of life for all people
4. however, proponents of the existing health care model argue that the private model provides incentives for people to work harder, thus creating a better economy
   a. they also argue that the quality of care will diminish if the implementation of the government-controlled health care system occurs
5. since the proposed government system will jeopardize the quality of care for all patients, the existing health care system should remain instituted

Body: support "private"

1. because the current health care system provides incentives for individuals to work, a stronger economy results
2. if these incentives did not exist, then people would not contribute to society
3. with the private health care model, employees strive to succeed
4. people understand that more prestigious positions offer additional benefits;
   a. consequently, people further exert themselves in order to achieve these goals
   b. when employees exhibit increased dedication, both an augmented production for the company and a stimulation of the economy result
5. in addition, the wealthy individuals of society argue that since they pay the majority of the taxes, everyone would receive health care at their expense if the government changed the system;
   a. however, the few should not have to support the many

    b. consequently, the poor should not receive treatment if they do not contribute anything to society

  6. because everyone must learn to provide for himself, the current system must remain employed

Body: refute government

1. adversaries of the current health care system contest that the government should change the model to create a governmentally controlled one in which no one has to pay

    a. they believe that this new model would produce an equal chance and better quality of care for all people, thus creating a healthier and more productive workforce

2. in reality, however, the quality of care would diminish

3. because an insufficient amount of time/manpower exists to treat everyone equally, the number of personnel and treatments needed would soon overwhelm the hospitals

4. even though many people contest that everyone deserves an equal chance to receive health care, equality will never exist

5. for instance, even though a patient's name may appear at the bottom of the waiting list, health care providers will treat this person first if he waves a $100 bill in the air

6. because the affluent still reign, this action defeats the whole purpose of creating a system of equality

Conclusion:

1. in today's society, many people argue that a change needs to occur within the health care system from a private system to a governmentally controlled system

2. although these opponents to the existing system argue that the new system will create equality, society has demonstrated that true equality will never exist because the wealthy and strong will always dominate

3. because the current system provides incentives to individuals creating a stronger economy, the system must continue to function, and health care must remain a privilege, not a right to people

SAMPLE PAPER

The Definition of Health Care

The United States' health care model exists today as a privilege, not a right, to citizens. Through this model, individuals receive insurance from job benefits. Because all individuals do not have equal chances to receive health care, many people contend that this model creates inequality in the health care system. These challengers wish to amend the issue of health care from a privilege to a right in order to create a better quality of life for all people. However, proponents of the existing health care model argue that the private model provides incentives for people to work harder. They also argue that the quality of care will diminish if the implementation of the government-controlled health care system occurs. Since the proposed governmental system will jeopardize the quality of care for all patients, the existing health care system should remain, and health care is a privilege, not a right.

Since the current health care system provides incentives for individuals to work, a stronger economy results. If these incentives did not exist, then people would not contribute. With the private health care model, employees strive towards a goal. People understand that more prestigious positions offer additional benefits; consequently, people exert themselves harder in order to achieve these goals. When employees exhibit increased dedication, both an augmented production for the company and a stimulation of the economy result. In addition, the wealthy individuals of society argue that since they pay the majority of the taxes, everyone would receive health care at their expense if the government changed the system; however, the few should not have to support the many. Consequently, the poor should not receive treatment if they do not contribute anything to society. Because everyone must learn to provide for himself, the current system must remain employed.

Adversaries of the current health care system argue that government should change the model to create a governmentally controlled one in which no one has to pay. They believe that this new model would produce an equal chance and better quality of care for all people, thus creating a healthier and more productive workforce, creating a stronger society. In reality, however, the quality of care would not increase but rather diminish. Because an insufficient amount of time and manpower exists to treat everyone equally, the number of personnel and treatments needed would soon overwhelm the hospital. Even though many people contest that everyone deserves an equal chance to obtain health care, equality will never exist. For instance, health care providers will always treat an individual waving a $100 bill in front of his face before anyone else, even though that person's name may appear at the bottom of the waiting list. Because the affluent still reign in our society, this action defeats the whole purpose of creating a system of equality.

In today's society, many people argue that a change should occur within the health care system from a private system to a government-controlled system. Although these opponents to the existing system argue that the new system will create equality, society has demonstrated that true equality will never exist because the wealthy and strong will always dominate. Additionally, the current system not only provides incentives to individuals but also creates a stronger economy. Because of this, the present system must continue to exist.

Causal Arguments

A **causal argument** is one in which the writer explains the causes for an event or how one event or series of events creates another. In the following example, the argument follows a causal pattern.

> In the summer of 2001, a vast area of Lake Erie became unable to support fish life. This dead zone was caused, according to freshwater biologists, by zebra mussels. The biologists' reports indicated that the zebra mussel filtered the lake water, which allowed light to penetrate to the depths of the lake. The infusion of light to the lake bottom helped aquatic plants grow, and these plants depleted the water of oxygen, which killed off the fish living in that area.

This example follows the causal pattern in that the result, Lake Erie's dead zone, was caused by the introduction of a simple mollusk. The argument hinges on the biologists' abilities to identify a chain of events that explain the problem in reasonable and rational terms.

Scientists have been interested in causal analyses to explain human behavior. For example, what causes anorexia nervosa? Some people feel that television is the cause. To support this concept, the task of the writer is to delineate the chain of events involved:

> Television promotes body styles that are unattainable for most young people, particularly females. In a sample of young girls with anorexia, researchers discovered that all of them devoted at least one hour of their day to watching television shows, particularly MTV. Seeing models and actresses on television who are very thin, the girls reacted accordingly to meet those body-type expectations. They dieted to an extreme to become like the characters they saw on television. Consequently, when they could not meet these high demands, they starved themselves and suffered physical and psychological ramifications from their efforts. In essence, some may argue, television causes anorexia.

In both of these examples, the issue of causation is studied. In the first example, causation is studied as a single event. In the second, causation is studied to determine reasons for a continuing trend. However, one uses a direct causal link and the other employs a form of inductive reasoning. Both of these methods can be used to prove a causal analysis, but the direct link is the more effective.

In the first example, the biologists writing about the zebra mussel discuss the direct consequences of zebra mussel behavior. The zebra mussel filters water at an alarming rate of 1 liter per day. Zebra mussels reproduce rapidly and can often cover the bottom of the waterway in which they reside. As they populate and filter the water, the water clarity improves. As the water becomes clearer, the ability for sunlight to penetrate deeper into the lake is enhanced. Since sunlight encourages plant growth through photosynthesis, the plants at the bottom of the lake that would normally not receive large doses of sunlight receive more sunlight, which encourages growth. These plants grow rapidly and reach the end of their life cycle at a faster rate. They die and fall to the bottom, where they decompose. The decomposition of plant material absorbs oxygen at great rates, which deprives the water of the necessary means to support fish life. In this example, the direct connection between the links (zebra mussels, plant growth, oxygen depletion) and the event (the dead zone in the lake) is clear.

Consider the other example, which uses a causal link by inductive reasoning. In this example, the high rate of anorexia is said to be caused by television. The sample of patients suffering from the disorder admitted to watching several hours of television per day. Consequently, the argument rests on the inductive reasoning that the representative sample can explain the causes of anorexia for all patients.

This type of reasoning does not employ the direct causal link—and it cannot, because it concentrates on human behavior. Human behavior is often difficult to connect to causality, since many variables can exist in determining our actions. Furthermore, this is the weakness of causality proved through inductive means. Induction attempts to prove that all are the same as the representative sample. This cannot be true in the case of anorexia. In fact, many other factors can contribute to the disorder of anorexia. Consequently, the few in this study do not represent the whole. Such inductive reasoning can prove only a high probability or merely identify a contributing factor. In most cases, it does not prove the effect in its entirety.

Examining the Weaknesses of Causal Arguments

In arguing for a causal connection made by a chain of events, the obvious area of scrutiny is the chain. In the foregoing example of the zebra mussel, the existence of the dead zone is not challenged. It exists. However, the causes of the dead zone can be varied. Consequently, the causes can be argued. Additionally, in terms of the chain of events, the argument seems logical, but other factors could intervene in the chain to cause the dead zone. For example, the existence of zebra mussels may not be the problem; the dense population of zebra mussels could be the contributing factor for these environmental changes. In fact, high levels of phosphates, usually from soaps and cleansers in wastewater from industries, contribute to the increase in zebra mussel reproduction. In essence, then, the causal chain is faulty. The dead zone in Lake Erie is not caused by zebra mussels but by infusion of high levels of phosphates into the lake.

In the causal argument based on inductive reasoning, the anorexia case, the inherent weaknesses of the argument rest in the results and the sample. For example, in the anorexia example, a counterargument could be made that not all women appearing on television are unnaturally thin, and therefore, the girls affected by the disorder model their behavior after others.' In this case, the results are faulty. Likewise, the counterargument could be made that television does not cause anorexia by itself, but anorexia derives from contributing factors such as low self-esteem. Additionally, the sample can be faulty. Although all the girls polled listed television as a major activity in their lives, other girls who suffer from anorexia may not watch television. Consequently, the sample is not representative; it represents only an example of probability.

Again, the weaknesses to any argument should be recognized by the writer to guard against mistakes in logic and reasoning.

Sample Student Essay
CAUSAL ANALYSIS

In recent years, the popularity of baseball has declined. Attendance at the ballparks is down by double-digit figures, and television ratings have consistently dropped. The causes of this decline have been argued. Many feel that the game is too slow for today's young people. Others argue that the salaries of ballplayers and the demands of their union have taken the fun out of the game and made the players and owners businessmen who are cutthroat aggressive in getting their way. Some have even claimed that the differences in the two leagues have lead to a division in styles of play that cannot be rectified when the World Series is played. This is evident in the argument over the designated hitter (DH).

Major league baseball consists of two leagues: the American League (AL) and the National League (NL). In 1973, the AL enacted the DH rule (Miller, 1998), which instigated a continuing debate. NL enthusiasts detest the DH rule because they claim it generates poor game quality and a lack of excitement. Among other benefits, AL devotees argue that the DH rule amplifies the quality of play and provides the exhilaration that the fans desire. Overall, the presence of the DH rule enhances baseball's appeal. The DH rule is not the cause of baseball's decline.

To augment offense, the AL instituted the DH rule in 1973. While the DH rule did boost offense, 12 pitchers in the AL won 20 games. Baseball's current power-hitting renaissance commenced in 1993, not in 1973, as it would if the DH rule caused it. Between 1993 and 1998, major league baseball expanded from 26 teams to 30 teams. The number of proficient hitters exceeds the number of superior pitchers, so when expansion occurs, pitching suffers and hitting flourishes. Since 1993, the AL and the NL possessed high slugging percentages—the percent of multibase hits relative to overall hits—of over .400 for 9 years and 8 years, respectively, due to the lack of quality pitching, not the DH rule.

DH rule antagonists attribute the inflated offense to the rule because stereotypical DHs hit frequent home runs. Opponents claim National Leaguers smack fewer home runs and mobilize strategy beyond American Leaguers. Rivals also aver that no additional stimulation or fascination exists in AL baseball due to the DH rule.

Unlike the AL style of play, the present NL style of play centers on home runs. The number of home runs hit in the NL, over the past four seasons, surpasses the number hit in the AL. In 1998, two NL sluggers blasted over 60 home runs, and another player whacked 73 home runs in 2001. Until 1998, no player hit more than 61 home runs in a single season. Advanced training techniques, enhanced bats, innovative technology, and nutritional supplements stimulated the offensive explosion.

Traditional thinking alleges that hitting pitchers impose the exploitation of stratagems, but with excessive home runs flying out of NL parks, the AL metamorphosed into the strategic league. Out of the 10 players who finished in the top 10 for batting average and home runs, 6 played in the NL. Once home run–centered, NL strategy lost its vigor. Instead of manufacturing runs by stringing together hits, teams wait to attack their challengers with three-run home runs. AL teams employ hit-and-runs, stolen bases, double steals, and bunts to spur their offense, constituting an exciting game for the players as well as for the fans.

Hearts pound with anticipation as fans watch hit-and-runs unfold. It invokes feelings of promise, like the potential of a profitable inning. While exciting to watch, home runs leave no players on base and no expectation of more to come. While home runs invoke ebullition, long strings of hits draw uninterested spectators into the action.

Retaining one player as an offensive player affords their manager an effortless mission of figuring out his lineup or any changes that may occur during the game. Beyond that of an AL manager, an NL manager reflects before changing pitchers because the pitcher bats. When necessary, the insertion of a relief pitcher follows the removal of the starting pitcher. Relief pitchers refrain from taking batting practice; thus, they seldom hit during games. In order for relief pitchers to refrain from hitting during games, the manager applies a double switch. A bench player replaces a starting defensive player, who departs from the game along with the starting pitcher. The new pitcher occupies the position player's vacated batting spot. The double switch ensures that pitchers do not hit in the NL after the deletion of the starting pitcher; therefore, the NL turns into the AL after eliminating the starting pitcher.

While most pitchers covet the opportunity to contribute to their team's offense, they realize that their team would be better served with a DH hitting for them. Pitchers recognize that hitting negatively effects their pitching because pitchers tire after hitting and running the base paths. When they commence pitching, their legs enervate, and their endurance suffers. Most pitchers use their legs to generate force and velocity, and when their legs fatigue, their velocity declines. Along with a decline in velocity, pitchers suffer losses in their control and command of the strike zone. Skilled hitters recognize this and take full advantage by getting a hit. AL pitchers do not hit; hence, they remain strong and effective throughout the game.

The presence of the DH rule prompts exciting play in the AL because DHs, along with all other hitters, evolved into blended hitters who hit for average, lay down bunts, steal bases, walk, and hit for power. An extra player, who contributes on multiple offensive levels, adds a new dimension to AL baseball. Pitchers seldom hit home runs, and their managers and teammates distrust pitchers to hit on a consistent basis. The DH rule allows the manipulation of multiple strategies. Pitchers accomplish one outcome in two ways: They can yield an unproductive out, or they can construct a productive out. This extra facet makes AL baseball more exciting than NL baseball.

Injured players profit from the existence of a DH rule because injured players can return earlier by performing offense and excluding defense. Playing offense, without defense, allows injured players to avoid dangerous movements such as quick side-to-side movements, twisting, and abrupt stops and starts. This grants the return of a player with a lower extremity injury quicker than usual.

The DH rule also extends the careers of older players by a few years. Various people cite this as an argument against the DH rule, because if a player contributes to merely half the game, then they do not deserve to play. Older players often become DHs because they posses subpar speed and defensive skills. Older players may lose their ability on defense, but they still boast plenty of aptitude for hitting.

Playing DH near the end of their careers allowed Hall of Fame players like Paul Molitor and Dave Winfield to stretch their employment. An older NL player, who suffers from back problems, would retire because of an inability to bend down, even if he could contribute as an offensive weapon for his team. Mark McGuire retired after the 2001 season because of chronic back and knee pain. If he played in the AL, he could have continued his career as a DH. Numerous people paid to watch Mark McGuire thump home runs as a first baseman, and countless more fans would pay to see him blast home runs as a DH.

For the 29 years of the DH rule's existence, baseball purists doubted its success and considered it an experiment that would fade out. Barring any unforeseen complications, the DH rule will subsist for another 29 years and continue to draw fans to baseball.

Exercise

WRITING AN ARGUMENT

Directions: Read the following topics and think about choosing a side and defending it for an argument essay. You must choose one side and defend and/or refute the opposition.

Organization

Introduction: Provides background. Show that a situation exists that has two (or more) sides. For your thesis, provide the side you want to defend.

Body: Provides evidence. Support your claims here with evidence and then use separate paragraphs to show why the opposition's claim is invalid.

Conclusion: Restates your claim. Be sure that your position has been supported and that your claim is clear.

1. In a time of managed care, hospital mergers, stagnant salaries, and downsizing, is moving all professional programs to 6-year graduate-level studies the best for the profession?

2. Should physical therapists (PTs) be allowed to diagnose and dispense physical therapy care without the referral of a physician? This is the case in many (35 I think) states, yet most of the insurance companies in these states do not reimburse for these "unprescribed" services. Should there be a "tenure period" before PTs can practice without referral (for example, 2 years with referral, then direct-access privileges granted)? Should physicians be allowed to own their own PT clinics and refer to them for their own profit?

3. Should PTs be reimbursed for delivering interventions for which we do not have sound evidence (research foundation) of their efficacy? Is this practice ethical? If it is not, we have a problem, as most of what is done in medicine, including PT, is based in anecdotal evidence, not any hard outcome data.

Paper Topics or Issues to Consider for Argument

Consider any of the following controversies to help you formulate a paper.

1. When should you break the patient's confidentiality, if ever?

2. Should a health practitioner lie if it does not harm the patient or promotes some good feeling?

3. If you mistakenly prescribe the wrong medication, but its effects are harmless to the patient, should you notify superiors or the patient?

4. What are your obligations to your profession or colleague if you suspect he or she is abusing drugs or alcohol?

5. Is medical treatment or health care a right or a luxury?

6. If a rape victim seeks treatment but does not want the police involved, what are your obligations?

7. Someone with deep religious convictions refuses medical treatment that could save his or her life. What should you do?

8. If a patient threatens suicide but asks you to keep this information confidential, what are your obligations?

9. What is your role in alerting authorities to patients presenting issues with incest or child abuse?

10. A wife seeks medical treatment for a sexually transmitted disease but claims she is not promiscuous. Is it your responsibility to have her confront her husband for treatment?

11. Can informed consent be given with a blink of the eye?

12. A woman carrying a late-term fetus wants to try a new medication that will help her clear a skin condition. The medication, however, could cause a serious defect in the baby. She wants to take the risk. What do you do?

13. Some diseases are degenerative in nature, and patients will never regain their functional status unless some breakthrough treatment is discovered. Parkinson's disease patients, for example, suffer from degenerative muscle problems, but physical therapy treatments will provide no long-term rewards. Can you recommend treatment and, consequently, insurance coverage for a patient in this condition?

14. After a shootout on the street, three patients arrive in your emergency department with only two beds available in the intensive care unit. Two are policemen, and the other is a drug dealer. Which two get the beds?

15. Can health care providers serve society's needs for medical treatment and still serve their business needs to make (or not lose) money?

16. Many patients seek transplants, and organs are scarce. Who decides which patient gets one and when? If one person needs a liver and is an alcoholic, and another person needs a liver because she lost hers in a car accident, who receives the liver? If one person can pay more for his transplant than another, is he entitled to move up on the list, considering the high costs of the procedure?

17. Most Medicare dollars are spent on patients who are in their last months of life. If a computer program was developed to calculate the life expectancy of these patients, could medical professionals refuse treatment of some to aid the good of the rest?

REVISING YOUR ARGUMENT: CRITICAL READING AND REASONING

Once the document is written, you must re-examine the work through a critical analysis. In the introductory chapters about the writing process, critical reading and writing were addressed. Here, the same principles apply, but the approach is unique. In writing, reading, and revising your arguments, you must be able to read your work as a supporter of the cause and as a dissenter. Reading from these two perspectives will help you formulate a clean argument that does not operate under lapses in logic.

Supporter Perspective

As you write your drafts of the argument essay, you will no doubt read and revise your work as a supporter of your cause. When you have finished the final draft, you must reexamine the text to assure your readers that you have reached your goal. The most important element to remember is that, because you are the one formulating the argument, you may not be able to visualize the argument—you may be too closely tied to it. In other words, you may not read the text as an objective reader, responding to your claims and evidence with a purpose. Look at each paragraph in terms of the thesis, and then ask yourself if the purpose of the paragraph directly supports the claim or thesis. Adding clarifying sentences that connect to your thesis or reinventing your paragraph to meet the needs of the thesis will make your document coherent and unified.

Dissenter Perspective

Not only should you read your own work with the eye of a supporter, but you must also read as a dissenter. This approach will encourage you to challenge your thinking on all fronts. When you read, write comments in the margins of your text. Challenge the claims you make, the evidence you use to support them, and the patterns of reasoning to connect the claims with the evidence. Just as you were instructed to ask questions about varying subjects when you read the work of others, ask the same kinds of questions about your own work. Suggest alternatives to each element of the argument. Can alternative claims be made about the subject? Can alternative evidence be applied here that will make the claim inaccurate? Can alternative forms of reasoning be applied to best shape the argument?

Assessing the Strength of the Argument—Lapses in Logic

Ultimately, the argument is based on value systems or beliefs, and these are debatable. How you support your beliefs with facts and reason will dictate the success of your position. Consequently, be sure that your facts are accurate. In terms of research, be sure that your evidence is authoritative and also well supported by the field. If volumes of research contradict your source, you should understand why and incorporate this thinking into your document. If you challenge the research, you will be inclined to investigate further and solidify your position with additional research and thinking.

Additionally, examine your patterns of reasoning. If you have created lapses in logic, how can you fix them? To understand how lapses in logic occur, read the following list and apply each to your methods of reasoning.

- **Hasty generalization:** a faulty reasoning pattern that results when a claim is made with insufficient evidence. The support for the claim has not been fully verified. For example, a prospective candidate walks into the Youngstown Yacht Club to ask for a membership application. She is greeted by a desk clerk who is rude and abrupt in his comments. The candidate walks out of the club and claims that the yacht club is full of snobs and that she will never consider joining. Her claim is made on the basis of the behavior of one employee, not the group of employees or the membership. Her claim is faulty because of a limited scope of evidence supplied.

- **Agenda-based claims:** a dangerous strategy used frequently in advertising and politics. The argument presents a position or claim, but the claim is based on promoting a specific agenda. For example, chondroitin and glucosamine have been under fire from medical practitioners because the evidence to support the effectiveness of these supplements is not apparent. Accordingly, an argument could claim that the benefits claimed for supplements are not proved, so that consumers should beware of the fact that such supplements may not be efficacious. However, in an agenda-based claim, a rival manufacturer of a drug with similar effects might assert that supplements are not effective and dangerous and should be banned from the marketplace. This claim asserts that the supplements are not effective, which may not be true—the evidence is not in. However, to assert that they are dangerous is another matter. No evidence supports the fact that they are dangerous. The hidden agenda here is to scare the consumer away from the product to protect territory.

- **Circular reasoning:** an error in logic in which the evidence used to support the claim is essentially the claim itself. For example, a student submitted a paper arguing that prayer is just as effective for patient recovery from illness as any other form of treatment. When asked for proof, she responded by asserting that since she believes in prayer, it works. Prayer in itself is part of a belief system. Consequently, her argument as she delineated it is as follows: "Prayer works because I believe prayer works"—an example of circular reasoning.

- **Non sequitur:** a Latin term meaning "it does not follow." Thus, a non sequitur is a statement or concept that does not logically follow what precedes it.

- **Red herring**: another lapse in logic created by misdirecting the reader to support other causes, not the original claim. For example, orthopedic physicians argue that supplements such as glucosamine and chondroitin will not lessen the joint pain caused by osteoarthritis. In support of this claim, the writer may assert that manufacturers of dietary supplements are trying to compete with drug companies for a share of the market, and to protect their share, they will market their products using false information. The information supplied here may or may not be true, but this is not the issue. The purpose of the argument is to prove the effectiveness or ineffectiveness of supplements on osteoarthritis pain. The claim is not supported by the evidence, but the writer attempts to sway readers' opinions by vilifying the opposition. The original claim attempts to convey the message that supplements are not effective; the evidence supplied attempts to achieve the same purpose, but the ideas are not connected. This can also be considered a case of incoherence, or lack of a unified message (covered earlier in Section 1).

Ultimately, these lapses in logic are the result of poor thinking and planning. They can be avoided by recognizing the principles of rational argument and checking your work against reason. Logic is the cornerstone of good writing, and this issue has been covered in several areas of this text, such as in the sections on coherence and unity in Chapter 1 and in the section on critical thinking and reading in Chapter 5. The principles of effective writing are based in logic and reason.

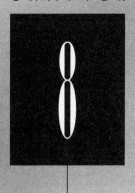

Writing to Inform:

The Research Paper

Key Terms

Authoritative source material Generally accepted by the profession and published in referenced publications

Block quote Direct quotes of more than 40 words, requiring format change

"Cut and paste job" Relying on the words of others to produce the flow of ideas in the text

Direct quote Information taken directly from a source and indicated with quotation marks

Paraphrase Information used that is reinvented in the writer's own language; not a direct quote

Plagiarism Using the works, ideas, or words of others without providing appropriate reference or citation; allowing the reader to assume that borrowed knowledge belongs to the author

Primary research Gathering data and performing experiments to create conclusions

Scholarly research Seeks to use information to launch original thinking

Secondary research Using the published works of others to support claims

Summary A short description of a text's main points or message

Summary research Seeks only to gather information from a variety of sources and synthesize

Synthesis Summaries of texts combined into a paper

chapter objectives

On completion of this chapter, the reader should be able to

1. Understand the differences between primary and secondary research projects.

2. Utilize the appropriate style manuals and meet industry standards for the writing of research papers.

3. Know how to avoid plagiarism.

4. Target a specific audience for scholarly research.

5. Formulate a research question, later to be transformed to a working thesis statement.

6. Create a plan to gather research and assess the authority of researchable material.

7. Define different types of support for research.

8. Develop patterns of reasoning in support of thesis.

9. Borrow information and present it in the appropriate form dictated by the American Psychological Association (APA): paraphrase, direct quote, or block quote.

10. Build a "References" section according to standards dictated by the APA.

11. Understand the need for direct quotes, paraphrasing, and summarizing and implement when appropriate.

12. Demonstrate an ability to quote borrowed material to accurately represent its meaning and tenor.

13. Utilize marks of punctuation to integrate the words of others into the text.

14. Demonstrate an ability to paraphrase borrowed information to accurately represent its meaning and to avoid using the language of the author to do so.

*E*xpository writing gives explanations or provides information. This information can derive from experts in the field or through your own experimentation. Ultimately, informative writing relies on facts and research and is most often used in professional environments.

Although informative or research writing is not organized like an argumentative essay, it does aim to convince. Most writing aims to influence the reader to accept what is written. Informative writing can serve to educate because it is based in fact and, as a result, is objective by nature. Conclusions can be reproduced or verified by others in the field or through the research the writer provides. Additionally, information must be accurate and correct.

Furthermore, since research or informative work is objective, it should be arranged in logical sequence and clearly written and presented. A discussion of the forms of reasoning, similar to the patterns introduced in Chapter 7, is presented in this chapter. Likewise, writing style should match the objective nature of your content.

This chapter explores subtle variations of the research-based writing you will perform for academic exploration and for professional development.

THE ACADEMIC RESEARCH PAPER

Research papers come in two species: summary and scholarly. Papers based on **summary research** are the type you have already written in high school or in introductory writing classes. For a summary research paper, you simply discover a topic, find some sources about the topic, and then synthesize this information into a paper to give an overview. This form of research writing will be used sparingly in your professional and academic writing pursuits. As you advance in your studies, you will be required to write papers that contribute to the field's scholarly dialogue. Simply synthesizing what others have said is no longer adequate. Instead, your

professors and mentors will expect that you read the research that is published and then contribute original thinking to it. This type of **scholarly research** will be expected for your thesis or dissertation and for articles that you publish in the future.

Follow the same recursive writing process when you write your research paper and draft it. You will, however, need to add additional steps in the planning stages to help you make progress. These additional steps are discussed next.

Purpose and Audience

The audience for your research papers is an educated group of scholars and colleagues. Write for their sake, but do not assume that all scholars know everything about every subject. This is an impossible expectation. You should also consider your instructor as your audience, not as a user of the specific scientific data you have collected but as the person responsible for assessing how well you manage this information. The term *manage* here indicates that you will gather appropriate source material and make sense of it for your professional or scholarly audience. Presentation also encompasses correctness and the ability to demonstrate competence in research paper formatting.

Writing research papers indicates that you are writing to find answers. Consequently, all researchers and writers begin with a question to answer. How you formulate this question or arrive at it is a unique process of reading and discovery that you as a writer must find. Formulating the question requires study and focus. As you formulate your research question, you will narrow your subject and give your paper direction. Think of it as a thesis statement.

Finding an appropriate thesis statement derived from a research question is difficult because not every question is a researchable subject. For example, the following research questions are *ineffective* because they leave open too many variables and lack focus:

Why is crime on the rise?

Why do high school students use drugs and alcohol?

Why do children fail to learn?

Such questions ask a writer merely to call attention to the problem instead of finding real answers, unless these are the questions that precede a dissertation or multivolume work on the subject.

Effective research questions are narrowly focused, have a single problem to address, or have clear boundaries. The following research questions are appropriately narrow in focus:

> Is physical therapy a viable treatment for Parkinson's disease?
>
> How does temporomandibular joint (TMJ) dysfunction occur and what are its short- and long-term effects?
>
> Is stuttering a physical or a psychological dilemma?

Developing a clear and narrowly focused research question arms you with a direction or purpose when you begin to gather research.

Gathering Research

Many students believe that the first step in writing a research paper is to enter the library and begin gathering texts or articles about a general category of study or interest—to conduct **secondary research**. If you approach the paper in this manner, you will suffer from disorganization, and your paper will consume most of your waking time.

> *General Rule: Find a problem that interests you and formulate a question to be answered before you begin gathering source material.*

Regarding research as a quest for an answer gives you your focus. You cannot know whether you have found useful material unless you know for what you are looking.

Your purpose is to provide information and give answers, but this may not always be possible. You may be forced to conduct **primary research**, or the original experiments, to find the best answers to your question. If you fail to find appropriate research or fail to find definitive answers, you have not failed in your writing. Some research papers indicate that little research has been completed on a subject, and that certain questions or issues need to be addressed. Other papers show that a simple answer cannot be provided. Still others raise

more questions and set up the basis for further or future research. If you find no information and feel yourself wasting time, abandon the topic, but give it serious consideration first.

Your ultimate purpose in gathering and writing research papers is to make yourself more informed about a particular subject. We, as scholars, cannot know everything about everything, but we can become knowledgeable in a certain area of study or specialize in a field. Find your interests, but, most important, demonstrate your expertise in the field by contributing original thoughts.

Evaluating Source Material

Gathering research data is often a process unique to each individual. We all have strategies that work for us or frustrate us, and we can choose which strategies to employ and which to ignore.

Various sources are available for research studies: library books, reference works, periodicals, government documents, electronic resources (databases, CD-ROMs, Internet sites), and interviews with professionals in the field. If you are unclear about the use of any of these sources, consult the APA style manual for help or seek help from your reference librarian. Your librarians are employed to help you. Use their expertise to help you locate sources and gather information.

This text will not assume that every writer of academic or professional research understands how to evaluate the source material they find for authority and reliability. Books, journal articles, and printed information you find in your library are acceptable for any or most research projects because the library acts as a filter to keep out illegitimate research. For journals, academicians, an editorial board, or other experts in the field review submissions to determine if the work is worthwhile and legitimate. These groups confer and accept or deny work that is submitted for publication. Working through this process, such groups establish what is acceptable as quality research and what is not. Many works are rejected for various reasons (see section on writing the journal article in Chapter 10).

Most, if not all, of the journals and books in your library are considered legitimate research tools, but the Internet has created confusion among students and aspiring scholars. The Internet poses unique problems because the World Wide Web hosts material that can appear on many different types of Web pages and in various formats. The polished appearance of such material may give the "feel" that the work is legitimate, but you need to be able to check it against some established standards. Most of your professors and scholars in the field will advise you against using any source material from the Web because the quality, authority, and reliability of the information there vary. The problem with the information that you find on the Web is that it appears to be *published*. Published information, as you now know, must be reviewed by a team of scholars or editors—but in fact, anyone can "post" anything to the Web. (*Publish* is not a term to be used with the Web because the word *publish* implies authority and reliability. More accurate terms are "post" and "upload.") As a general rule, do not borrow from any source that has a ".com" suffix. A ".com" Web address can be purchased by any party and used for any purpose. In fact, this is the essence of the problems created by the Web: People post false or misleading information, and readers accept it as truth. Consider also the radical sites that promote sexual deviance and/or ethnic bias. These sites dwell in the same world as many "research" sites or information storehouses.

You should avoid ".com" sites entirely, even if the sources posted there "look" legitimate—such as a journal article that has been reproduced—because the material may violate copyright law. As a professional, you do not want to promote work that infringes on the intellectual property rights of scholars in your field.

Although ".com" sites should be avoided, students may think that other sites ending in other prefixes are legitimate. This is not always true. Surf around the Web and look at some of the material on ".edu," ".gov," or ".org" Web sites. The information found on ".edu" sites you would think would be legitimate because it is posted on an educational institution's Web site. Many times, student papers, which are not accurate or reliable, are posted to discussion boards or are held up as examples of work well done. These are not reliable sources, obviously, but such papers may appear on the Web with the institution's Web address as the source. Often, professors who cannot publish their work in refereed venues (because of various reasons) will post their work to the Web as a means of self-publishing or self-promotion. Again, this information is not to be trusted because it is not refereed. Sources that derive from ".org" or ".gov" are more reliable, but put them to the tests of validity before using them.

Sadly, the storehouses of research papers, at sites like "cheat.com," must also be addressed. First, anyone who cheats will eventually be caught and punished. Second, the information and papers that are on these sites are generally weak work created by weak students. Your academic preparation will quickly reveal to you that these documents are not worth the time it takes to download them. Third, as technology increases in complexity, ways to cheat will increase in complexity; however, students who cheat fail to realize that technology advances on both sides. For every advance made by cheaters, academics and scholars create better and more effective ways to catch them. Scholars and instructors have access to Internet technology that helps verify whether a paper is plagiarized or stolen. Suspect papers can be submitted to services that scan all on-line documents to match words and phrases with the sources from which they came. Technology advances make cheating more difficult. Do your work and engage the process to better yourself and learn.

Determining Authority in Resources

Use the following guidelines to help you determine if a source is a legitimate one:

1. Reliable source material: A source is reliable if it is published in a venue that is refereed by scholars or professional editorial staff members of the field. Anything published in university presses, in scholarly journals, or by presses specializing in scholarly work is acceptable. Information published in weekly news magazines and newspapers

should be checked for accuracy since many of these are written with strong political or social slant.

To check the reliability of material found on line:

- Check to see if authors, dates, publishing places, or other publication data are presented. If they are not, do not use the source, or find the original source of publication before using it.

- Be aware of sites that intend to incite action or to sway opinion on issues of controversy. Usually, these are persuasive essays and not research-based essays and therefore are not reliable.

2. **Authoritative source material:** A source is authoritative if it is a part of the field's scholarly dialogue. Check to see if the article is referenced by other scholars in their work or in bibliographies about the subject.

To check the authority of material found on line:

- Find the author's name on the source. If the author's name is omitted, do not use.

- If the author is named on the site, check for credentials. Be sure that the author is considered an expert in the field. Assess such background information by identifying the author's advanced degree or position at universities, colleges, or research institutions.

- Check to see that borrowed information is documented according to a standard style manual and that conclusions are well reasoned and clearly supported.

3. On-line materials to avoid:
   E-mail
   Usenet groups
   Chat rooms
   SPAM

Be judicious in the material used for support of your research. You jeopardize your standing as a professional by using illegitimate resources. Your profession expects you to police your ranks, and your instructors do as well.

Supporting Ideas

Once researchers gather the appropriate information, they must find ways to express and prove their ideas in the context of the research paper. Supporting material is the content that fits into the established framework and gives the writer's claim the support it needs to make it valid to any reader.

Supporting material exists in many forms, but the most relevant forms to the research writing experience are the following:

- Explanation: the supporting rationale for any claim that answers questions about what, how, and why. Usually, this information is found in researchable material such as theoretical developments or in like experiments.

- Statistics: the use of numbers to show tendencies. Statistics can be used to demonstrate trends (such as conditions occurring over time: "the number of ADHD-diagnosed children has jumped X% in the last 10 years"), magnitude (such as amounts by comparison: "New York is the highest taxed state in the country, compared with California, Massachusetts, and New Jersey"), or segments (such as breaking down a whole to examine the parts: "percentages of obese versus malnourished children in the United States").

- Examples: illustrations of the point being made. They can be factual or hypothetical, detailed or undeveloped, depending on the needs of the audience.

- Testimony: the opinions or conclusions of others. Expert opinions often carry the most weight, but common opinion, such as those demonstrated in polls, is often used to discuss trends in thinking or acting. In either case, the issue of credibility is important. Determining what sources influence your audience is governed by the subject or purpose.

Patterns of Reasoning

In any research writing experience, the author/writer asserts a claim and supports it with verifiable supporting evidence. However, in many cases, the most important element of critical thinking is ignored: reasoning. Reasoning is the element of thinking that links the support to the claim and allows the reader to draw conclusions.

Reasoning patterns that are generally accepted by critical thinkers and writers of research papers are (1) deductive reasoning, (2) inductive reasoning, (3) causal reasoning, (4) reasoning from sign, (5) reasoning from parallel case, (6) reasoning by analogy, and (7) reasoning from authority.

Deductive Reasoning, or Reasoning from Generalization

The generalization begins with a generally accepted premise and applies that premise to a specific instance:

Premise: Excessive consumption of saturated fats is unhealthy.

Instance: Cheese contains high levels of saturated fats.

Conclusion: We should limit our intake of cheese to remain healthy.

Inductive Reasoning, or Reasoning from Example

Examine a set of specific facts, circumstances, or instances and draw a conclusion from the sample. Thus, analysis of specific examples leads to a conclusion about the whole.

Fact 1: The University of Buffalo has not recruited class A players for its basketball program this year.

Fact 2: St. Bonaventure University has not recruited class A players for its basketball program this year.

Fact 3: Niagara University has not recruited class A players for its basketball program this year.

Conclusion: Quality recruiting is a problem for Western New York colleges.

In inductive reasoning, the conclusion is only as effective as the depth of the examples. Consequently, to be fair when using this type of reasoning in research, the samples must be representative and typical and be taken from a wide variety of sources or population.

Causal Reasoning

In causal reasoning, the writer relies on the assumption that the world and its functioning parts are predictable. The writer connects an event, A, with an event that follows it, B, and determines that B is the result or consequence of A.

Event A: School violence has increased in the last ten years.

Event B: Video games with violent content have increased in popularity in the last ten years.

Conclusion: Video games with violent content are the cause of increased school violence.

The problem with this type of reasoning is that many writers oversimplify the process or make generalizations. They fail to consider other factors that contribute to, influence, or cause the event. For example, in the foregoing sample, the causes of increased school violence can be far reaching. Simply pinning the problems of violence among young people on the use of video games is not reasonable because too many factors influence the actions of young people. In this sample, the research argument would be better served by concluding that video games may be a contributing factor, not the sole cause.

Reasoning from Sign

An observable mark indicates that a condition exists. If the water in my backyard ice rink is frozen, then I can conclude that the temperature has fallen below 32° Fahrenheit. In business, economic indicators are examples of reasoning from sign. When market indexes are up, they indicate a strong economy.

For medical practitioners, reasoning from sign is used most often. A practitioner will use an observable mark as evidence for a certain state or condition. For example, presenting symptoms such as a "runny nose," sore throat, and persistent cough, indicate that the patient has a cold.

Reasoning from Parallel Case

Parallel case reasoning compares two subjects and concludes that if the two share similar characteristics, then they must also share others. For example, the writer may state that Niagara University should implement a program to fund apartment-style dorms because St. Bonaventure University implemented a successful program to fund its new, apartment-style dorms. The strength of this connection resides in the degree of similarity between the two entities being compared. In this case, Niagara and St. Bonaventure are both small, private, Catholic colleges in Western New York with similar programs, enrollment criteria, and numbers.

Consider the weakness of the following parallel case reasoning: Buffalo should develop its waterfront into a shopping and restaurant mall because Baltimore has developed its waterfront successfully in this manner. Baltimore and Buffalo are cities with similar histories, but their waterfronts are not similar and their climates are dissimilar. Consequently, to be sure of logical reasoning, compare similarities and differences of the two items or issues being discussed and be sure that you are comparing apples with apples.

Reasoning by Analogy

Like the parallel case form, reasoning by analogy compares two things, but the items in comparison are different. For example, I often compare my daughter to a squirrel because she hides food in her cheeks. Thus, the use of analogy may be weakened when the items compared are too dissimilar to make a valid conclusion. My daughter exhibits only that one characteristic of a squirrel. She does not dart around the room in a haphazard motion nor does she climb trees or dart out into traffic. Ultimately, analogies are used to clarify or provide insight rather than argue.

Reasoning from Authority

The issue of authority is most used in the writing of research papers. The validity of any claim made by a student writer is often dependent on the sources used to reach those conclu-

sions. If the sources come from experts in their fields, then their conclusions are generally accepted because the reader will assume that the researchers have done their job well.

Consider the following example:

> According to Albert Bigelow Paine, the biographer of Samuel Clemmens, the author-persona Mark Twain died a miserable man because of many failed business ventures.

As readers, we accept the fact that Twain died a miserable man not because we know Twain's history but because we know that Paine has established himself as an expert in the field if he is the biographer. Often, the issue of authority is not challenged, however, and this can lead to horrible mistakes that can be spread across time. For example, Edgar Allan Poe's biographer was an enemy who invented the depraved, notorious character that many people know. Not until 1941, with the reassessment of Poe's letters and documents, was the record set straight. However, the myth of Poe's depravity was exciting to the reading public, and the stories have stayed with him until this day.

The validity of this type of claim rests with the true authority of the source. Be sure of your author's expertise by checking for credentials and expertise. Also, a good researcher will determine any biases the author might hold after reading other published works by that author.

Do not assume that anyone who is in the public eye is an expert. Many students hear Hollywood stars voice their concerns about political or social issues. Such people are not experts; they are using their celebrity to further a cause in which they believe.

CITING SOURCES IN APA STYLE

Borrowing information, as you know, requires you to credit the authors from whom you have borrowed. When you borrow, you present the information as a quote, as a summary, or as a **paraphrase**. For every piece of information borrowed, you must provide an in-text citation according to the format established by the APA or another style manual stipulated by your professors.

In the APA format, the author listing is most important. It is the element of your work that leads your reader to the appropriate source (in your "References" section) for further reading or for evaluation of source material. If you fail to provide the correct name, your reader will not be able to find the source you listed in your "References," which lists all of the works you have cited. If you have an in-text citation that refers to nothing in your "References," the accuracy, authority, and reliability of your work become immediately suspect.

Forms of In-Text Citations

Paraphrased Information

The APA requires you to list the author and year of publication after any information that is borrowed in paraphrased form.

> Rugby is played on a pitch and not on a field (Jones, 1987).

Notice the format here that must be followed. After the end of the borrowed information in paraphrase form, skip one space and insert an opening parenthesis. Type the author's name, a comma, and the date of publication, and then type a closing parenthesis. The period of the sentence then appears *after* the in-text citation.

If you mention the author's name in the context of your written work, you can create the citation in the following manner:

> According to Jones (1987), rugby players compete on a pitch and not on a field.

Directly Quoted Information

Information that is rewritten in its original form also must be attributed to the author, but additional information is required. First, place all words borrowed directly from the source within quotation marks, providing that you have not quoted more than 40 words in consecutive order (40 words or more appear as a **block quote**, formatted as described in the next section). Second, the in-text citation now requires the author's last name, date of publication, *and* page number from source, listed as *p.* and then the number. A single space separates all the elements of the in-text citation and/or after all marks of punctuation, and the period to terminate the sentence is placed after the citation.

> Rugby is "played on a pitch 110 yards long and 75 yards across" (Jones, 1987, p. 20).

If you introduce the author within the context of your written work, you do not need to duplicate the author's name in the in-text citation.

> According to Jones, rugby is "played on a pitch 110 yards long and 75 yards across" (1987, p. 20).

It could also be written as follows:

> According to Jones (1987), rugby is "played on a pitch 110 yards long and 75 yards across" (p. 20).

Variations in sentence structure and presentation can result when the writer decides to offer additional information about the author, such as credentials, or about the source material, such as place of publication.

> According to Jones (1987), who was a member of the World Cup championship team and whose work appears in *Rugby Magazine*, rugby is "played on a pitch 110 yards long and 75 yards across" (p. 20).

Block Quotes

If you cite 40 or more continuous words from one source, you should present your information in a block quote. A block quote is distinguishable from a running **direct quote** in three ways:

1. Block quotes begin a new line, and all lines of the quote are indented 5 spaces from the left margin (lines up with paragraph indentation).

2. Block quotes use no quotation marks.

3. Block quotes require that the terminal mark of punctuation at its end be placed *before* the in-text citation.

EXAMPLE:

According to an article in *Rugby Magazine*, the future of rugby in the United States looks promising:

> Rubgy is played on a pitch 110 yards long and 75 yards across. This is roughly the size of an American football field, which makes playing facilities easy to locate. Furthermore, fewer injuries occur in rugby than in football, basketball, or lacrosse. Surprisingly, more head injuries occur in soccer than in rugby. (Jones, 1987, p. 20)

Such statistics surprise many parents, but most still feel that the sport is barbaric, and they keep their children away from contact sports.

Variations in In-Text Citations

Citing a Work by Title

When the author's name is not known, use an abbreviated form of the title that includes the first word that would normally indicate its place in the alphabetized References page. The following information is from an article with the title "Paving the Way for Rugby in America."

> Rugby injuries are far less severe than in other contact sports ("Paving the Way . . . ," 1987).

Citing Multiple Authors

To cite multiple authors, use the following conventions:

Two different sources indicating the same evidence:

> (Jones, 1987; Smith, 1990)

Two authors of one source:

> (Jones & Smith, 1987)

Three, four, or five authors of one source:

> First instance:
> (Jones, Smith, Wells, & Carver, 1999)
> Second and subsequent occurrences:
> (Jones et al., 1999)

Six or more authors of one source:

> All instances:
> (Jones et al., 1999)

Note: All questions about variations can be addressed through the APA style manual.

The References Section

General Concerns

- Alphabetize your entries according to the last name of the author(s). If no author is available, use the first significant word of the title.

- Double-space all entries.

- Use hanging style indentation. First line is full width. All others are indented.

- All punctuation marks require only ONE space following their insertion.

- Author entries include last name, first initial, and middle initial, if offered.

- Use an ampersand before the last author in the list (e.g., "Glenns, Jones, & Smith").

Format Considerations for Books

Jones, D., & Smith, K. (1999). The new rules of rugby. New York: Corrigan & Wells.

- Capitalize only the first word of a book's title, proper nouns in the title, or the first word following a colon.

- Underline the title of the book.

- Give city of publication if it is recognizable as a large city in the United States. If it is not, offer the city and the two-letter abbreviation of the state:

  Lewiston, NY:

- Eliminate words such as *Co.*, *Inc.*, or *Publishers*" from the publication data, but include *Press* if offered.

Format Considerations for Journal Articles

Jones, D., & Smith, K. (1999). Paving the way for rugby in America. Rugby Magazine, 44, 20–24.

- Titles of articles are not underlined or italicized.

- Capitalize only the first word of an article's title, proper nouns in the title, or the first word following a colon.

- Capitalize the titles of journals as you would any title and underline.

- Use a continuous underscore from the title of the journal through the volume number and the comma after the volume number.

- No *p.* or *pp.* is necessary for pagination listing.

Electronic Resources

Jones, D. & Smith, K. (1999). Paving the way for rugby in America. Rugby Magazine, 44, 20–24. [Database] EBSCO Host: Academic Search Full Text Elite.

- After the publication information, include in brackets a description of the source. This could also include "CD-ROM" or other variations of information storehouses.

- Include the name of the database hosting service as well as the source in which the article appears. The Web address is not necessary here because typing in the address from the Web will not lead your reader into a password-secured database. If your reader wants to access the information, he or she can find the original or search the database with the information provided.

Jones, D., & Smith, K. (August 1999). Paving the way for rugby in America. The Buffalo News, p. A-6/ [On-line newspaper]. Retrieved October 7, 2000 from the World Wide Web: http://www.buffalonews.com/rugby/america

- The date listed after the author is the date the information was posted to the Web.

- The brackets indicate the type of on-line source, which could also be "On-line journal," "Electronic version," and so on.

- The date of retrieval is self-explanatory but does not appear in any other entry type.

- No period ends the Web address unless it is part of the Web address.

As always, check the APA manual for variations or problems.

Exercise

BUILDING THE REFERENCES SECTION

Directions: Reinvent the following list of references according to an acceptable style manual format. Identify what type of source is listed; then apply the appropriate format. Be sure to identify and change problems in mechanics (capitalization, underlining) as well as simple formatting.

1. Lanshire, Phillip. "Why We Need Direct Access" Home page: http://www.chass.com
2. Snyder, Peter and Diane Olsen. "A Pore Segment: DEG in Channels." Journal of Biological Sciences, 1999, 24, p. 74. Chem Abstracts database, May 24, 2000, www.Chemabstracts.com/pore/
3. Bowling, A. (1997). Research Methods in Health: an Investigation of the Brain. Buckingham, Open Univ. Press.
4. Measuring Disease. Handbook of qualitative research. 2000. pp. 47-59.
5. Publication Manual of the American Psychological Association. (your edition)
6. Lewitus, A.J., R.V. Jesien, T.W. Kana, E. May, M. Herzog, J.H. Hawkins, and R.S. Cone. 1990. Species distribution of Ulcerative Lesions of Pimlico Sound Fish. Journal of Aquatic Research, 22, 1304.

QUOTING, SUMMARIZING, AND PARAPHRASING

To successfully participate in the field's scholarly dialogue, any writer or researcher must understand the methods of incorporating other scholars' work into their own writing. Citing borrowed information most often provides support for claims or adds credibility to your writing by demonstrating the ideas you are presenting derive from serious scholars and their work. Documentation is a way of telling your reader that you are standing on the shoulders of some bright people who have created these studies before you. However, citing borrowed information can also help you demonstrate a timeline of previous research that dictates that your work is the logical next step. Citing information from others allows you to provide your readers with examples of various perspectives on a subject. In fact, expert researchers often use dissenting opinions to formulate an argument regarding the subject and to further represent that their views are different for a reason. To become an expert researcher, incorporate the following mechanisms into your work.

Direct Quotations

The earlier section "Directly Quoted Information" delineates how to quote directly, but a paper filled with direct quotes does not always result in good writing. Have a reason to quote someone directly. If the words are exceptionally strong, use them, but do not dominate your paper with direct quotes (some authorities call for less than 10% of the paper or document to be directly quoted). Direct quotations are simple reproductions of the writers' words you have borrowed, but a paper filled with quotations begins to lose its authorial voice. In other words, you are no longer the voice dominating the paper; the voice of the borrowed information takes over, and your voice is lost. Research work that borrows direct quotes too often is called a "**cut and paste job**."

Such "cut and paste" papers will often earn poor marks, if not failing grades, because someone else has done your work for you. The paper that quotes heavily but depends on only one source is even weaker. This type of paper lacks original thinking or relies on the work of another author, which defeats the purpose of your writing altogether. Your job is to assimilate others' ideas and springboard from them into some original thinking of your own.

Original thinking is the key to writing a research paper. Many students who are not clear in their purpose will rush to the library, find a few texts on a particular subject, and then select an idea that can fit into a paper. This type of research is called **synthesis** and does not constitute the type of scholarly work that is necessary for research at an advanced level of study. Syntheses can be used for parts of a

paper (called summaries), but the real thinking and original ideas come from you and not another source. Have something original to say, and your focus will naturally rest on your ideas, not on another's. Use sources to back up what you claim, use them as a springboard to take the study further, or apply them to another situation. When you use information in this manner, you will want to condense borrowed information in order to get to your ideas and presentation. Much of this type of writing is done through the use of the paraphrase.

Paraphrases

Paraphrased material borrows someone else's ideas and presents them in your own words, but the paraphrase still requires the in-text citation, according to APA style. Paraphrasing is not a method of changing a few words or substituting synonyms to call the words your own even though the ideas are not your own. Read the later section, "How to Avoid Plagiarism," to fully understand the methods of paraphrasing.

Summaries

To summarize an article, reduce the text to its major findings in one or two sentences. The **summary** is a generalization concerning the major point the article makes or determines the reason the article was written. The summary most often is used as an introductory element to research writing critiques or as the foundation to longer research projects (thesis or dissertation) such as literature reviews. Literature reviews are important to the viability of major research undertakings in that they establish the history of previously completed research, thereby establishing your work in the line of necessary research.

HOW TO AVOID PLAGIARISM

To successfully compete in any academic setting, writers must know how to cite material borrowed from sources or else be faced with charges of plagiarism. **Plagiarism**, or using another's ideas or words without acknowledging them, is often the source of many stumbling blocks for writers. Most writers would not copy someone else's paper and put their name on it. This is the most obvious—and most easily detected—form of plagiarism. Instead, in most cases, plagiarism occurs out of ignorance of the rules of writing and attribution. Many writers who are penalized for plagiarism (by a failing grade for the assignment or for the course, or presentation before a judiciary board for expulsion) do not know that they have broken the law, but ignorance of the law does not excuse them from being held to it. Many do not realize that they have borrowed "too closely," yet the charges and punishments remain the same.

This section demonstrates how to avoid the actions that lead to inadvertent plagiarism.

Direct Quotes

Information that is directly quoted must be placed in quotation marks and provided with an in-text citation. Most important, the quotation must be exactly as the author has written it. To avoid any confusion about who owns the information presented, always introduce your author or source somewhere in the sentence. You do not need to conceal the fact that you are borrowing information—in fact, be forthcoming about it.

Changes to the quote, including removing words or changing the tenses of verbs for readability, must be noted with the use of indicators such as the ellipsis (three dots) or brackets.

The Ellipsis

For a smooth transition between borrowed words and your own, you may be required to eliminate some words from the original. In other cases, you may need to eliminate unnecessary information from a quote. For these situations, use the ellipsis.

Integrating your words with the direct quote will help build cohesion and unity within your text. When you eliminate words or entire sentences from a quote, you must indicate that you have altered the direct quote because now it

does not appear exactly as it does in the original source. The ellipsis is the indicator you will use, and to create one, type three periods and skip spaces between them. An ellipsis that ends a sentence still requires a terminal mark of punctuation. Be sure to skip a space after the last ellipsis period, and then type the terminating period. Consider the following example:

> **ORIGINAL:** "Mary had a little lamb, little lamb, little lamb; Mary had a little lamb whose fleece was white as snow" (Goose, 1803, p. 4).

> **WORDS OMITTED:** "Mary had a little lamb . . . whose fleece was white as snow" (Goose, 1803, p. 4).

Understanding how quotations create coherence breaks is the sign of a mature writer. You cannot simply insert quotes into your text and expect your reader to make leaps across breaks in coherence. You must provide transitional elements or integrate the quotes into your work smoothly. Integrating your quotes into *your* words makes the borrowed information easily manageable by your reader and allows you to maintain authority over the borrowed information and the direction of your paper.

> According to Mother Goose, one of Mary's ewes birthed a lamb and its "fleece was white . . . " (Goose, 1803, p. 4).

Brackets

Use brackets to indicate that you have added words or any other elements of the sentence for readability or to indicate incorrectness.

> **ORIGINAL:** Looking over the side of the bridge created a dizzying affect in his behaviour, as he stumbled and fell.

> **REVISED:** "Looking over the side of the bridge created a dizzying [e]ffect in his behaviour, as he stumbled and fell."

> **ORIGINAL:** Looking over the side of the bridge "can effect behaviour," as he stumbled and fell.

> **REVISED:** Looking over the side of the bridge "[a]ffect[ed his] behaviour," as he stumbled and fell.

If, for instance, the spelling of a word or the grammar used was incorrect in the original, you could indicate the problem within the quote by using [sic].

EXAMPLE: Looking over the side of the bridge created a dizzying [e]ffect in his behaviour [sic], as he stumbled and fell.

Acceptable and Unacceptable Uses of Direct Quotations

Read the following passage from an article entitled "A Brand-New Olmsted" from the April 2001 edition of *The Atlantic* (p. 26). Then assess the comments that follow the passage to determine problems in direct quotation.

ORIGINAL

The Scranton Public Library, also known as the Albright Memorial Building, was built thanks to the generosity of John Joseph Albright, a Buffalo financier who had grown up in Scranton and made a vast fortune in the coal-shipping business. In 1890 he and his three siblings donated the land, which was the site of the family homestead, and Albright pledged to pay for the construction of the new building. He knew exactly what he wanted, specifying that the building should be designed by his Buffalo architect, Edward B. Green, and that the grounds should be landscaped by the Brookline, Massachusetts, firm of Olmsted, Olmsted and Eliot.

COMMENTS

1. The Scranton Public Library's gardens were designed by Federick Law Olmsted in 1890. "He knew exactly what he wanted." *(Quote does not relate clearly to rest)*

2. Albright wanted the Library "designed by Edward B. Green and the ground landscaped by Olmsted, Olmsted, and Eliot." *(Words omitted from quote without indication)*

3. Albright's legacy in Scranton is the public library, with "its grounds should be landscaped by the Brookline, Massachusetts, firm of Olmsted, Olmsted and Eliot." *(Verb shift)*

Steps to Creating Acceptable Paraphrasing

A paraphrase expresses the essential information from a source but does so in your own words. This technique will help you reduce the amount of directly quoted material in your text (avoid the "cut and paste"), and it will help you build consistency in the presentation of ideas in

your document. Paraphrasing does not mean that you can simply change a few words, reverse word order, or provide synonyms. An effective paraphrase presents the information in a manner that is consistent with your style of writing and demonstrates your full grasp of the material.

To create an effectively written paraphrase, follow these steps:

1. Read, reread, digest, and reread the original passage to gain a full and complete understanding of the information presented.

2. Distance yourself from the original. If you have to, turn over the paper or close the book from which you are citing. This will force you to come to terms with the information by using your own words. *(Keeping the text in your line of vision will invariably tempt you to look at the words used by the author and use them as your own. This is not an effective method and leads to plagiarism.)*

3. Write on the top of your note paper a few key words or phrases that will help you organize your thinking. Create the passage.

4. Compare your paraphrase with the original for accuracy in information presented. Be sure that your words indicate the exact message that the author conveys.

5. Check your paper for words or phrases that have been borrowed. Sometimes, our understanding of a text or passage derives from the fact that we memorize key words or phrases from the text that have meaning for us. Invariably, if this occurs, you will use those terms in your paraphrase. If you must use words from the original because the phrases or terms are extraordinary or unique to your field, place those words or phrases in quotation marks and follow the rules for citing information in direct quotes.

6. Place the appropriate citation at the end of the paraphrase: author and date of publication.

Acceptable and Unacceptable Forms of Paraphrasing

Read the following passage again and then compare the acceptable and unacceptable versions of the original in the subsequent para-phrases. Examine documentation style and method as well, and look for inconsistencies.

ORIGINAL

The Scranton Public Library, also known as the Albright Memorial Building, was built thanks to the generosity of John Joseph Albright, a Buffalo financier who had grown up in Scranton and made a vast fortune in the coal-shipping business. In 1890 he and his three siblings donated the land, which was the site of the family homestead, and Albright pledged to pay for the construction of the new building. He knew exactly what he wanted, specifying that the building should be designed by his Buffalo architect, Edward B. Green, and that the grounds should be land-scaped by the Brookline, Massachusetts, firm of Olmsted, Olmsted and Eliot.

UNACCEPTABLE VERSION

The Public Library in Scranton, Pennsylvania, was donated by the generous John Joseph Albright, a millionaire who made his fortune in the coal-shipping industry. In 1890, Albright and his broth-ers donated the family homestead for the library, and Albright paid for the entire project. He knew exactly what the building should look like, so he hired Buffalo architect Edward B. Green to design the building and the firm of Olmsted, Olmsted and Eliot to design the grounds. (*The Atlantic*, 2001)

ACCEPTABLE VERSION

According to *The Atlantic*, John Joseph Albright and his brothers donated some of their family's land in 1890 to build the public library in Scran-ton, Pennsylvania. Albright wanted the building to reflect his style; consequently, since he had worked with both in the past, he hired Edward B. Green as his architect and Frederick Law Olm-sted's design firm to develop the gardens and courtyards (*The Atlantic*, 2001).

Exercise

PARAPHRASING

Directions: Read the following passages and then write acceptable paraphrases of each.

1. The University of Michigan time-analysis data confer that traditional college-aged students spent the bulk of their lives in structured, adult-oriented activities. They are the most honed and supervised generation in human history. If they are group-oriented, deferential to authority, and achievement-obsessed, it is because we achievement-besotted adults have trained them to be. We have devoted our prodigious energies to imposing a sort of order and responsibility on our kids' lives that we never experienced ourselves. [from Brooks, D. (April 2001). The organizational kid. <u>The Atlantic</u>, <u>287</u>(4): 40–54.]

2. Opiate poisoning is easily treated and reversed with naloxone. Large doses of naloxone may be needed to treat massive opiate overdoses because it has a short half-life of only 15–20 minutes. Treating opiate overdose in chronic opiate user can precipitate acute withdrawal. Classic symptoms of acute withdrawal include vomiting, cramping, and yawning, and sweating. [from Salyer, S. W. & Battista, R. (2001). Managing the acutely poisoned patient. <u>Physician Assistant</u>, <u>25</u>(6): 41–49.]

3. Following the fall salmon run, steelhead trout enter the Niagara River, feeding greedily on the millions of eggs deposited by the spawn-ing salmon. Steelhead are a silvery lake-run version of rainbow trout, and the best time to fish for these hard fighters is December through March. Fishing is done with small "kwikfish" lures or by drifting egg skeins near the river bottom. [from Raykovicz, M. (2001). Niagara: River of opportunity. <u>New York State Conservationist</u>, <u>55</u>(6): 19–21.]

Exercise

WRITING A RESEARCH PAPER

Directions: At this point, you have written papers that demonstrate your position on a controversial topic. Your next assignment asks that you support your position with verifiable and appropriate research.

Step 1: Choose one paper or topic and revise the document to meet the professional writing standards. If necessary, reinvent the paper (start over) to allow for the addition of evidence or research.

Step 2: Research your topic thoroughly by ref-erencing appropriate journals, textbooks, or electronic source material. Remember that your resources must be appropriate for professional writing. Consequently, do not depend on ".com" Web sites to support your material or magazines that slant material to one political/social opinion. *(Note: If you must use Web resources, make sure that you verify the legitimacy of ".edu" or ".org" suffixes.)* Electronic databases are best for secondary resources. See your librarians for help.

Step 3: Add research to your argument. Maintain your argument throughout the paper, and support it with verifiable evidence from your legitimate resources (research). The arguments you present should stress *your* position. Do not allow another source to write your paper for you.

Step 4: Follow the guidelines of the APA style manual for appropriate citation of your source material (in-text citations).

Step 5: If possible, refute the argument of the opposition by referencing researchable material, which supports the opposition, and arguing against the authors' claims. This process will require strong thinking and an ability to thoroughly examine your subject.

Step 6: Edit the paper for continuity, coherence, and clarity.

Sample Research Paper
APPLICATION OF APA-SPECIFIC METHODS

The Effectiveness of Aquatic Therapy as a Treatment for Children with Neuromuscular Diseases

INTRODUCTION

Neuromuscular diseases, including multiple sclerosis and cerebral palsy, usually include a demyelinization of axons in the central nervous system (Gehlsen, Grigsby, & Winant, 1984).[1] Transmitting information from the brain to the muscular system, axons play a crucial role in mobility and muscle strength (Gehlsen et al., 1984).[2] The degree of myelinization determines the speed at which the nerve conducts the impulses from the brain. As a result, affected individuals exhibit decreased speed of movement and decreased muscle strength. A majority of neuromuscular diseases have no true treatment to improve the physical

condition of the patient; physicians cannot reverse the demyelinization process, which causes most of the symptoms associated with the diseases. Many researchers have conducted studies examining the effects of various treatment methods on patients with neuromuscular diseases, but in a majority of cases, the subjects were adults. For children with neuromuscular diseases, researchers have put forth little effort to investigate possible methods of treatment (Dumas & Francesconi, 2001).[3] More research focused on pediatrics would help find ways to improve the quality of life for patients at an earlier age, and an early start in treatment would create greater benefits for those individuals throughout adolescence and into adulthood. Searching for treatment methods for such diseases has led researchers and medical professionals away from traditional treatment in order to explore some alternative methods. Researchers have investigated aquatic therapy as a possible treatment for individuals, particularly children, with neuromuscular diseases. Findings indicate that an aquatic therapy regimen results in many short-term improvements such as increased "muscle strength and functional mobility" (Duvall, R., & Roberts, P., as quoted in Dumas & Francesconi, 2001, p. 69).[4] However, a need for more research on the long-term effects of aquatic therapy is necessary before any absolute claims can be made regarding the benefits of an aquatic treatment program.

DISCUSSION

Aquatic therapy provides a more active form of treatment for patients, whereas hydrotherapy, another popular water treatment implemented by therapists, refers to a passive form of treatment (Dumas & Francesconi, 2001).[5] Through research, therapists discovered the natural therapeutic effects of water in treating patients, in both aquatic therapy and hydrotherapy. In aquatic therapy, therapists utilize the properties of water to their advantage to increase treatment possibilities for individuals with debilitating neuromuscular diseases. To reduce the adverse effects of the patient's body mass during exercise, therapists use the buoyancy of the water so patients can perform more weight-bearing tasks in which they do not have to also resist their own body mass (Dumas & Francesconi, 2001).[6] In addition to buoyancy, the high viscosity associated with water benefits the patient by producing gradual resistance as the patient moves through the pool (Hutzler et al., 1998).[7] Since the resistance of water does not equal that provided by normal land therapy equipment, the water enables the patient to perform a greater variety of exercises with a greater range of movement and with a decreased risk of stress on the patient. Finding a way to reduce stress for the patients while providing therapy that still provides benefits has been a main goal of therapists working with patients with neuromuscular diseases. Water temperature provides yet another benefit specifically to patients with neuromuscular diseases. The water can achieve various temperatures warmer than the normal air in a land-based therapy room. From the water, the patient's body temperature can rise slightly, and this rise in body temperature reduces the occurrence of spasms and other involuntary movements characteristic of patients with this type of disease (Hutzler et al., 1998).[8] From such information, one can conclude that the properties of water alone qualify aquatic therapy as a topic of research as a possible treatment for children with neuromuscular diseases.

By using aquatic therapy as a treatment method for neuromuscular diseases, therapists can help improve the degree of muscle strength in patients. Neuromuscular diseases normally result in muscle atrophy because a decreased myelinization of axons innervating skeletal muscles decreases the ability of the muscle to reach the maximum level of activity. Focusing on improving muscle strength helps increase the quality of living for patients by allowing a more active and independent lifestyle. To restore muscle strength to an acceptable level, therapists can use an aquatic environment and the properties of the water to provide resistance with minimal physical stress on the patient (Hutzler et al., 1998).[9] Decreasing stress levels in the patients plays an important role in treatment because extensive stress will result in fatigue, another characteristic of neuromuscular diseases, and the onset of fatigue may prove harmful to the patient. In a study by Peterson (2001), a patient with multiple sclerosis engaged in an aquatic therapy program that increased the muscle strength of the lower extremities by a significant degree.[10] Upon entry into the program, the patient required assistance to transfer from wheelchair to bed and could not ambulate, but following treatment, she could ambulate with minimal assistance in shallow water (Peterson, 2001).[11] The increased mobility and muscle strength achieved in water can later transfer to land activity. Therefore, aquatic therapy

can serve as the first step in rehabilitation and make the process of land rehabilitation easier for the patient.

In addition to increased muscle strength, an aquatic therapy exercise program can improve range of motion in both the upper and lower extremities of the patient. The buoyancy of the water decreases the weight of the limbs, enabling the patient to move with greater ease; however, the water's natural resistance still provides enough force to make the patient work and thus improve range of motion. Allowing the patient to create movements more representative of everyday motions, the aquatic environment better prepares the patient for activities of daily living (Prins & Cutner, 1999).[12] In a situation such as this, aquatic therapy has obvious advantages over a land-based program. Standard therapy equipment allows for somewhat rigid motions that do not permit the most natural movements. In the case of individuals with neuromuscular diseases, the goals of the therapists center on improving the functional abilities and activities of daily living for the patients, not achieving maximal muscle capacity and providing the patient with a lifestyle equivalent to individuals without a neuromuscular disease. Therefore, if an aquatic therapy program provides the results desired by the therapists, it should receive consideration as a treatment method, even if in combination with a traditional land-based therapy program.

When designing treatment programs for individuals with neuromuscular diseases, therapists must consider fatigue as a determining factor in the rehabilitation, and after assessing the patient's initial level of fatigue, the therapists can decide which exercises the patient can perform and the level of intensity at which the patient can perform these exercises. Experiencing muscle atrophy makes patients with neuromuscular diseases more susceptible to fatigue than other patients of physical therapy. Therefore, researchers must consider fatigue when investigating the effectiveness of the aquatic therapy program for patients with neuromuscular diseases. More specifically, children will fatigue faster than adults with the same diagnosis, so the combination of age and the symptoms characteristic of the disease affect the method of treatment. In a study conducted by Gehlsen et al. (1984), patients with multiple sclerosis participated in an aquatic therapy program, to examine the effects of the program on fatigue and other factors.[13] Focusing on the lower extremities, the researchers found that the fatigue measurements for the participants decreased almost 2%, a significant decline (Gehlsen et al., 1984).[14] The buoyancy of the water removes much of the unwanted weight on the patient, increases breathing ability, and reduces the perception of pain (Wade, J., as quoted in Dumas & Francesconi, 2001).[15] With increased levels of oxygen obtained from increased respiration, the muscles have a greater source of energy and can work longer, increasing the time exercise is possible without the patient's experiencing fatigue. Increasing the period of time over which the patient can perform exercises can reduce some treatment time since patients can exercise longer during a single treatment session. In terms of dealing with fatigue in the therapy program, an aquatic environment helps reduce the adverse effects of fatigue and shows more potential benefits for children with neuromuscular diseases.

Aside from the physical and quantitative benefits accompanying an aquatic therapy treatment, some researchers suggest that an aquatic environment can provide psychological benefits for children with neuromuscular diseases. By allowing for more work with less fatigue and stress, an aquatic environment permits greater advances in a shorter period of time than are possible with land-based therapy. Along with the noticeable physical improvements, the children feel a sense of accomplishment and pride in the work they have done (Wade, J., as quoted in Dumas & Francesconi, 2001);[16] the feelings of success provide greater motivation to continue work, thus increasing the chances for improvement of their original condition (Wade, J., as quoted in Dumas & Francesconi, 2001).[17] When treating children, physical therapists should acknowledge the importance of motivation and self-image in the treatment process. Children, especially those born with neuromuscular diseases, cannot comprehend any other way of life aside from their current condition. As a result, motivation and determination may be lacking in the treatment process because the children cannot realize the importance of rehabilitation and how physical therapy can improve their quality of life. An aquatic environment provides the ideal setting for children to engage in physical therapy exercises; they may see only the entertainment aspect and forget the actual benefits of

the rehabilitation. In some cases, patients can participate in the design of the treatment program, thus improving their self-image and encouraging continuation in the program (Peganoff, S. A., as quoted in Dumas & Francesconi, 2001).[18]

CONCLUSION

Aquatic therapy provides many benefits in the treatment of neuromuscular diseases, in adults as well as in children. However, little research exists as to the definitive benefits of an aquatic program, especially in the field of pediatric physical therapy. In all of the foregoing studies cited, the researchers and therapists incorporated the aquatic therapy program into the patient's normal land-based therapy program, so researchers do not attribute all of the patient improvements to the aquatic therapy alone. According to most of the data collected by researchers, an aquatic therapy program results in improvements in muscle strength and fatigue, but a lack of research exists on the long-term effects of an aquatic program. Although existing research shows trends toward establishing aquatic therapy as a viable treatment, therapists must conduct further studies examining the effectiveness of aquatic therapy as a treatment method for children suffering from neuromuscular diseases before physical therapists will begin implementing such a program.

References

Dumas, H., & Francesconi, S. (2001). Aquatic therapy in pediatrics: Annotated bibliography [Abstract]. *Physical & Occupational Therapy in Pediatrics, 20*, 63–78.[19]

Ghelsen, D. M., Grigsby, S. A., & Winant, D. M. (1984). Effects of an aquatic fitness program on the muscular strength and endurance of patients with multiple sclerosis. *Physical Therapy, 64*(5), 653–657.[20]

Hutzler, Y., Cacham, A., Bergman, U., & Szeinberg, A. (1998). Effects of a movement and swimming program on vital capacity and water orientation skills of children with cerebral palsy. *Developmental Medicine and Child Neurology, 40*, 176–181.[21]

Peterson, C. (2001). Exercise in 94°F water for a patient with multiple sclerosis. *Physical Therapy, 81*(4), 1049–1058.[22]

Prins, J., & Cutner, D. (1999). Aquatic therapy in the rehabilitation of athletic injuries. *Clinics in Sports Medicine, 18*, 447–461.[23]

COMMENTS

1. The in-text citation for this sentence includes the last names of the authors and the year of publication. This citation indicates a paraphrase; the sentence included in the paper includes information from an outside source but uses wording from the author of the paper.

2. The citation for this sentence also refers to a paraphrase. However, the citation only includes the last name of one author followed by *et al.* For a reference with more than two authors, the last name of the first author can be followed by *et al.* once all of the names have been included in one previous citation.

3. The citation indicates a paraphrased sentence and includes the last name of the two authors and the year of publication.

4. The passage to which this citation refers is a direct quote. The authors of the paper have used the exact words of the authors of the original source. Therefore, the citation must include the last names of the authors, the year of publication, and the page from which the quote was taken. The citation is located after the end quotation marks but before the period ending the sentence. This citation also includes two sets of last names because the source that the authors of the paper cite cites yet another source. Therefore, all of the names are mentioned.

5. Again, this sentence uses information from another source, but the author of the paper uses his or her own words. Therefore, the last names of the two authors and the year of publication are included in the citation.

6. This citation refers to another paraphrase and includes the last names of the authors and the year of publication.

7. This paraphrase citation includes an improper citation. It makes use of *et al.* but the last names of the next three authors have not already been written out once.

8. Again, this citation indicates a paraphrase because it includes the last name of one author followed by *et al.* and the year of publication.

9. This citation also indicates a paraphrase because it includes the last name of one author followed by *et al.* and the year of publication.

10. In this citation, only the year of publication is found in parentheses. The author's last name is mentioned within the content of the sentence and therefore does not need to be included in the citation. Including the author's name in the sentence adds some variety to paraphrased sentences.

11. This paraphrase citation includes only one author's last name and the year of publication.

12. Since the preceding sentence was paraphrased from an outside source, the authors' last names and the year of publication are included in the citation.

13. In this paraphrase, the last name of one author and *et al.* are included in the content of the sentence, so the citation includes only the year of publication.

14. This citation for a paraphrase includes one author's last name followed by *et al.* (because the other authors have been mentioned once already) and the year of publication.

15. The citation follows the format for a paraphrase by including the authors' last names and the year of publication. However, another name is mentioned and followed by *as quoted in.* This phrase means that the source document has quoted another individual, and the piece of information included in this paper is from that other source.

16. The citation follows the format for a paraphrase by including the authors' last names and the year of publication. However, another name is mentioned and followed by *as quoted in.* This phrase means that the source document has quoted another individual, and the piece of information included in this paper is from that other source.

17. The citation follows the format for a paraphrase by including the authors' last names

and the year of publication. However, another name is mentioned and followed by *as quoted in*. This phrase means that the source document has quoted another individual, and the piece of information included in this paper is from that other source.

18. Again, the authors of the source document have cited another publication in their work, and that author's name is included in the citation.

References

19. Abstract as an original source. A reference such as this includes the last name(s) and initial(s) of the author(s), the year of publication, the title of the article followed by the word *Abstract* in brackets, the name of the journal, the volume, and the page numbers.

20. Journal article with three authors. The reference includes the last names and initials of the authors, the year of publication, the title of the journal article, the journal from which the article was retrieved, the volume number, the issue number, and the page numbers.

21. Journal article with four authors. The reference includes the last names and initials of the authors, the year of publication, the title of the journal article, the journal from which the article was retrieved, the volume number, and the page numbers. I should also note that the ordering of the authors within a single reference should match the ordering on the article itself. Oftentimes, as in this case, the authors' names are not listed alphabetically. The ordering reflects the degree of involvement of each author in the research.

22. Journal article with one author. The reference includes the last name and initial of the author, the year of publication, the title of the journal article, the journal from which the article was retrieved, the volume number, and the page numbers.

23. Journal article with two authors. The reference includes the last names and initials of the authors, the year of publication, the title of the journal article, the journal from which the article was retrieved, the volume number, and the page numbers.

Exercise

REVISING THE RESEARCH PAPER

Directions: Revise and rewrite the following proposal to make it an acceptable document for standard, academic writing by employing any and all strategies that we have addressed thus far in this text. You must address writing issues on several levels: essay, paragraph, sentence, and word. You should also add or delete information when appropriate or reorganize the essay as needed to meet demands of logic and proportion. Additionally, the "References" section does not meet the standards presented by the APA style manual or any other style manual. Make the appropriate changes, and also change the inaccurate information in the in-text citations.

Title: Media Effects on Body Image in College-Aged Women

Today, according to mass mediums, a thin fat-free body is seen as the ideal body in our culture. In a body image survey conducted by Psychology today, it was revealed that 15% of woman say they would sacrifice more than five years of their lives to be at their desired weight. (Spitzer et al 1999) Anything from soap operas to film to popular magazines are influencing women to set for what the most part is unrealistic and unattainable goals for how they want to see themselves. Which is called the Cinderella Syndrome. The ideal body weight portrayed by the media is one that is 13–19% below what is considered healthy (Schell 1998) yet it is one that woman use as a standard for comparing themselves. (Wilcox and Laird 2000) Body dissatisfaction and a desire to loose weight has become a norm for collage age woman which begins a lifetime of that thinking and feeling. Advertising, their friends, magazines, their mother, movies and their romantic partner are rated by Collage woman as more influential of their ideas about attractiveness then did men in a study done by Reed in 1998. Overall adolescent and collage-age woman are at the highest risk as their body fat and weight concern competes with biological reality. (Owen & Laurel-Seller 2000) Even with these alarming statistics role models in the media follows the trends of the Miss America Pageant winners, since the 1950's these woman's body sizes have decreased significantly as well as Playboy centerfolds; of whom one-third meet the

Body Mass Index criterion for anorexia nervousa. In my study I plan on trying to find out if there is any relationship between brief media exposure and a decreased body satisfaction, drive for thinness and perfectionism. I also plan on comparing their Eating Disorder Inventory results with the participant's actual weight to see if there any that are overweight and if that has any affect on their perceptions. I plan to use clips from this years Miss America Pageant; to see if watching these woman on TV has an affect on their body image and satisfaction which I made up. There is also a control that I use half will watch a clip from the popular TV show The Price is Right. I am hoping to find that even brief exposure to these "skinny" woman can have affects on one's thoughts and feelings about their own body. I will use a measure of eating disorders, the Eating Disorder Inventory (EDI) before the participant watches the video clip and then I will question the participants after the video clip regarding drive for thinness and body satisfaction. I think I will find a relationship between woman who have a low score on body satisfaction, and also have some characteristics of having a eating disorder. I have enclosed the Eating Disorder Inventory. Members of Daemen College faculty have used this in the past, and find it a reputable measure.

Works Cited

Spitzer, D. and Jones, Michael, and Slade, Samuel. (1999). The Cinderella Syndrome. Psychology Today. Vol. 25. Number 6. Pages: 25–35

Reed, Marian (1998). Women and Men in College. Bantam, NY, pp. 215, 217, 299, and 306.

Schell, David. (1998). Media Measures and The Ideal Body. Journal of Adolescent Psychology, 2.6 (February): pages 6–12.

Wilcox, F. & Laird, Sandra. (2000). The Eating Disorder Inventory: theory and application. Eating Disorders Quarterly. Vol 6. Num. 1. Pages: 117–119.

Owen, William and Laurel, Seller. (2000). Eating Disorders and the Adolescent. Prentice Hall. 2000. New York and Tokyo. Pages 200–209.

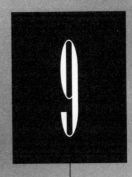
Writing the Thesis

Key Terms

Appendices   Sections of text, outside of the standard chapters, that hold large bodies of information that cannot fit logically into the flow of text; often in the forms of charts, graphs, and tables

Delimitations   Considerations in determining the merits of the results and the application of the results to other avenues of research or practice

Discussion   The meaning of the results

Informed consent   A method of protecting the subjects' rights by providing subjects with clear instructions and options for participation or withdrawal

Limitations   Outside forces that have been placed on the study and influenced results

Literature review   Summary of researchable material that directly influences the writer's research and/or experimentation

Methods   Principles used to gather data or conduct research

References   The list of bibliographic entries used as a basis for the research

Results   The evidence that allows the author to make a claim

Chapter Objectives

On completion of this chapter, the reader should be able to

1. Understand the categories of organization for the thesis.

2. Develop a topic and a workable thesis.

3. Write a proposal, including its integral parts, according to standard research writing procedures.

4. Propose and conduct research according to the standards that protect subjects' rights.

5. Develop a proposal suitable for submission to any body governing research.

6. Develop a consent form to be used or modified to protect subjects' rights.

7. Convert a thesis question into a thesis statement.

8. Follow a protocol and develop categories of discussion to create chapters of the thesis.

The thesis is your contribution to the scholarly dialogue. Instead of relying on the works of others to supply opinions or positions, as you have done in standard research papers, you will use the works of others to launch you into your own study. Ultimately, the thesis demonstrates your ability to gather secondary research and generate primary data and then blend the two into a paper that adds to the scholarly conversations in your field or profession.

This chapter addresses the blending of secondary research and primary data into a coherent and generally accepted form. The headings and categories provided are not necessarily exhaustive, nor do they represent an "industry standard." Certain professions or academic disciplines require other categories of discussion that may not be listed here. You should recognize that the ultimate authority in the formation of your thesis is your committee and thesis advisor.

Additionally, as the format is subject specific, so too may be the documentation style. Certain professions require APA style for the thesis, but the standard for journal writing may be American Medical Association (AMA) or Council of Biology Editors (CSE) style. Again, the authority in this subject is your thesis committee.

THESIS PROPOSAL

The thesis you will write for an advanced degree requires a proposal. Proposals provide a specific research question, a general discussion of research about the topic, and a reasonable outline of how you plan to answer the question. These issues are addressed accordingly in the subheadings that follow.

Each thesis must be proposed to a mentoring faculty member or group of faculty for approval. Through this process, faculty can help guide students to narrow topics, find adequate research materials, and meet the required format for writing in the discipline. As with any research project, the advice and guidance of your mentor or overseeing professor are invaluable. Seek the advice of a professional to help start your journey.

Generating a Topic

Finding a suitable research topic will be the result of months, if not years, of steady reading and thinking about various subjects. Consequently, you will write a thesis about a subject that you know well from previous studies or investigation. You will not wake up one day and decide to write about a particular subject without contemplating the subject first to determine if it is a viable research subject. Often, suitable research projects for a thesis derive from the work of professors or other ongoing research. Involve yourself with your professors and find a mentoring relationship with one who suits your needs and tastes. The product of this relationship will be satisfying.

Crafting a Research Question

Once you begin to narrow your subject, you will ultimately be asked to formulate your thesis around a research question or statement of problem. This is a daunting task: to reduce your overwhelming amount of thinking and research into one question.

The research question should completely demonstrate your purpose of the paper. This sounds elementary, but many students do not understand the difficulty of narrowing the focus of their work. They often consider topics too broad for a reasonable study. For example, no one can reasonably attempt to answer, in a single thesis, why adolescents choose to use drugs and alcohol. The answers are various and could be unlimited. Many other students fail to actually present a discoverable problem, such as how something functions or how one element relates to others and the interactions caused by the relationship. Some scientists may consider the following a good starting point for a research project thesis: the relationship between children who use English as a second language (ESL) and poor standardized test scores. This statement has variables (test scores) that can be measured and relationships that can be analyzed (native English speakers versus nonnative speakers of English). It is not a question yet, but the foundation is set.

Furthermore, your research question should also include language that reveals your answer to the dilemma presented. In the following example, "culturally congruent instruction" must be defined, but the term constitutes valid language in your thesis.

Can culturally congruent classroom instruction improve standardized test scores in ESL students?

The study group can then be narrowed to a specific culture or group, and the test scores data can focus on ACT or SAT scores.

Many instructors prefer that you present the research question in bold language instead of trying to conceal it in an introductory paragraph or discussion. Feel free to use phrases such as "In this study, I plan to . . ." or "This research project intends to . . . ," but use this method in the proposal only. Such language will not be appropriate for the final research paper.

Writing the Introduction

With the research question established, you can now provide general background information and rationale for undertaking the study in an introductory passage. The introduction you write here may be tweaked later for use as the introduction to your thesis since both will have the same focus and purpose: to introduce your topic, provide background information (or a literature review—discussed next), and explain why you chose to accomplish work on this topic.

By stating the problem first, the writer can explain the issues relevant to the discussion following, and the writer can anticipate the results of the study or negative reactions to the work and explain. With the problem stated and the options explained, the writer can then focus on hypotheses that help answer the question or solve the problem. Such presuppositions will be based on research that is presented either here or in the "Literature Review" section.

Literature Review

A **literature review** allows your reader to understand the breadth of knowledge and accomplishment already directed to your study. You will provide short summaries of the works published that have an impact on or relationship to your work. To successfully complete this part of the proposal, you will need to break down your research topic into elements of researchable topics and then attack each variable. Once the research is collected and summarized, you will organize your summaries into a unified essay addressing the topics of research. Building transitions between sections of research or between articles requires steady and constant revision and rewriting.

At some colleges and universities, the literature review is absorbed into the introductory section and consequently eliminated as a subheading in the proposal. As always, check with your professor(s) for guidance here.

See the later section entitled "Outline for Writing the Review of Literature" for a detailed description of this phase.

Proposed Method

You should understand that your proposal will not fully explain your methods because the study has not yet commenced. However, you will be required to offer a sketch of the types of studies you plan to incorporate and the rationale for using each. You should also provide your readers with samples of how you plan to present the data that you have collected. You can offer sample tables, charts, graphs, or text boxes associated with graphics.

References

Some committees require that following the "Literature Review," you list the references you used in bibliographic form according to the style that governs your thesis, such as APA style.

Ultimately, the emphasis in the proposal is on the introductory section and the review of associated literature. Your reader wants to know why you have undertaken the study, the factors that make your work unique or other background information, your proposed hypothesis to explain the answers you may have found, and the literature that has been published about all facets of your topic.

HUMAN SUBJECTS RESEARCH REVIEW PROPOSAL AND CONSENT FORM

Proposal

The human subjects research review proposal ensures that all research involving human subjects is appropriately reviewed in accordance with pertinent legal and ethical requirements. Specifically, the subjects cannot be put in danger, nor can their legal rights be circumvented for the purposes of the study. Additionally, research that studies humans must be accompanied by information fully explaining the purpose of the study in language that can be understood by the subjects. The proposal, then, is an abbreviated form of the thesis focusing on the use of information gathered from subjects assuring the field of science that the rights of the human subjects are protected.

The researcher may wish to consult the federal regulations at the following Web address: http://ohsr.od.nih.gov/mpa/45cfr46.php3#subparta.

The purpose of the human subjects research review proposal is to minimize risk to subjects and to guard the researcher against litigation if an injury occurs during the data collection phase. The subjects are exposed to minimal risk if the researchers use procedures that are consistent with the principles of scientific research. Additionally, the rights of the subjects must be preserved in the selection process. For example, members of populations who cannot legitimately recognize the advantages and disadvantages of such research are avoided (children or the developmentally challenged), unless the risks outweigh the rewards, such as in the case of studying ways to improve treatment methods for mental retardation, for example. Other pop-

ulations are protected as well to assure the field of science that certain groups are not unfairly used as laboratory rats (economically or educationally underserved populations). Finally, the rights of certain groups are protected for their own safety, such as pregnant women.

To protect the rights of the researchers and the subjects, the researchers will maintain the data for purposes of the research project only and monitor the data. To assure any subject of confidentiality and privacy, the subjects may have access to such records at any time.

The following list of headings should be addressed in the writing of any human subjects research review proposal to maintain scientific integrity of the experiment:

Title of the project

Names and contact information of researchers and faculty advisors (if necessary)

Statement of purpose

Significance of study

Risks

Research methodology

Data collection procedure

Informed Consent Form

To protect the subjects' rights, no researcher may involve a human being as a subject in research unless the researcher has obtained the **informed consent** of the subject or from the subject's legally authorized representative.

The elements of the informed consent document for study projects should follow the following proposed categories:

Names and contact information of researchers and faculty advisor (if applicable)

Names and contact information for questions about subjects' rights or research

Title of study

Statement indicating research will be done and for what purposes

Description of procedures, including expected duration, experimental elements, and so on

Description of possible risks and benefits to the subjects

Description of alternative procedures that could benefit the subjects

Statement of conditions and procedures of confidentiality and anonymity

Statement indicating that participation is voluntary

Statement that refusal to participate will not result in penalty or loss

Statement that subject may withdraw at any time

Statement that documentation has been provided to prove that the subject is over 18

This form should then provide a place where the subjects can sign and date the implied consent form. Additionally, the researchers and a witness should also sign the document in the presence of the subjects to ensure the integrity of the research.

THESIS CHAPTER ONE: INTRODUCTION TO THE PROBLEM

During the writing of your proposal, you thought about a particular subject and developed central ideas that needed researchable evidence to prove your position. In the introduction of the proposal, you focused your position into a research question and provided the necessary background information to explain the details surrounding your issue. This introduction, used in your proposal, can serve as the foundation to the introduction you will write for the body of your thesis.

The thesis introduction should indicate to your reader why your project was undertaken. It should again describe the problem and its relationship to the field, but instead of developing a research question, you will develop a research statement. You will convert your original question to a statement—for example:

PROPOSAL QUESTION: Can culturally congruent classroom instruction improve standardized test scores in ESL students?

THESIS STATEMENT: Culturally congruent classroom instruction improved/did not improve standardized test scores in ESL students.

In some cases, your investigation into your subject may reveal that your original hypothesis was misguided or that your attempt to prove one issue led you to consider other issues. Here is your chance to revise your purpose statement to reflect your true aim.

REVISED THESIS STATEMENT: Culturally congruent classroom instruction improved SAT scores in Hispanic students.

The remainder of the thesis should be written in response to the hypothesis or thesis statement. In fact, once you make your claim, the remainder of the text in the introduction should attempt to explain what you did as a researcher and gatherer of physical evidence, and how you reveal your strategies for proving your point.

The introduction, as any writer knows, serves as the foundation of the paper or research project. In the thesis, it serves a specific function covering a variety of subjects. The subjects covered in the following discussion represent a standard used at many colleges and universities. This standard should be checked against what your advisors recommend. Also, the introduction, in most cases, does not provide researched information. It may establish that certain studies were conducted that lead you, the writer of the thesis, to this subject, but, as with any thesis, research (or evidence) belongs in a specific location, usually the middle chapters.

Introductory Statement

The introductory statement should provide a brief and direct overview of the subject and explain why such a project is worthy of a book-length research study. Essentially, this statement provides the purpose of the thesis, but it does not state the problem. This section of the thesis can be a single paragraph or a few paragraphs in length.

EXAMPLE
The theory of plyometrics was founded upon the idea that muscle, if elongated immediately before it contracts, would produce a more powerful and stronger contraction. Given this basic premise of plyometric theory, little research or documented scientific analysis has been published to support this notion.

Statement of the Problem or Research Question

The formal "Statement of the Problem" explains that a problem exists. This section should establish the reasoning for your venture into this subject area. Many students find that this section easily accommodates background information or that it explains significant research that has led you to this point. Some disciplines require the thesis writer to produce a specific research question. This is a useful pursuit in that it gives the researcher/writer specific charges or purpose.

EXAMPLE

All recently published studies on plyometrics were conducted using some form of long-term training, such as aerobic exercise or sport-specific training. Although these studies have shown an increase in the participants' capabilities, they have failed to support the notion that basic plyometrics is capable of increasing muscle power and strength. Therefore, inclusion of aerobics and other supplemental techniques may undermine the foundations of basic plyometric theory.

Purpose of the Study

In light of the background information that has been established, this subsection establishes the specific direction of the paper. In fact, this subsection, in a statement or a paragraph, is considered the thesis statement that explains to your reader what you are attempting to accomplish.

EXAMPLE

Attempting to form a better understanding of plyometrics, the researchers of this study concluded that prior studies failed to support the basic plyometric theory. In response, they attempted to prove if plyometrics is relative to the immediate storage and release of energy from the muscle fiber tissue that produces an immediate effect on the muscle, showing increased power output through vertical jumps.

Significance of the Study

Once you have established that a problem exists or that a question needs to be answered, and you have provided your reader with your plan to do so, you now need to explain to the reader why anyone would care. Put your project in perspective. Consider the effects on the profession or other researchers, and consider the scope of influence your project may have. This section is an important consideration in that the relevance of your work, to the world or readers out there, is thoroughly analyzed.

EXAMPLE

This study may help support the notion that plyometrics does, in fact, improve muscle strength and power. Additionally, this study may support plyometrics as a beneficial method of training for patients of physical therapists and the general public.

Delimitations of the Study

In considering **delimitations**, the researcher must consider the limits of the results and application of the results to other avenues of research or practice. It is important to identify for the reader those factors that hinder the researcher's ability to generalize the results. In other words, ask this question: Why are these results significant only to this body of researchable material or group of subjects? If I performed this study on another group, would the results be the same in all circumstances?

EXAMPLE

The variables that limit the researchers' abilities to generalize results are the following:

- the age of the subject compared with that of the rehabilitation population
- the physical ability of subjects compared with that of the rehabilitation population
- the small sample size used in this study.

The researchers attempted to eliminate variables from affecting the results of this study by allowing the subjects to act as their own controls. The following variables were eliminated: gender, body weight, lever arm of the lower extremities, and height.

Limitations of the Study

Just as the researcher must consider the limits of the results and application of those results, the researcher must also explain the **limitations** that have been placed on the study. Obviously, given a bottomless pit of money, researchers can produce specific results. However, in the real world, limits on financial resources and funding often keep the researchers from moving forward with specific charges. Consider other factors as well, such as a limited population pool, the limits of time, and the limits of the organization that is sponsoring such research.

EXAMPLE

The study may not provide acceptable results secondary to the following:

- Financial resources were limited.
- The length of the study was constricted to 1 year.
- The number of and diversity of subjects were limited.

Assumptions

All research, no matter how thorough, relies on assumptions of some kind. For example, researchers often use mechanisms for testing, and sometimes, machinery can be faulty or the measurements gathered can be skewed by factors outside of the writer's control or knowledge. A thorough researcher will understand that assumptions are a factor and explain their possible influence. An admission of such assumptions does not weaken the thesis, as many students may believe. This only establishes the writer's integrity.

EXAMPLE

This study is based on the assumption that all of the subjects jumped from the ground to the 41-cm box in the same general manner each time they performed a jump. The reliability and validity of the testing measurement depend on the researchers' ability to read a tape measure accurately and with consistent use of the region of the fingertip for measuring.

Definition of Terms

In any study, writers and researchers will use terminology that may not be familiar to their audience. As a matter of convenience, place those definitions here instead of interrupting the flow of your paper in other sections with diversions that simply define. Define unfamiliar terms here, and also, use this section to define how familiar terms are used in unfamiliar or unique ways.

EXAMPLE

Plyometrics: a quick, powerful movement involving prestretching the muscle to activating the stretch-shortening cycle to produce a subsequently stronger concentric concentration.

Depth jump (drop jump): a vertical jump that is started from a surface higher than ground level. The subject jumps to the ground and then springs up as high as he or she can in one motion.

Adequate range of motion: within 10° of normal values for hip flexion and extension, knee flexion and extension, and ankle dorsiflexion and plantarflexion.

Hypothesis

The hypothesis establishes, in a shortened form, your results. Establish what you expect to discover here. You set out to prove something; explain it.

EXAMPLE

Vertical jump height is enhanced immediately with a plyometric jump.

Conclusion

A formal "Conclusion" is optional, but it can serve a useful purpose. Provide, here, a brief summary of the preceding chapters, and then provide a brief preview of the chapters that will follow. This will allow the reader to build expectations that you are sure to follow.

THESIS CHAPTER TWO: WRITING THE LITERATURE REVIEW

The "Review of Literature" should establish for your reader that you comprehend the work of others who have researched and written about topics related to your investigation. In embarking on this quest to answer a question or to solve a problem, you will stand on the shoulders of some important people who came before you. In other words, others have poured a foundation of knowledge on which you now stand. To qualify your work as legitimate, you must demonstrate that you understand how these researchers and their writings have influenced your work.

This part of the research paper is a struggle for most students because they will be tempted to simply list their sources and provide a one- or two-sentence summary of the work. They will continue in this fashion until they exhaust their bibliography. This is not the proper approach. Remember, the literature review is an essay explaining the genesis of your research and thinking. Explain to your reader the topics that led you to your discoveries and formulate passages that explain which texts or articles were influential in establishing these topics in the body of research that you uncovered and how they relate to your topic of investigation.

The following list will help you keep this perspective and help you present these ideas in a form that resembles writing, not a list.

Understanding the Literature Review

1. Know your purpose: Discuss the scholarly writings that influence your work.
   - Have the proper psychological orientation: Discuss what others have written in relation to what you plan to do (to see your effort in terms of the scholars who have written before you).
   - Be aware of relationships between authors' ideas and your own.
   - See your work and others' in new ways.

2. Have a plan: Organization and structure help keep the reader focused.
   - Consider creating an outline.
   - Write for your purpose. At the top, write your research problem (as you would a thesis statement).
   - Write your paragraphs around a topic— not a list of your sources. Build *coherence* by providing *structural* signals and *transitional* sentences.
   - Other considerations for organization: Start with broad categories of discussion and move to more narrow ones (think of an inverted pyramid). Consider the classic or groundbreaking studies first to provide a historical perspective.

3. Emphasize relatedness: Always relate your ideas back to your purpose.
   - Literature reviews should never be a chain of isolated summaries (Jones says . . . , Smith says . . . ,). In this form, no attempt is made to demonstrate the connection between the source and your topic.
   - Clearly demonstrate how the source relates to your topic or subtopics.

4. *Review* the literature; do not reproduce it.
   - Present the ideas of others and cite the information you borrow.
   - Know how to use direct quotations and paraphrasing techniques.
   - Discuss the works of others in relation to your topic. The important issue here is not the findings of such work, but how the work relates to your ideas.

5. Summarize the works: What does it all mean?
   - Write a concluding section that describes how all of the research you have performed relates to the research question you have proposed.

6. Edit and revise; this is the most important step.
   - Review the structural foundation.
   - Build coherence by connecting ideas.
   - Create grammatically correct sentences.
   - Form the citations accurately.
   - Proofread and edit again.
   - Use an editor to help revise—again.

Outline for Writing the Review of Literature

The Literature Review surveys all of the resources that are relevant to your research problem or question. It should indicate the significance of the following types of research material that have affected your subject and your findings. Accordingly, it should be organized into sections that define the research performed in specific areas of your project:

Theoretical framework: Every major research project depends on a specific angle or theoretical approach. The philosophical position of the writer must be established to orient the reader to the findings. To this end, the "Review of Literature" section must examine the philosophical or theoretical undertakings that support the task. Such orientation requires summaries of texts and theories proposed in those texts.

Related research: All research that supports the writer's findings are summarized here. Most likely, studies have been conducted in the field that parallel the writer's project or have been used by the writer to establish a foundation in thinking. All researchers depend on the work of great people who came before them. This section establishes that the research findings provided do not exist in a vacuum; they are dependent on the research that the field has accepted.

Methods summary: This section provides summaries of the research concerning the mechanisms to gather and analyze data. In order for the thesis writer's work to be accepted, he or she must prove that the methods used have been established as acceptable by the field. This section describes the tools used to gather data, instruments used for measurement, and methodology used. These issues must be fortified with the standard research documents, as such research will lend credibility to the findings.

Summary paragraph: The summary paragraph presents a conclusion about the varieties of research used and the influence they have on the researcher's work and findings.

Student Sample Essay
REVIEW OF RELATED LITERATURE FOR PRIMARY RESEARCH PROJECT

Force and power generation problems exist with novice sport, orthopedic, and rehabilitation populations. An inability to produce adequate power will decrease a person's ability to perform functionally in everyday activities. Certain people have activities of daily living that naturally call for a greater power production. This regular exertion of energy cannot be completed if the person suffers from decreased endurance as a result of a functional or organ compromise.

Several patient populations fall into the category of having declined force/power-generating capac-

ity. Multiple sclerosis and stroke patients experience progressive deconditioning. Postoperative patients or those compromised by immobilization must be allotted adequate healing time, as the body will decondition and tissue quality will change with inactivity. Traumatic brain injury and pediatric patients may have power generation problems that contribute to motor planning issues.

Research shows that several plyometric techniques are advantageous to athletes when used as part of their training. Matavulj et al. (2001) coupled regular, mid-season high school basketball practice of 90 minutes, 6 times per week, for 6 weeks, with either a 50-cm or a 100-cm drop jump. Matavulj et al. found that the experimental group performing the 50-cm drop jump recorded an increase of 4.8 cm in post-test measurements. The experimental group completing training with the 100-cm drop jump recorded an additional 5.6 cm in their vertical jump post-test measurements. The control group showed no significant increases in their vertical jump heights.

Gehri et al. (1998) described the counter-motion jump (CMJ), a form of plyometrics, as a smooth flexion of the hips, knees, and ankles simultaneously followed by a rapid extension at these joints, resulting in a vertical jump that is initiated and completed from the same ground location. In this study, training consisted of 12 weeks of aerobic exercise combined with increasing sets of 8 repetitions of CMJs. The researchers oversaw a population that consisted of equal numbers of male and female subjects, who were not participating in any competitive sport at the time. They concluded that, when a squat is performed before a vertical jump, height increased by 113.61%. When CMJ was performed, an increase of 108.04% was recorded. After the drop jump was completed, the resultant height was increased to 110.95%.

Matavulj et al. measured subjects prior to the 6-week study and again 2 days post training. Measurement of flight times were obtained using the Ergojump system with the best of three jumps recorded. A similar device was used to measure heights reached by subjects who performed CMJs in other studies.

The researchers in these studies were searching for an optimal height where muscles are able to release the most energy. Some discovered that height changes were detrimental to performance, and others attempted to support the inclusion of plyometric training in athletes' programs. The best method for allowing muscles to release their stored energy has not been determined.

References

Gehri, D., Ricard, M., Kleiner, D., & Kirkendall, D. (1998). A comparison of plyometric training techniques for improving vertical jump ability and energy production. *Journal of Strength and Conditioning Research, 12*(2), 85–89.

Matavulj, D., et al. (2001). Effects of plyometric training on jumping performance in junior basketball players. *Journal of Sports Medicine and Physical Fitness, 41,* 159–164.

Sample Student Essay
REVIEW OF RELATED LITERATURE FOR SECONDARY RESEARCH PROJECT

INTRODUCTION

Consisting of a multitude of long collagen strands woven together to permit forces up to 500 pounds, the anterior cruciate ligament (ACL) helps to maintain the alignment of the femoral and tibial condyles of the tibiofemoral articulation by limiting anterior and posterior movement of the femur (*Caring for the Knee,* 2000). Since people today engage in more rigorous physical activities than in the past, the knee joint has become one of the most used and abused joints in the human body, and as a result, knee ligament injuries have increased by 172% over the past 15 years (*Caring . . . ,* 2000). Most of these ACL injuries result from a twisting motion of the knee, common in contact sports, such as football, and pivoting sports, such as skiing or soccer. Although most ACL tears require surgery, some patients can evade surgery by avoiding activities such as jumping or pivoting, which cause instability. In order to strengthen the knee to prevent further injury, these patients may develop their quadriceps and hamstring muscles to help create additional natural stability for the knee (*Caring . . . ,* 2000).

In most cases, however, the amount of instability and the magnitude of the patient's symptoms require surgery to reconstruct the damaged ligament. When surgeons recommend surgery, three different reconstructive techniques using two different types of grafts exist for patients. In the autograft method, surgeons use the patient's own tissue as a source for the replacement ligament (*Caring . . . ,* 2000), and they most often use patellar or hamstring tendon autografts for this procedure. Using the patellar tendon autograft technique, surgeons remove the middle third of the patellar tendon, which connects the tibia to the patella, with small bony plugs at the ends of the tendon (Stone, Walgenbach, & Mullin, 2001). After making a small incision in the knee, sur-

geons drill small tunnels into the bone and then feed the newly constructed patellar tendon ACL through the tunnels, securing it with a staple-and-buckle system (Stone, Walgenbach, & Mullin, 2001). Fastening the graft in this manner allows new blood vessels to grow into the transferred graft, causing increased healing. In the second autograft technique, the surgeons use the semitendinosus-gracilis tendons, or hamstring tendons, which connect the muscles in the posterior portion of the thigh to the lower leg. After a fraction of these two tendons is removed from a small incision in the leg, surgical fixation of the tendons within the knee is achieved to form a new, strong ACL (Aglietti & Buzzi, 1994). In the allograft technique, however, which is similar to organ transplantation and less common than the autograft technique, surgeons use tissue from either a cadaver or a tissue bank to serve as a replacement for the torn ACL (*Caring . . . ,* 2000); in this procedure, a donated Achilles tendon functions as a common allograft substitute.

Since many forms of replacement procedures exist today, researchers and experts continually debate which technique produces the most successful results for the recovering ACL patient. However, because it " . . . provide[s] better knee stability in the long term compared with the two other surgical repair methods . . . " (Andrish, 2001, p. 3), the patellar tendon autograft technique produces the most success for patients undergoing surgery.

LITERATURE REVIEW

The purpose of Hiemstra, Webber, and MacDonald's study entitled "Knee strength deficits after hamstring tendon and patellar tendon anterior cruciate ligament reconstruction" " . . . was to examine the strength of the knee flexors and knee extensors after two surgical techniques of ACL reconstruction and compare them with an age and activity level matched control group" (Hiemstra, Webber, & MacDonald, 2000, p. 1472). In this study, Hiemstra, Webber, and MacDonald hypothesized that the hamstring reconstruction group would exhibit a graft-dependent knee flexor strength deficit, while the patellar tendon reconstruction group would reveal a greater magnitude of knee extensor strength deficit, when compared with the hamstring group. To obtain proper results in this study, the researchers compared 24 active ACL-reconstructed patients with a 30-person control group, using the universal goniometer to assess range of motion (ROM), the 10-cm VAS to assess pain, and the KT-1000 arthrometer to assess tibial-femoral displacement. After analyzing the results at the end of the study, the researchers found that they had correctly hypothesized the results prior to the outcome of the study. In fact, by the end of the study, researchers concluded that regional strength deficits of the knee flexors and extensors following reconstruction depended on the autograft donor site and also determined that knee extensor strength exists as a prerequisite to a functional recovery after ACL reconstruction.

In the "Anterior cruciate ligament graft fixation comparison of hamstring and patellar tendon grafts" study, Steiner and Hecker not only compared the biomechanical properties of the hamstring and patellar tendon ACL reconstructions but also identified the graft fixation techniques that produced ACL reconstructions similar to the intact ACL control group. To achieve these results, the researchers assessed the tensile properties of two reconstruction techniques of ACL reconstruction in 18 pairs of cadaver knees with an average age of 69.5 years. After analyzing each knee using four different semitendinosus-gracilis tendon reconstructive techniques, Steiner and Hecker removed the hamstring grafts, replacing them with four different patellar tendon grafts, and then they tested the new grafts, recording the yield load, tensile strength, displacement, and stiffness for each technique. Testing these techniques allowed the researchers to conclude that the strongest hamstring tendon graft fixation with the double tendons secured with soft tissue washers yielded the highest strength, 103% of the intact ACL, while the patellar tendon graft fixations produced the highest degree of stiffness. Based on the results from this study, researchers concluded that the best graft techniques available for patients having to undergo ACL reconstruction include the doubled-hamstring tendon graft, which uses washers to fix the looped tendons around the post on the tibia, and the patellar tendon graft, which uses interference screws for fixation.

In the study "Patellar tendon versus doubled semitendinosus and gracilis tendons for anterior cruciate ligament reconstruction," Aglietti and Buzzi sought to determine both the advantages and disadvantages of the patellar tendon and hamstring tendon reconstruction techniques by comparing them with a control group. To compare results of patients 28 months after ACL surgery using two different types of grafts, the researchers used the Cybex II isokinetic dynamometer to assess both extensor and flexor muscle strength and the KT-2000 arthrometer to test side-to-side displacement for the 60 patients with chronic knee injuries. After reviewing the data obtained from this study, the researchers recommended that surgeons

should perform patellar tendon reconstruction on younger, more motivated patients with higher demands and use the hamstring tendon method in older, less motivated patients.

References

Aglietti, P., & Buzzi, R. (1994). Patellar tendon versus doubled semitendinosus and gracilis tendons for anterior cruciate ligament reconstruction. *American Journal of Sports Medicine*, *22*(2), 211–219. [Database]. Ebsco Host: Health Source: Nursing/Academic Edition.

Andrish, J. T. (2001). Comparing ACL reconstruction methods. *Physician and Sports Medicine*, *29*(10), 3–5. [Database]. Ebsco Host: MasterFILE Premier.

Caring for the knee. (2000). Retrieved February 7, 2002, from University of Philadelphia Medical Center, Sports Medicine Web site: http://www.upmc.edu/SportsMedCenter/repair-treat-rehab-knee.htm

Hiemstra, L. A., Webber, S., & MacDonald, P. B. (2000). Knee strength deficits after hamstring tendon and patellar tendon anterior cruciate ligament reconstruction. *Medicine and Science in Sports and Exercise*, *32*(8), 1472–1479.

Steiner, M. E., & Hecker, A. T. (1994). Anterior cruciate ligament graft fixation comparison of hamstring and patellar tendon grafts. *American Journal of Sports Medicine*, *22*(2), 240–248. [Database]. Ebsco Host: Health Source: Nursing/Academic Edition.

Stone, K., Walgenbach, A., & Mullin, M. (2001). Anterior cruciate ligament repair. Retrieved February 7, 2002, from http://www.stone-clinic.com/aclrep.htm

THESIS CHAPTER THREE: PROCEDURES, METHODOLOGY, AND MATERIALS AND METHODS

In the formal "Proposal," you provided your reader with a brief discussion of the plan intended to develop a research strategy. In the actual thesis, you will provide the detailed plan of attack that you used. This section is an important part of the thesis in that it allows your readers the opportunity to judge the validity of your **methods**—the principles used to gather data or conduct research. In other words, anyone who was interested could duplicate your results if they followed the same formula you present. Additionally, your methods will indicate that your rationale for discovery yields the conclusions that you will develop in the "Results" section of the thesis. In short, this section presents the methodology used in the study examining how you actually researched your problem. It demonstrates, according to specific topics, the steps you took to answer your research question or prove your thesis statement. *(Note: Since the procedures for performing the research and gathering data will have been completed in the past, use past-tense verbs to describe your methods.)*

Using headings and subheading formats outlined for you in your APA style manual, present the following groups of information. Under each heading, provide a complete description of actual incidents as they occurred and facts surrounding the methods.

Introduction/Consent

An optional component, the "Introduction/Consent" section should outline the general principles of gathering your research data. It should also include a brief description of the researchers' attempt to meet the expectations and qualifications of human subjects research review.

EXAMPLE

Before being able to participate in this study, each subject received a verbal explanation of the study's intention, and each willingly signed a consent form (Appendix X-1). Prior to participating, participants were asked a series of six questions, and several measurements of their lower extremities were taken (Appendix X-2) to clear them for participation. All subjects were informed that they could ask questions or withdraw from the study at any time.

Subjects

Describe the population of subjects used. The number of subjects usually indicates how well the study population relates to the general population. Additionally, you will want to explain how you collected your sample of subjects to perform such a study. Your aim is to gather subjects through a method that is free from bias, but this is, in most cases, impossible. Consequently, you may want to provide an explanation of how bias works itself into the study and may affect results. If you have not included a separate heading to provide assurances that human subjects' rights have not been violated, you should do so here. Often, a separate document, registered with the college, serves this purpose, and a simple statement of compliance will suffice.

EXAMPLE

Twenty subjects participated in this study as well as random volunteers. By being compared only with themselves, all subjects acted as controls. The study consisted of 13 males and 7 females as well as 10 athletes and 10 nonathletes, who were all 18 years of age or older. All 20 subjects had not experienced any lower extremity pathologies, including muscle strains, within the last 6 months, nor did any have balance problems or any form of plyometric training before their participation in this study. Adequate range of motion in bilateral lower extremities was measured in all subjects.

Setting

Describe from where you gathered your test subjects and the facilities in which you performed the tests used to gather data. This section provides the reader with assurances that the subjects were chosen using a scientifically based method and that the facilities were appropriate to gather such data from this population.

Design: Method of Collecting Data

Describe the experimental design as a blueprint of your strategy: clinical trial, controlled or random, and so on. It also outlines the plan you used to create or determine variables in your study. Include all instructions, time of data collection, equipment used, and number of trials.

Tests and Descriptions

Describe the material used to gather evidence: surveys, equipment to perform therapy, measuring devices, instruments, and so forth.

*Validity and Reliability of Measurements
or Procedures*

Prove that your measurements and procedures are valid by explaining thoroughly the task performed, the outcome gained, and the progressions or changes as expected in the scheme of your study. You may also want to describe how you analyzed your data.

EXAMPLE

This study required several instruments to be used, but only one was directly relative to reliability and validity: a tape measure and the researchers' ability to read the measure accurately and consistently. Other instruments used were black paper taped to the gym wall, white chalk, a wooden box 41 cm in height, a clock, a scale, and a goniometer.

The researchers attempted to validate this study by accounting for all 20 participants in both the validation and the study group. Each subject would be compared with themselves rather than the others, to eliminate variables. The vertical heights measured from the ground are considered the validation group; the vertical heights measured from the drop jump are considered the study group.

Procedure: Method of Data Analysis

Describe the elements of the experiment on which the study hinges, such as treatments provided to each group or subgroup and the control group. Explain what you plan to do with the data once collected. Furthermore, you must be specific about the type of statistical analysis you have used and discuss the field's acceptance of this type of data analysis.

EXAMPLE

The height in centimeters that each subject jumped, starting at ground level, was compared with the height jumped from the drop jump for the same subject. Data were analyzed using a paired t-test. The statistical test was used to determine significant difference ($p < 0.05$) between the two heights for each subject.

Below are other topics to include in this section, at the direction of your advisor:

Consent forms

Test instrument

Validation group

Study group

Study design

Intervention format and presentation

THESIS CHAPTER FOUR: ANALYSIS AND RESULTS

The "Results" chapter simply provides your **results**—outcomes of the study performed. It describes what was found. This part of the thesis should be written without rambling explanation or commentary. Simply provide the end product of the science employed. In other words, the "Results" section should reflect the research problem presented and provide the evidence for making your claim.

Often, the "Results" section of the thesis can be reduced to tables, charts, or graphs that logically compare data. Remember not to simply duplicate in writing what the tables, charts, or graphs already represent. Your written comments should extrapolate the important elements of the graphics for the reader and relate them to the findings of the study.

Any "Results" section should delineate differences between primary or secondary evidence. Primary evidence describes the results; secondary evidence draws inferences from the primary.

The information provided in this chapter can be presented by using the following subcategories for organization. Include the subcategories that are relevant to your work, and omit those that are not.

Subjects

Test instrument

General analysis

Results

A "Discussion" section, however, always is necessary.

Discussion

In the **discussion**, you should, in a straightforward manner, answer the research question or provide full and articulate answers or support for your thesis statement. More important, you will discuss the meaning of your results. Explain how the results have meaning to the field and what you have learned from the experiment. Present your data and results, and make generalized conclusions from them. Expound on the correlation you found between groups or explain how some expected outcomes never materialized. This is the place to discuss controversy or reveal anomalous results.

Your purpose in the "Discussion" section is to assure yourself that your reader will make the correct assumptions or interpretations that you have. You should not make unfounded conclusions or speculate without solid research to support your claims. You can, however, mention that certain questions have not been addressed or answered, and consequently, more research should follow in this direction.

Finally, you should examine how your study relates to the scholarly dialogue that is continuing in the field under this category or how your study can be used through practical application in the profession.

First, the discussion should explain why you obtained the results you did. Second, it should provide a clear description of the correlation between your findings and findings of other studies.

Sample Student Essay
DISCUSSION FOR PRIMARY RESEARCH PROJECT

Twenty subjects began the study, but only seventeen completed: six females, eleven males, eight athletes, and nine nonathletes. The three subjects who withdrew gave no reason for doing so.

A paired t-test was performed on the data collected (Table 1), using an alpha level of $p < 0.05$. Each subject participated in three trials, with the mean height drawn from the three trials. When comparing the mean for each condition using the paired t-test and alpha level, a significant difference was found at $p = 0.0002$.

Subjects as individuals showed a difference between two heights (Graph 1); however, by examining the average heights for all subjects, an obvious difference is apparent (Graph 2).

DISCUSSION

The results of this study showed a significant difference between the two heights for each individual subject. The data from Table 1 indicates that six subjects experienced a difference of 1 to 2 cm, four showed a difference of 3 to 5 cm, two experienced an 8-cm difference, three increased by 10 cm, and one by 16 cm. The results showed that only one subject lost difference between the two heights (–0.085 cm).

From these results, the researchers suggest that the energy and its release is not related to participating in a sport. These issues are related to the difference between muscle fibers of each individual. Additionally, leg length and body weight were measured, and no relationship was found between these measurements and the results with respect to outcomes. Our study's findings suggest that neither a person's athletic prowess nor his or her physical training influences the effect of plyometrics.

Sample Student Essay
DISCUSSION FOR SECONDARY RESEARCH PROJECT

DISCUSSION

According to the results in each of these three studies, the patellar tendon autograft technique has proved superior to the hamstring tendon autograft technique. Using peak moment and multiple velocity measurements, Hiemstra, Webber, and MacDonald (2000) established that while both the hamstring and patellar tendon groups demonstrated similar knee extensor strength deficits of 25.5% in comparison with the control group, the hamstring tendon group demonstrated a significantly greater knee flexor strength deficit of 17%, on average, across all velocities and contraction types when compared with the control group (2000). Researchers have found these knee flexors especially important in the recovery of ACL-reconstructed patients. In fact, since the knee joint uses the flexors for stabilization and deceleration of the leg motion, an increased risk of ACL graft rupture, injury, or interference in returning to previous levels of function exists secondary to the compromised ability of the knee flexors (Hiemstra, Webber, & MacDonald, 2000). Therefore, because evidence has shown that the hamstring tendon reconstruction substantially compromises the ability of these knee flexors more often than the patellar tendon reconstruction technique, failure of the hamstring tendon graft more often occurs in recovering patients. For this reason, " . . . patients who participate in sports that require prominent use of the biarticular hamstring muscle group may want to avoid the possibility of a knee flexor deficit" (Hiemstra, Webber, & MacDonald, 2000, p. 1475). Since the patellar tendon autograft does not compromise the ability of the knee flexors and does not create increased graft rupture and failure, this graft fixation technique proves more advantageous than the hamstring tendon technique.

In Steiner and Hecker's study "Anterior cruciate ligament graft fixation comparison of hamstring and patellar tendon grafts," the researchers found that ACL reconstruction success depends highly on secure graft fixation (Steiner & Hecker, 1994). In fact, "[t]he goal of graft fixation is to prevent overstretching or failure at graft fixation sites, and thereby to permit early motion and early weight bearing without the loss of stability" (Steiner & Hecker, 1994, p. 241). Therefore, if a fixation technique demonstrates greater stiffness, superior strength and success follow. Regardless of the technique tested in Steiner and Hecker's study, all of the reconstructions using hamstring autograft tendon resulted in significant decreased stiffness when compared with the control group (1994). In fact, most of the hamstring tendon techniques produced values less than half of the control group values. Once again, this decrease in stiffness produces an increased instability of the knee joint. Conversely, the patellar tendon fixation techniques not only revealed significantly higher stiffness values than the hamstring group but also produced stiffness values similar to those for the intact ACL group (Steiner & Hecker, 1994). Therefore, in order to achieve maximum final strength, Hiemstra, Webber, and MacDonald concluded that a successful outcome of the ACL reconstruction procedure depends on the amount of stiffness produced by the fixation technique (1994), and in order to achieve the greatest stiffness for the reconstructed knee, patients should choose the patellar tendon autograft fixation technique.

In addition, Steiner and Hecker also substantiated that all of the hamstring reconstruction techniques revealed relatively weak attachment sites owing to the slow tearing from their tibial insertions, causing increased limitations for the patient (1994). In fact, with prolonged pullouts, these hamstring tendon autografts also demonstrated increased suture fixation failure (Steiner & Hecker, 1994); conversely, the patellar tendon autografts did not demonstrate graft failure with prolonged pullouts, thus proving, yet again, to be the better fixation technique. Furthermore, during displacement test-

ing, Steiner and Hecker found that all of the hamstring grafts failed at higher average displacements than those for the original ACL, while the patellar tendon grafts, on average, failed at shorter displacements in comparison with the hamstring group (1994). Additionally, these patellar tendon patients did not show a significant difference from the intact ACL in terms of displacement, demonstrating further benefits to the patellar tendon autograft use (Steiner & Hecker, 1994). Therefore, because the hamstring tendon group succumbs more to failure, the patellar tendon technique surpasses the hamstring tendon technique in producing the most successful recovery for patients.

Supporting Steiner and Hecker's findings, Aglietti and Buzzi (1994) concluded that patellar tendon patients achieved better stability but increased extension loss and patellar problems. Conversely, with the use of the hamstring tendon replacement technique, patients obtained less stability but demonstrated a decrease in patellar and motion problems (Aglietti & Buzzi, 1994). Despite the minor extension loss in the patellar tendon group, these researchers concluded that athletes returned more frequently to sports participation with patellar tendon reconstruction than did the hamstring group, at rates of 80% and 43%, respectively (Aglietti & Buzzi, 1994). The researchers attribute this accelerated return to the increased stiffness, which causes increased stability, found in the patellar tendon autograft patients. In fact, like Steiner and Hecker's study, the patellar tendon autograft produced greater stiffness when compared with both the original and hamstring tendon–reconstructed knees, thus increasing stability for the patient (Aglietti & Buzzi, 1994).

Additionally, Aglietti and Buzzi attribute many other weaknesses to hamstring tendon use, making the patellar tendon autograft superior. For instance, crepitation, crackling within the joint, developed repeatedly in the hamstring reconstructions. In addition, Aglietti and Buzzi also found increased side-to-side anterior displacement, causing greater limitations and instability for the patient undergoing the hamstring tendon reconstruction technique (Aglietti & Buzzi, 1994). Even after the surgeon affixes the soft tissues of the hamstring tendon to the bone during reconstruction, an increased rate of failure and instability of the hamstring graft becomes apparent (Aglietti & Buzzi, 1994). Therefore, researchers advise a less accelerated rehabilitation program for these hamstring tendon patients (Aglietti & Buzzi, 1994). Since the patellar tendon graft displayed better stability than the hamstring tendon, the researchers also recommended the use of the patellar tendon for reconstruction of chronic ACL-deficient knees (Aglietti & Buzzi, 1994). Based on the data obtained from Aglietti and Buzzi's study, researchers routinely use patellar tendon grafts more often for athletes and first-time ACL patients, while older patients, patients with preexisting patellofemoral problems, and patients with failed patella tendon autografts prefer the hamstring tendon reconstruction. In conclusion, when researchers asked patients to express their satisfaction or dissatisfaction with their operated knee in comparison with their normal knee at the conclusion of the study, the patellar group reported higher ratings, thus revealing the patellar tendon autograft technique, yet again, as the most beneficial reconstruction choice for patients (Aglietti & Buzzi, 1994).

References

Aglietti, P., & Buzzi, R. (1994). Patellar tendon versus doubled semitendinosus and gracilis tendons for anterior cruciate ligament reconstruction. *American Journal of Sports Medicine, 22*(2), 211–219. [Database]. Ebsco Host: Health Source: Nursing/Academic Edition.

Andrish, J. T. (2001). Comparing ACL reconstruction methods. *Physician and Sports Medicine, 29*(10), 3–5. [Database]. Ebsco Host: MasterFILE Premier.

Caring for the knee. (2000). Retrieved February 7, 2002, from University of Philadelphia Medical Center, Sports Medicine Web site: http://www.upmc.edu/SportsMedCenter/repair-treat-rehab-knee.htm

Hiemstra, L. A., Webber, S., MacDonald, P. B. (2000). Knee strength deficits after hamstring tendon and patellar tendon anterior cruciate ligament reconstruction. *Medicine and Science in Sports and Exercise, 32*(8), 1472–1479.

Steiner, M. E., & Hecker, A. T. (1994). Anterior cruciate ligament graft fixation comparison of hamstring and patellar tendon grafts. *American Journal of Sports Medicine, 22*(2), 240–248. [Database]. Ebsco Host: Health Source: Nursing/Academic Edition.

Stone, K., Walgenbach, A., & Mullin, M. (2001). Anterior Cruciate Ligament Repair. Retrieved February 7, 2002, from http://www.stone-clinic.com/aclrep.htm

THESIS CHAPTER FIVE: SUMMARY, CONCLUSIONS, AND RECOMMENDATIONS

Obviously, like any concluding chapter, this chapter should present a summary of the study conducted and discuss, in a broad sense, the conclusions drawn from the results. As a matter of contributing to the field's scholarly dialogue, you should offer recommendations for the uses of the conclusions. Offer specific descriptions of or practical applications to which the conclusions can be applied. Finally, as any good researcher will do, supply the reader with the open-ended issues that your study generates. Your work obviously cannot be the end of the research line in your subject area. Discuss the avenues of possible research to be conducted in this field as a result of your work. In other words, ask the next valid research questions.

At the end of your thesis project, you will supply your reader with any necessary **appendices** —text sections outside of standard chapters that present additional information, often in graphs, charts, and tables.

Finally, your **references**—containing the sources you have cited—should adhere to the standard format specified by your instructors.

EXAMPLE

Past studies regarding plyometrics have attempted to prove that plyometrics is a beneficial technique of exercise. Several studies combined plyometrics with a long-term training program consisting of aerobic exercise or sport-specific training. These combinations allowed the researchers of this study to question the results of past studies, since the results of past studies may have been derivative of pure conditioning or the effects of plyometrics. These studies failed to support the notion that basic plyometrics is capable of increasing muscle power and strength without being combined with other forms of training.

This study concluded that muscle fibers can efficiently store and release energy as power. Through mechanisms of negative work and positive work, a patient can increase the amount of force and power available for use.

The following list delineates possible recommendations for future research. We suggest that future studies investigate the relationship associated with microscopic organisms responsible for plyometrics. We also advocate the continuation of this study using new technology.

Sample Student Essay
CONCLUSION AND REFERENCES FOR SECONDARY RESEARCH PROJECT

CONCLUSION

Since these studies indicate that the patellar tendon autograft causes increased stability and stiffness for the knee joint, the patellar tendon autograft remains the best option for most patients, especially for those who are physically active. In fact, because the hamstring reconstruction technique compromises the ability of the flexors in the knee, which help in knee stability, patients with the patellar tendon reconstruction demonstrate a decreased chance of graft rupture in comparison with the hamstring tendon technique.

However, as in all studies, many factors may have limited the research in these particular studies, preventing researchers from expanding their research fully. For instance, many studies, including "Knee strength deficits after hamstring tendon and patellar tendon anterior cruciate ligament surgery," use the contralateral knee as a comparison for the reconstructed knee. However, this method does not give an accurate measure of the exact deficit of the reconstructed knee (Hiemstra, Webber, & MacDonald, 2000). For example, when a patient undergoes reconstructive surgery on one knee, the other knee suffers and undergoes a deficit also; therefore, the deficit measured by comparing the reconstructed leg with the normal leg does not accurately represent the actual deficit of the reconstruction itself. In Steiner and Hecker's study, researchers tested only cadaver knees from persons aged 48 to 79, even though teens and younger adults constitute most ACL injuries (1994). Once again, researchers cannot necessarily expand the findings from the knees of older bodies with those of physically active adolescents and young adults. In fact, aging individuals function at different levels and engage in many different activities compared with young adults, and therefore, the needs from the outcome of surgery between a 72-year-old senior citizen and a 21-year-old college soccer player contrast greatly. In order to get a complete understanding of the effects of a reconstruction technique, researchers should examine patients of both genders, all ages, and a wide range of physical activeness to get an accurate measure. In addition, none of these studies examined the effects of the allograft technique compared with the autograft technique. Once again, in order to get a complete picture of what the best option for a patient should be, all techniques should be researched in order to find a reconstruction technique that best meets the patient's needs.

References

Aglietti, P., & Buzzi, R. (1994). Patellar tendon versus doubled semitendinosus and gracilis tendons for anterior cruciate ligament reconstruction. *American Journal of Sports Medicine*, 22(2), 211–219. [Database]. Ebsco Host: Health Source: Nursing/Academic Edition.

Andrish, J. T. (2001). Comparing ACL reconstruction methods. *Physician and Sports Medicine*, 29(10), 3–5. [Database]. Ebsco Host: MasterFILE Premier.

Caring for the knee. (2000). Retrieved February 7, 2002, from University of Philadelphia Medical Center, Sports Medicine Web site: http://www.upmc.edu/SportsMedCenter/repair-treat-rehab-knee.htm.

Hiemstra, L. A., Webber, S., MacDonald, P. B. (2000). Knee strength deficits after hamstring tendon and patellar tendon anterior cruciate ligament reconstruction. *Medicine and Science in Sports and Exercise*, 32(8), 1472–1479.

Steiner, M. E., & Hecker, A. T. (1994). Anterior cruciate ligament graft fixation comparison of hamstring and patellar tendon grafts. *American Journal of Sports Medicine*, 22(2), 240–248. [Database]. Ebsco Host: Health Source: Nursing/Academic Edition.

Stone, K., Walgenbach, A., & Mullin, M. (2001). Anterior Cruciate Ligament Repair. Retrieved February 7, 2002, from http://www.stone-clinic.com/aclrep.htm

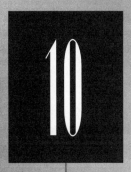
Writing for Publication

Key Terms

Abstract A short description of the ensuing article

Descriptive review A summary of studies or research; most often used in literature reviews

Direct patient education literature Specific instructions written for a specific patient

Editorial An informed opinion solicited by a publication

Evaluative review A separate publication that evaluates the science of published information

General patient population literature Documents prepared that anticipate patients' concerns and frequently asked questions

Journals Publications in specific fields that are governed by editorial boards and committees that referee submissions

Review A component of the scholarly dialogue that assesses the value of published information

Scholarly dialogue The "conversation" that exists between professionals to debate pertinent issues

chapter objectives

On completion of this chapter, the reader should be able to

1. Understand the protocol used for judging submissions for publication.
2. Develop text and/or research appropriate for publication.
3. Understand the need for quality assessment of other scientists' work.
4. Create text that uses appropriate voice, terminology, and organization principles for nonacademic audiences.

*P*ublishing is an important process for academicians, who sometimes fully depend on filling a curriculum vitae (CV) with journal article publications and book titles for promotion considerations. For practitioners in the field, publishing may not appear to be an important part of job responsibilities, but it can be vitally important. According to recent statistics, over 50% of those practitioners who published were promoted over their counterparts. Employers see employees who publish as those who stay current with changes in the field and become active participants in the process of change.

Writing an article, however, does not guarantee its publication. More than a third of articles submitted to nationally recognized **journals** are rejected, with higher rates of rejection for more prestigious journals. Moreover, rejections are not usually based on volume; in other words, journals will not reject a good article because they have too many in queue. Most journals will stockpile the good submissions for later distribution.

The reasons for rejection vary, but the most common reason is that the article does not fit the focus or purpose of the targeted journal. To avoid this pitfall, read the editorial remarks on the title page of the journal and gather the instruction information carefully, such as type of articles the journal accepts and the format in which articles should be presented. With the overflow of articles pouring onto their desks, editors can easily reject an article that does match style and content in favor of one that does.

Other articles are rejected because of substantive problems in research and presentation. For example, an article that contains weak data or describes a poorly constructed study is easy to reject. Writing concerns should also be considered here. Many articles are rejected not because the study was poorly constructed but because the writer failed to delineate his or her purpose clearly. As a result, the article seems to swerve from its purpose, and no article that has a weak purpose will be published. Other writing problems have led to rejection as well. For example, poor grammar and mechanics alone can be sufficiently distracting that the reader loses concentration on the message. Editors regularly reject manuscripts for basic writing problems. Editors want to work with professionals and people who value their work enough to put effort into communicating their cause accurately.

Although the task for publishing is daunting, it should be every writer's goal and the goal of every practitioner. This chapter reviews the different types of writing that are most often publishable.

LETTERS AND EDITORIALS

Letters to the Editor

Letters to the editor may not seem important to the depth and scope of what a journal offers, but letters often are read most frequently by the journal's readership. Many people enjoy the pithy comments of astute readers, but others see the value in the **scholarly dialogue**. Many articles are published, and not all editorial boards can make guarantees that an article will be infallible. Sometimes, practitioners in the field can make assessments of the published work and offer commentary. In some cases, the letter can demonstrate points of contention with the published results or methods; in others, the letter can support or even offer new or variant ways to approach the subject. Thus, the letter serves as a mechanism that allows the scholarly dialogue to persist.

The key to publishing a letter is objectivity and brevity. No one can disagree or agree unless he or she has evidence or proof to support a claim, and no one wants to read unsubstantiated claims. Furthermore, if you have a claim to make, make it by offering your perspective in a brief format. Lead in by addressing the background information offered and the title and publication data of the article or subject. Provide a body paragraph or sentences that make your point clearly and without rambling. Get to the point, offer your evidence, and then offer a conclusion that pulls the letter together. Most journals will require that you submit your name, position or title, address, and E-mail address to verify your position or standing in the field. These may also be helpful to writers who want to contact you about your scholarly position.

Letters to the editor often take a specific form or have specific instructions attached. As always, know the format and function that the journal's editors require.

Editorials

The **editorial** is yet another forum for continuing the field's scholarly dialogue. Often written by established professionals in the field, editorials usually address a new or emerging topic and present an expert's position on the issues. Additionally, editorials are unique in that they provide little if any research. Most often, the journal solicits the opinion of the expert to take a side in a conflict, to present a conflict's opposing sides, or to simply demonstrate the impact that new and developing issues have on the field.

Editorials at the local level (newspapers, newsletters, or pamphlets) serve the same purpose, but they are far less prestigious. Often, they constitute a starting point for other research, or they present a group's position on a divisive issue. Most recently, the types of editorials that dominate the local scene are from practitioners battling HMOs or managed care facilities, and the arguments stem from issues of autonomy to revenues. Although editorials and letters to the editor will not serve to add weight to your publications list, they do demonstrate activity in the field and present an informed opinion. Begin some of your professional writing projects with submissions to local newspapers and newsletters within your field or organization. These editorials can give you the necessary practice of writing for other professionals in your field and exercise your ability to analyze your situation and to articulate your position. Often, what begins as a simple letter turns into a conference presentation, a journal article, or even the premise for the start of a book-length work.

CRITIQUING THE WORK OF OTHERS: WRITING THE ARTICLE REVIEW

Scholars often compare studies or analyze the work of others because many varieties of research exist. Furthermore, studies and their results can also be manipulated to suit the desired outcomes of the researchers. Consequently, the potential for problems necessitates close scrutiny of any text in any profession. This process of assessment of the value of published information—formal **review**—is part of the scholarly dialogue within the profession. Review articles provide a quick assessment of the work and its value to the field and to non-professionals as well. Two types of review articles exist: descriptive and evaluative.

Descriptive Reviews

The **descriptive review** assesses changes in the field and provides a link to the document in the history of previous research. This type of review most often is used in literature reviews or to build the introductory sections of a thesis or dissertation. The reader of a longer work will want to understand the processes of background research that have been engaged and to determine if studies have been neglected or ignored that might refute the writer's findings. The literature review offers a quick analysis of multiple studies and their major findings as they relate to the author's research subject. Likewise, literature reviews are usually no more than a few pages in length, and in some cases, they are reduced to a few paragraphs or a single paragraph for each entry.

Evaluative Reviews

The **evaluative review** helps assess the answers to questions provided by research. This type of review is seen most commonly as a separate publication in journals, not in dissertations and theses. Since the author of the article to be reviewed has offered a question to be resolved, the evaluative review should assess the answers provided, rather than focus on a conflicting opinion. A conflicting opinion should be supported with solid research and methods and then written as a separate article for publication. Evaluative reviews examine the methodology and results of published works.

To write a critique or review of an article or chapter, choose an article from a scholarly journal or publishing house. An understanding of the importance of using scholarly texts is essential. Teams of scholars and critics in the field, who generally accept the article's worth in the field's continuing dialogue, referee scholarly publications. As a result, your review challenges or supports their decision to include the work in the field's scholarly dialogue. Critiquing less scholarly work, for example from a newspaper or news magazine, is moot in that these works are intended not for critical analysis but for consumer digestion. As you would evaluate a source for research, apply the same principles here.

Once you have chosen an article for review, read the document several times carefully and thoroughly. Your goal is to completely understand the material as well as the methods, results, and conclusion sections. Address also the audience and purpose. Once you have mastered the content, scrutinize the work by asking questions about the entirety of the work:

- Why does the author undertake the study?

- Do certain pressures from society, medicine, or culture dictate that the study be completed? To whom and for what purpose was it written?

- What questions are asked and how does the author (intend to) answer them?

- What are the results of the study? Are the results a logical end to the methods and materials used? What methods did you use to determine if the primary research is accurate?

- What questions remain unanswered? What further research needs to be completed as a result of this study? What research might also derive from future considerations of the subject?

Writing the Evaluative Review

Once you have answered these questions and formulated an evaluation and assessment of the work, you are ready to begin writing the critique. The critique contains three sections: the citation, the summary, and the evaluation.

At the top of the page, place the bibliographic entry for the source in the format appropriate to your field. APA style is generally accepted in most allied health and medical fields.

To write the summary, provide a few sentences of background information concerning the reasons for the study's publication and the questions that the researchers aimed to answer or address. In the same paragraph, provide a transition to the materials and methods used to complete the study, and then state the authors' major findings. The summary should be brief and concise. Too much information distracts the reader from your purpose, which is the assessment.

In the assessment or evaluation paragraph, provide your analysis of the study's weaknesses. Determine if the results are a logical extension of the data presented or if the authors have made generalizations that reach beyond the scope of the study. Examine the materials and methods employed, and assess general research techniques and data gathering. Assess the conclusions of the study and the impact on the field or future research.

In the assessment section, many writers will feel licensed to criticize. Criticism that is devastating and not constructive, however, is both unprofessional and inappropriate. Your goal here is not to bash the author but to provide constructive criticism and assessment to better the next study. Also, your goal is not to place wholesale value judgments on the text. Writing that the article is "worthless" or "should not be read" makes the *reviewer* look unprofessional, not the author. An editorial board of professionals has decided that the article has worth. You may reveal your ignorance in offering such harsh criticism.

Likewise, offering meaningless and trite fluff in your assessment is also not recommended. Phrases such as "I really enjoyed the article" frustrate your reader because they are empty praise. Your reader does not care about what you do or do not enjoy. Also, phrases such as "the research was well done" tell the reader nothing. Give substantive comments.

In some cases, you may want to assess writing techniques if poor writing interferes with the communication of the message. Making statements about writing style, misuse of terms, poor grammar and mechanics, or incoherence is useful because it may send a message to the editorial staff about professionalism, or it may heighten other readers' awareness of writing problems in the field.

If your critique is part of a larger document, such as a literature review, you do not need to include a conclusion, but if it is a stand-alone document, a conclusion should be included.

Sample Student Essay
EVALUATIVE REVIEW

> Lewek, M., Stevens, J., & Snyder-Mackler, L. (2001). The use of electrical stimulation to increase quadriceps femoris muscle force in all elderly patients following a total knee arthroplasty [Electronic version]. *Physical Therapy*, *81*, 1565–1573. Retrieved November 11, 2002, from Health Reference Center Academic database.

Lewek, Stevens, and Snyder-Mackler organized a case study in response to previous research, which noted that older patients experienced excessive loss of force strength in their quadriceps femoris muscles. Such losses result in decreased range of motion (ROM), decreased strength, and increased functional limitations of the elderly individuals. The case study completed by Lewek et al. measured the effects of neuromuscular electric stimulation (NMES) on the force strength of the quadriceps femoris muscles in a 66-year-old man who received a total knee arthroplasty. Although researchers performed numerous experiments measuring the effects of NMES in younger patients, the case study completed by Lewek et al. is one of the few measuring the effects in elderly patients.

Lewek et al. based the case study on several previous experiments. The article describing and clarifying the purpose of, methods used for, and result acquired from the NMES case study credits these researchers as sources for several tests and methodologies. While explaining every aspect of the case study, Lewek et al. noted that some of the tests and data lacked accuracy. Despite the emphasis on reliability and accuracy, certain measurements remain questionable within the study owing to inadequate equipment. Much of the study remains questionable because of the fact that the study consisted of only one male patient and lacked any experimental controls. The patient within the study performed outpatient therapy consisting of exercises at home and at the clinic without any restrictions or controls. Within the article, Lewek et al. established the need for a controlled study containing numerous participants in order to verify the effectiveness of NMES treatment. The article included a "discussion" section that not only summarized the findings but also stated many of the limitations and inadequacies of the study. Containing possibilities for further improvements on the case study, the "discussion" section of the article substantiated the different possibilities for use of NMES in certain patients.

Well-written and comprehensible, the "discussion" section of the article correlated the data found to the content of the rest of the article. Written for an educated audience, the article incorporated medical terminology with the basic explanations allowing the content to be easily understood yet professional. The article regarding the case study consisted of varied sentence structures, grammatically correct sentences, and a verb-based writing style. One of the few exceptions to the consistently impressive grammar was in the title of the article; Lewek et al. wrote "all" where the word "an" should be. Despite the few mechanical discrepancies, Lewek et al. presented a well-composed, concise, and logical article.

Lewek et al. created a succinct article that consolidated the most important information about the assessments, methodologies, and results from the case study. In the final paragraphs, the article notes that the study produced the expected results in the elderly man, yet without the proper experimental environment, accurate results remain unattainable.

Sample Student Essay
DESCRIPTIVE REVIEW

The mind is a strong element used in the road to recovery after an illness or physical problem. Even though the mind is an amazing tool used during healing, it is not the cure-all answer to all the problems in the human body. In addition to other medical rehabilitation and treatments, alternative medicine forms such as prayer, meditation, herbal treatments, and massage therapy may aid in the restoration of one's well-being, but these alternative medicine forms, on their own, cannot completely heal medical problems. Instead, the mind works with the body to heal.

Intercessory prayer is a technique in which an outside person prays for the health and well-being of another who is ill. The effectiveness of this alternative medicine form is questionable. In Randolph C. Byrd's 1988 study, the control group "required ventilatory assistance, antibiotics, and diuretics more frequently than patients in the IP group," and therefore, Byrd concluded that intercessory prayer is a beneficial technique that should be used in the curative process (Murphy, 2001). Murphy, the author of the article "Innocent Bystander," countered these findings stating that Byrd's study was not complete and questioned, "How does one interpret the fact that many people in the IP groups didn't show any improvement at all?" (Murphy, 2001). In other words, if intercessory prayer is reportedly beneficial, then everyone should experience improved health, which is not the case in Byrd's study. Murphy states, "Personal prayer can be a healthful activity," but it should not be the only form of treatment that should be administered to a patient (Murphy, 2001). This is supported by the 1965 study by C. R. B. Joyce and R. M. C. Welldone, who discovered no real clear correlation between the hospitalized patients who were prayed for and those who were not. However, even though intercessory prayer has not been proved to be 100% effective in recovery efforts, it should not be eliminated entirely in the improvement process. Instead, intercessory prayer should be used hand in hand with other medical techniques. Because prayer is an extremely powerful device, it is also involved in the placebo effect. If a patient knows that others are praying for him to get well, he will have a firm faith that God will come through for him and aid in his recovery. With this thought, the patient becomes more positive in his outlook, and his condition may even start to improve, allowing the patient to believe that his recovery is the direct result of the prayers.

Both massage therapy and meditation are two other forms of alternative medicine. Meditation, for example, is a calming mental exercise that is proved to help reduce stress, tension, panic, and anxiety. Besides these soothing effects, meditation is also a scientifically verified way to relieve chronic pain and reduce high blood pressure and may even be helpful for both headaches and respiratory problems, including asthma. Like meditation, massage therapy also provides relief from the symptoms of anxiety, stress, insomnia, depression, and tension as well as headaches, muscle pain, and back pain, but it is not capable of curing any serious or life-threatening medical disorders. Just as prayer allegedly does, meditation and massage both help to alleviate some of the other factors that are related to the illness but do not eliminate the underlying cause. Once these factors or symptoms are eliminated by the alternative medicine mind relaxation techniques, the patient, his body, and medical practitioners can all work together to cure the primary root of the problem. Because the mind and body work so closely together, both forms of treatment are more effective if practiced together.

Herbal remedies, which have become quite popular in the last decade, are one final form of alternative medicine that act on the placebo effect and do not necessarily give promising results. In fact, British alternative medicine researcher Dr. Edzard Ernst conducted a study in which he tested gingko biloba, St. John's wort, *Echinacea*, ginseng, and several other herbs that constitute over $590 million in sales annually in the United States alone (Bouchez, 2002). After carrying out sixteen well-conducted clinical trials, Ernst found no support that ginseng is an effective way to treat any condition (Bouchez, 2002). In actuality, his research indicated many potential side effects including insomnia, severe headaches, hypertension, nausea, and diarrhea. Despite these findings, people still continue to utilize these herbs. These sustained actions have to do with the placebo effect. People who take herbs are convinced that these herbs, such as ginseng, have life-altering effects that can help promote a healthy lifestyle. Believing what the labels and advertisements say, their minds believe it to be true and trick their body into thinking the same. Like the other forms of alternative medicines, however, these herbs do not remove the underlying cause of a person's illness.

In times of illness or physical distress, the mind tends to take over and makes the body believe something that may not actually be true. For this, the mind is truly a magnificent instrument used on the road to wellness. However, the emphasis that the mind is the main healing factor is false. While it is true that practices such as prayer and herbs improve the mind and relieve other symptoms of an illness, they do not make a bone mend any faster or make rheumatoid arthritis disappear. Instead, medical intervention is needed to yield successful recoveries in these examples. If both the mind and medical involvement are intertwined, however, the healing process will occur at a more rapid pace.

THE JOURNAL ARTICLE

The journal article is often a shortened version of the thesis, meaning that it should be presented in a similar format, including an introduction, sections on methods and results, and a discussion, as well as another component called the **abstract**. Here is a list of the components of the journal article, with their functions.

Abstract: Summarizes the ensuing article

Introduction: Explains why the research is necessary

Methods: Explains the process used to find the results

Results: Presents the actual findings from the data used

Discussion: Provides a clear explanation of the results in terms of your research problem

Writing for publication may offer different challenges from those posed by writing a thesis in that the article or journal publication requires you as the writer or researcher to condense massive amounts of material into a form that is easily digestible by your audience. Your audience does not want to relive the agony of the research and writing process with you; they simply want to recognize good science, good research, and conclusive and logical results. Write for their needs, and you will find yourself editing large sections of explanation from a thesis-length work.

Consider also that visuals and graphics help your reader digest information more readily. Work to make them user friendly, and provide the necessary explanation of each without duplicating the data in the written word.

Your purpose in writing for publication is to join the field's scholarly dialogue in order to present information that is useful to the profession. You must also remember to explain how your work fits into the world of research already published in this field and to explain how your findings relate to the status under which the profession already operates.

PATIENT EDUCATION LITERATURE

Patient education literature is a challenge to write for most health professionals because it requires that the practitioner communicate directly with the patient through the written word. In this context, effective communication requires that practitioners know what terms their patients understand to comprehend what is written. You know your patients best and are best suited to make these judgments.

Patient education literature not only serves its obvious purpose, to educate, but also can be used for other, not so obvious reasons. First, educating your patients through handouts or literature can save you time. You will not be required to repeat the same lessons. Additionally, as you save time, you can also save money. Your time is money, but also, your education materials may prompt a patient to carry out a healthy lifestyle that saves everyone money.

Additionally, preparing documents yourself that address patient concerns shows that you are genuinely interested in the lives of your patients enough to take the time to produce something for them. Also, this type of commitment from you will generate a further and necessary commitment from them as well. Patients who feel that their practitioner is looking out for their best interests will be more compliant and more willing to work with the practitioner. A patient who is compliant is not apprehensive. Apprehension derives from fears and the anxiety that they generate. Patient education literature can alleviate those fears and ultimately serve as a personal public relations tool. If you show that you care, the patient will respond accordingly.

Two types of patient education literature exist: **direct patient education literature** and **general patient population literature**.

Direct Patient Education Literature

Communicating with patients directly may be the easiest form of patient education literature to write because you understand your audience well. You know the patient's condition, history, and level of comprehension. For example, if you produce a document that explains the procedures of a home exercise program, you may be able to assume that your patient understands terms, positions, or symbols used, and you can supplement these written instructions with verbal cues.

The drawback to individualized documents is that they take time to create. Support staff may help here, but ultimately, the practitioner governs the knowledge that guides the document. Be prepared to take the necessary time to create such documents.

When producing the document, remember to make it reader friendly. In other words, do not create a document that is unclear and wordy. Consider any set of instructions you receive when you open a new product. If you are faced with cramped words on the page and small print, you are most likely to resist reading about the procedure. If the words are generously spaced and separated with visual cues for organization, you are more likely to engage the process readily. Also, be sure that the grammar and mechanics are correct. You do not want to jeopardize your standing in any community by demonstrating your ignorance. Proofread these documents as if they were intended for publication among your peers.

General Patient Population Literature

Anticipate the anxieties, concerns, questions, and general lack of knowledge in your patient population, and you will find fertile ground for producing general patient population literature. Consider generating flyers, posters, or handouts about common problems: endemic flu strains, anterior cruciate ligament tears, back pain, headaches, and so on, almost infinitely.

People who visit medical professionals want answers. They come to you for information because, if they had such information, they would most likely solve their problems on their own. For example, when patients reveal their symptoms and discuss the resultant problems, they ultimately want to know the answer to the

following question: "What's wrong with me?" Anticipate their questions that ultimately will follow:

"How did I get that?"

"How long will I be in this condition?"

"Am I going to die?"

"Is it curable?"

"What can I take to get back to normal?"

"Are you sure that is what I have? How do you know?"

"Will I need medication? surgery?"

"Will I be the same after this episode?"

Answering these questions for patients can stimulate interest in their health, leading them to a healthier lifestyle, and it can resolve their anxieties and fears. Your goal with such literature is to educate for a reason. You want the patient to understand the condition, treatment plan, and goals, and you also want to increase your standing with the community of patients and professionals with whom you make contact, either directly or indirectly.

General Guidelines for Producing Patient Education Literature

- Use bullets (for nonchronological listing) and lists (for chronological listing) to space out dense information.
- Use clearly identifiable and consistent headings and subheadings.
- Use brief paragraphs to leave generous amounts of white space and shorter sentences for ease in reading.
- Use diagrams or other visual aids whenever appropriate.
- Use appropriate language (shorter words that are easily understood).
- Use larger fonts for easy reading, especially for those with visual problems.
- Allow the patient to make contact with you or with office staff to ask questions. E-mail and phone numbers are best because they provide a sense of anonymity.

- Remember your audience. You are not creating this document for you or your colleagues; consequently, remove any unnecessary wording that might intimidate or confuse your reader.
- Be careful of warnings. Too severe language ("If you don't complete these tasks, you could die or . . . ") can lead to unnecessary anxiety for the patient. Be firm but understanding, cautious yet commanding.

- Identify yourself and personalize the patient's experience with you. Provide your office hours and other contacts in the office, and then provide a short biography or clips about your interests or specialization, as well as family or personal interests. Your patient wants to know that you are human; you should want your patients to know that you are human. Ultimately, they will have a better understanding of you.

3

Writing for Administrative Purposes

*A*nyone who enters the medical profession fully understands that 50% of any job is handling the formalities of operating within a business structure. Writing is usually that 50%. Ideally, you would like to treat your patients and hire someone else to manage the affairs of the office. Unfortunately, you cannot avoid paperwork.

Your primary writing responsibilities in the medical or allied health professions should be to chronicle your work to defend against litigation through malpractice or to document your work for reimbursement purposes. You must be able to demonstrate, in writing, that your treatments are within the standard scope of practice and that you want to be paid for services rendered. This is the purpose of documentation.

Additionally, you are in business to make a living, and you should be familiar with standard business procedures. For example, on your graduation, no one will be standing at the end of the stage offering you keys to your own office to begin your own practice. You must propose your ideas and provide business plans to receive loans. If you do not plan to open your own practice, you must be able to apply for jobs using a standard procedure.

Ultimately, other people will expect that you operate under the standards by which everyone else in the profession operates. This section outlines these expectations and formats to provide a reference for future activities in the real, not academic, world.

CHAPTER

11

Documentation

251

Key Terms

Discharge report Documentation chronicling the patient's progress to recovery or discharge from care

Documentation The strategies that practitioners use to chronicle their work

Initial evaluation The report form that outlines a practitioner's first clinical experience with a patient

Narrative The description of the events that take place between patient and practitioner; story form

Notes Brief sketches of procedures completed and conversations with patients, using a shorthand form of writing employing abbreviations and basic information

Progress report Documentation supporting patient assessments

Reimbursement Payment from a third party payer

SOAP note The accepted form for note taking, with four data categories: Subjective, Objective, Assessment, Plan

Third party payer An organization that pays health care providers for services rendered

Chapter Objectives

On completion of this chapter, the reader should be able to

1. Understand the legal and medical need for documentation and the processes of operation in the profession.

2. Use descriptive terms to explain a patient's functional progress by comparing that progress to specific, objective measurements.

3. Develop a strategy to prepare consistent documentation.

4. Develop notes in both SOAP form and narrative form.

*A*s with any form of writing in your profession, the methods and procedures of documenting your work are usually governed by a standard put forth by your employer. The methods listed here constitute a general guideline to the types of information that you should include in your **documentation** (any recording of the care you provide to a patient). You should recognize that this format and/or procedure will change according to the requirements of your workplace or the demands of your instructors.

Documentation may include initial evaluations, discharge and progress reports, notes or charts, and patient plans or instructional documents.

The Reasons for Documenting Your Work

If you think about the reasons you would want to document or chronicle your work, you should think about ways to create a paper trail of the work or care you provide for other practitioners to follow or to monitor the progress of your patients or your actions. Consequently, your primary goal for documenting your work is to communicate your methods to other practitioners in your field who might encounter your patient. They can then apply information from your analysis, plan of care, treatment modalities applied, success or failure with treatments, changes in patient performance or treatment outcomes, and short- and long-term goals. Documentation, in its simplest form, chronicles the path you have chosen so that others can follow.

Secondarily, your documentation is also the means to represent your work to your employers or to outside assessors. Many organizations or employers have set standards or procedures for practitioners to follow, and your documentation assures them that you have followed procedures accurately. Your work can then be scrutinized to ensure that you provided the best quality of care under the guidelines presented.

Documenting your work for the scrutiny of other organizations also helps the practitioner if the patient makes a legal claim against you and your work. Many health care professionals work with several patients every day, and you,

as one of these practitioners, cannot expect to remember every method or procedure you employed during a patient encounter several months previously. Your documentation is the paper trail that protects you from malpractice suits. It indicates your procedures and methods as they are measured by the standards set forth by your practice or health care organization.

As you protect yourself legally, your documentation can also help you protect yourself from health maintenance organizations (HMOs) or insurance companies that deny your claim for **reimbursement** for services rendered. You want to be paid for your work; consequently, your documentation will indicate that the work you performed was medically necessary and appropriate for the patient's condition. For more information on defending yourself legally or reimbursement issues, see the section "Legal Issues in Documentation" later on.

Finally, your documentation can be used for academic purposes, such as data gathering for a particular research project, but just as important is the fact that your documentation reflects your professional qualifications. Your ability to communicate with others—whether colleague, patient, lawyer, or **third party payer** (that reimburses you for services rendered)—may be the foundation to your success.

Preparing the Document

In every document you produce, attention to the details of writing well governs your success. You cannot reasonably expect anyone who reads your work to piece together a puzzle or to decipher hieroglyphics and still read your message as you intend it to be learned or read. Consequently, you should spend the necessary amount of time to assure yourself that your message is clearly communicated. Often, you may be required to convert your **notes** to a **narrative** describing your actions and the actions of the patient. The narrative forms are covered later in this chapter.

Your reader will digest information more readily if it is presented in groups of related data or in compartmentalized units of interest. The most helpful method of compartmentalizing your information is through the use of headings and subheadings. In many cases, you may be required to fill out forms, which suggests that the information you provide should be easily managed. See the APA style manual for specific instructions on headings, or you can create a system of your own. If you create a system of your own, be consistent within the document and within all other documents that you produce. Additionally, place the information in logical and chronological sequence.

Demonstrate your professionalism by proofreading your work for accuracy. If the information is not correct, do not expect to work in the profession for long. As you read for the accuracy of your content, read also for the accuracy of your wording. Often, inaccuracies result from poorly worded or weak descriptions of activity.

Providing precise wording requires that you know the language of your profession. This does not mean that you should fill your documents with jargon. Instead, the opposite is true. Consider that your audience may not know the precise meanings of terms you have used. Provide explanatory details to fully explain your methods and assessments. To do so, you should employ language that specifically delineates your message, not terms that you find convenient or language that is conversational. (See the section "Word Choice and Diction" in Chapter 3 for further help with this issue.) For example, a patient may tell you that she feels "numbness and tingling" in her right hand. These terms are imprecise for the medical profession. Instead, try: "Patient reports paresthesias in right upper extremity."

Conversational Language	Professional Terminology
"I passed out today."	Patient admits syncopal episode (time/date).
"I feel sick to my stomach."	Patient complains of nausea.
"I puked up blood with my lunch."	Patient reports hematemesis one time after eating (time/date).

Developing a strong grasp of medical terminology helps you be more precise in your documentation. Many of these terms you will use regularly as you enter the field, but every professional should be building a strong grasp on medical terminology in his or her particular field. In other cases, using the patient's words in quotation marks can be helpful in clarifying the condition described.

LEGAL ISSUES IN DOCUMENTATION

Documentation refers to a health care provider's written summary of his or her interaction with a patient. However, proper documentation also will record information relating to the time period before the patient presents to the provider: the patient's history and physical. It will also reflect all relevant details of the complete episode of treatment including the provider's discharge of the patient and the provider's submission of claims for reimbursement. Simply put, documentation is a health care provider's comprehensive written summary of his or her interaction with a patient through an episode of treatment. If done properly, documentation will capture a patient's history and physical, the provider's evaluation, assessment and diagnosis of the patient, the proposed treatment plan, treatment interventions, progress notes, the patient's outcome, and the bill or claim for reimbursement. Proper documentation will support the rationale for the proposed treatment, the medical necessity of the treatment, and the appropriateness of the intervention. It is the foundation of communication with patients, other providers, third party payers, and any other person or entity who or which may have reason to access a provider's documentation. Not only will documentation educate patients, other providers, and third party payers, but it is the central tool that supports the provider's claims for reimbursement. This section explains the importance of documentation: (1) as support for reimbursement in the health care delivery system, (2) to withstand reviews by third party payers, and (3) to avoid penalties and consequences for the failure to maintain adequate and proper documentation.

Documentation Supports Claims for Reimbursement

For health care providers, documentation provides the best evidence that a provider has rendered the correct treatment, at the right time, at the proper level of intensity, and in the most appropriate setting. If you meet these goals as a health care provider, you will have achieved the ultimate goal of providing quality health care to your patients. With proper care rendered to your patients, your next goal, then, is to receive reimbursement for the services you rendered. Not only will proper documentation show that you provided quality care to your patients, but it will support your request for reimbursement. This is important in today's health care industry, in which most patients do not pay you directly for your services; payment often comes from some third party—hence the term *third party payer*, which merely means that someone other than your patient will reimburse you for your services.

Since the third party payer was not present in your office when you treated the patient, your documentation will need to explain what you did, why you did it, how the patient benefited, and why your bill should be paid. If your documentation is not accurate, complete, descriptive, and legible, the third party payer will not have enough information to process and pay your claim, even if you performed the services. Your documentation must prove to the third party that you provided the services and that you are entitled to reimbursement. The audience who may read and review your documentation includes not only your patient or another health care provider but also third party payers such as Medicare, Medicaid, self-insured employers, third party administrators (TPAs), indemnity insurers, and HMOs. You should recognize that a large and diverse audience may review your documentation in order to process and pay your claims for reimbursement.

Documentation is often the first communication between you and a payer, and it is often the first document a payer will examine when deciding whether to pay for the services you have provided. Therefore, you should be mindful that the quality of the documentation you submit will give a payer a first impression of your approach to patient care. To make a good first impression, your documentation should be accurate, complete, truthful, descriptive, and legible and follow a logical progression.

Documentation should capture a patient's episode of care as accurately as possible. For example, if a physical therapist submits a claim for reimbursement to an insurance company with Current Procedural Terminology (CPT) code 97530, the therapist's records must be accurate to reflect that the patient's condition required that particular service and that the therapist actually performed that service. CPT 97530 is the code that describes therapeutic activities involving direct, one-on-one patient contact by the provider. If the therapist's documentation does not include a description that the therapist actually rendered this service as described, it is likely that the insurer will deny the claim, and the therapist will not be paid, even though he or she provided the service to the patient. If the documentation indicates that the service was rendered to the patient but does not include a description of the patient's condition or need for the service, reimbursement will be denied on that basis. Even if the provider has submitted complete and accurate documentation, reimbursement may be denied if the documentation is illegible and the payer cannot determine that payment is due. The burden is on the provider to submit complete and accurate documentation, in a legible form, to support the claim for payment. As explained later in this chapter, besides nonpayment, severe consequences and penalties exist for inaccurately documenting the performance of a service that was not actually performed, that cannot be clinically justified, or that is not supported by the provider's documentation.

The accuracy of a provider's documentation can be improved by using descriptive terms to explain a patient's functional progress as determined by specific objective measurements. In other words, you should carefully choose the terminology you use in your documentation so that it is as descriptive as possible and communicates the patient's health status before, during, and after your treatment intervention.

Although the use of descriptive terms can improve your communication with your patients and improve documentation submitted to third party payers, it can also provide a more efficient and accurate means to arrive at the correct diagnosis and treatment plan for your patient. Patients often fail to properly communicate their health care needs and often delve into topics unrelated to their care and treatment. By using descriptive terms and specific objective measurements in patient interactions, the provider can prevent patients from drifting into irrelevant conversations and can assist patients in accurately communicating their specific health care needs.

Consider the following two scenarios in which a patient presents to a provider's office with moderate pain in his lower back and a throbbing sensation in his left shoulder. In Scenario 1, the provider does not use any descriptive terms or specific objective measurements. In Scenario 2, the descriptive terms used are underlined and the specific objective measurements used are in bold.

SCENARIO 1

(without using descriptive terms or specific objective measurements)

Provider: "How do you feel?"

Patient: "Pretty good, but worse than normal."

Provider: "So what can we do for you today?"

Patient: "My back and my shoulder hurt."

Provider: "How do you think it happened?"

Patient: "I don't really know. I can't think of any one instance."

Provider: "Is it too painful for you to go to work or to sleep?"

Patient: "No, but sometimes my back and my shoulder really, really hurt."

Provider: "It doesn't sound like it's anything to worry about. I think we'll put you on some anti-inflammatory drugs and see you in a week."

SCENARIO 2

(with descriptive terms and specific objective measurements):

Provider: "On the health assessment form that you filled out in our waiting room this morning, you're complaining of pain in your back and shoulder, right?"

Patient: "That's right."

Provider: "Do you remember specifically hitting, bumping, or straining your back?"

Patient: "No, I just sort of woke up this way."

Provider: "Can you show me the area where you feel pain, such as the upper portion of your back, the middle portion, the lower portion, the left side, the right side, or any combination of those areas?"

Patient: "Yes, it seems that the pain is just in the lower back."

Provider: "Is it a sharp pain, a throbbing pain, a general soreness, or any other type of pain that you can describe to me?"

Patient: "It's not a sharp or a throbbing pain, but it's very sore, especially when I sit down or stand up."

Provider: "On **a scale of 1 to 10, 1 being very mild and 10 being a severe pain**, how would you rate the pain?"

Patient: "When I stand up or sit down, the pain is definitely intense, like an **8**, but at other times, the pain is more like a **4**."

Provider: "I think we can put you on some anti-inflammatory drugs and give you some stretching exercises to alleviate the pain in your back. We will see you in a week and consider a consult with an orthopaedist at that time. Now, with respect to your shoulder, is it your left or right shoulder?"

Patient: "Left."

Provider: "Can you exercise a full range of motion with your left arm and shoulder?"

Patient: "Yes."

Provider: "Do you remember specifically hitting, bumping, or straining your shoulder?"

Patient: "No, same thing, I just sort of woke up this way."

Provider: "Is the pain a <u>sharp</u> pain, a <u>throbbing</u> pain, a <u>general soreness</u>, or <u>any other type</u> of pain that you can describe to me?"

Patient: "It's a throbbing pain that comes and goes every so often."

Provider: "On **a scale of 1 to 10, 1 being very mild and 10 being a severe pain**, how would you rate the throbbing pain?"

Patient: "I would rate it at **2** when it throbs, but it's enough that I notice it."

Provider: "I'll give you some stretching exercises you can do on your own or you can have someone rub the area with a heat ointment and try to massage out the pain. I do not think that what you describe warrants any further intervention. You may have slept on it wrong. We will check your left shoulder next week when you come in for your visit to check your lower back. If anything comes up in the meantime, give me a call."

Although the foregoing scenarios are scripted and manufactured, they serve to illustrate how the use of descriptive terms and specific objective measurements, as in Scenario 2, can improve patient interaction and enable a provider to reach a more accurate diagnosis and plan of treatment. Descriptive terms and specific, objective measurements should also be used in a provider's documentation. Just as these words and phrases improve verbal communication with a patient, they improve a provider's written communication with third party payers. For example, documentation that describes a patient's condition as "patient complains his knee hurts when he walks down stairs" may not support the clinical need for arthroscopic knee surgery, and a payer may deny payment on the basis that the documentation did not support the need for surgery. However, a provider makes a much stronger case for reimbursement for performing arthroscopic knee surgery if his or her documentation reports that the "patient complains of moderate sharp pain on medial aspect of left knee when ambulating and of severe sharp pain on medial aspect of left knee when going down stairs; patient has been on anti-inflammatories for 6 weeks and has com-

pleted 6 weeks of intensive physical therapy with no improvement." This more complete documentation will at least justify the need for x-ray or magnetic resonance imaging (MRI) examination of the patient's knee, whereas the prior example of documentation fails to support any testing or clinical intervention. A provider should, however, be sure not to "lead" the patient.

In your practice, you may consider adopting checklists or worksheets that list a variety of descriptive terms to help identify specific areas of pain and types of pain that utilize a system of specific objective measurement such as classification of pain as "severe," "moderate," or "mild" or on a scale of 1 to 10, or range of motion described in degrees. Remember, however, that although checklists are helpful, they must be adhered to so that the completed checklist truly indicates the patient's condition.

Caution is indicated with the use of descriptive terms, checklists, or worksheets because one primary goal of documentation is to convey an accurate message. In other words, if you merely evaluate a patient and determine that there is no need to provide any skilled care, it would be inappropriate for you to use clinical terms in your documentation reflecting that you provided an "intervention." It is also important to verify that the terms or phrases you use are generally recognized by other health care providers and payers. The use of unrecognizable or nondescriptive terms may not accurately convey the treatment that you provided and may result in a delay or denial of your request for reimbursement. On a practical note, you should remember that although the use of medical, clinical terms will improve your documentation and communication with other providers and payers, patients are often confused by such terminology. Patients will better understand their condition, the treatment you have provided or plan to provide, and their prognosis if you avoid clinical terms and use common or layperson's terms in your discussions.

Your documentation should also follow a logical order and progression so that anyone reviewing the documentation can understand the progression of treatment in a chronological order. If a payer cannot follow the organization of your documentation or gets confused, the payer will not authorize reimbursement and will request from you further clarification. This results in delay of payment and also increases your administrative costs in retrieving patient files and attempting to reconstruct the care and treatment that may have been provided to a patient months before.

Remember that payers have countless numbers of claims and documentation to review every day; they will not spend time trying to determine the care you provided if it is not clear from the documentation. The burden is on you to provide adequate documentation to support the claim for reimbursement. It is recommended, therefore, that you document your treatment as you provide it. Contemporaneous record keeping is the best practice because your impressions are still fresh in your mind, and there is little risk you will confuse one patient with another.

This sounds like simple, commonsense advice, but it is surprising how many practitioners avoid their record-keeping responsibilities. A provider may procrastinate or altogether fail to keep adequate patient records for a variety of reasons. Maintaining adequate records is required by state licensing boards, which have little or no sympathy for providers who fail to abide by the law.

Consider the following case from New York State: A primary care physician, Dr. X, with a successful, busy practice received a request from a patient for a copy of his chart, as he had chosen a new primary care physician, Dr. A. Dr. X never responded. Dr. A then telephoned and wrote to Dr. X requesting copies of the chart without success. After 3 months, the patient's attorney telephoned and wrote to Dr. X, without receiving a response. The patient then filed a complaint with the New York State Department of Health, which sent several written demands to Dr. X to turn over the records. When the Department's investigators appeared at Dr. X's office, he told the investigators that the patient's records were in his car, which his wife had borrowed for the day. Dr. X said he would retrieve the records the following day. He later appeared before the judge with another excuse for not

having the records as the court had requested. Finally, the Department suspended Dr. X's license for 6 months, concluding that there was no patient chart. Dr. X was ordered to undergo psychiatric counseling because the Department concluded that no physician in his right mind could be so derelict in his duties. As a final note, the physician completed counseling, and the suspension of his license was lifted; however, six months later, he again refused to produce a patient's records, and the Department permanently revoked Dr. X's license.

The legibility of documentation also must not be overlooked. On reviewing a large number of hospital charts, one might conclude that some health care providers actually take pride in their cryptic and illegible handwriting. However, illegible documentation is not a badge of honor that should be worn proudly; it is an embarrassment that may result in denial of payment from a payer, may cause confusion among other health care providers, and may result in a patient's being discouraged by the provider's sloppiness and lack of attention to detail. From a payer's perspective, if he or she cannot read your writing, the payer will not authorize payment. Legible documentation and a clear presentation of patient care can reflect your level of professionalism and skill both to patients and to other providers and payers.

In general, as a provider, you will evaluate and treat a patient in your office and will dictate or write the diagnosis, the treatment recommended, and the treatment that you performed. Although accuracy and conciseness are the ultimate goals of documentation, it is important for a provider to justify the medical necessity for the service and to document that the service was actually performed. The rule to remember in patient documentation is that *more is more*. In general, most health insurance plans do not cover nonmedical, unskilled, or custodial care. Therefore, it is important that the provider's documentation justify and support the need for skilled, medically necessary care delivered by the provider to the patient. Documentation should also reveal that the treatment provided is safe and efficacious and that it will produce the desired result—the patient will get better.

Realities of Submitting Claims for Reimbursement

Health care providers are reminded that in order to make a career out of providing health care, two main goals need to be met: (1) provide quality care to patients and (2) receive payment for their services. HMOs, insurance companies, Medicaid and Medicare, and other third party payers have developed a set of reimbursement guidelines and requirements that need to be met by a provider before the processing and payment of the provider's claims. If these requirements are not met, your claims will be denied and returned to you, for resubmission in compliance with the payer's reimbursement requirements. While not all of the reimbursement methodologies and payment schemes that have been developed in the health care industry can be covered in this chapter, this section describes the general process employed by an individual health care provider in submitting claims and receiving reimbursement from third party payers.

Depending on your reimbursement agreement with a payer, such as an HMO, your office staff will review the patient chart and will submit one or more payment codes to the HMO. Most individual providers follow the CPT system of coding, a listing of descriptive terms and identifying codes for reporting medical services and procedures performed by physicians. Non-physician individual providers often use CPT codes because the CPT system is the most widely accepted billing terminology and coding system used in health care today. The codes themselves are composed of five digits that systematically designate procedures and services performed by individual providers. The codes simplify the reporting and billing for services. Each code represents a number of required components that must be met prior to the provider billing that CPT code. For example, if a provider sees a new patient in his or her office or other outpatient setting for evaluation and management, without an expanded or detailed history and examination, the provider's office would most likely bill CPT code 99201, which is considered a low-level code. In the billing, the HMO would receive the provider's name, the date the service was performed, CPT code 99201, and the provider's usual charge for that service.

Since CPT code 99201 is a low-level code for a procedure that does not involve complex decision making, diagnosis, or frankly, money, reimbursement will most likely be made without the review of backup documentation, unless the payer is aware that the procedure was not necessary or that the provider did not actually perform the service. By comparison, if a spine surgeon bills CPT code 63075, a very high-level code, for a procedure involving complex decision making, there is likely to be a thorough review of the provider's documentation, for before, during, and after the procedure was performed. Before authorizing payment for the service, the provider would most likely need to submit to the payer written documentation justifying the medical necessity to have the service performed in lieu of any other alternative therapy, and justifying why the present time is the most appropriate time to perform the procedure. If the provider's documentation is unclear, illegible, inaccurate, or incomplete, the payer will deny coverage for the procedure until the provider is able to justify the medical necessity of the service through his or her documentation. Conversely, if the provider's documentation is complete, accurate, and legible and supports the medical necessity of the treatment, the service will usually be covered in accordance with the reimbursement agreement between the provider and the payer. It is also important to mention that if the requested service is a medical emergency, the service is performed and covered by the payer without prior authorization. There may be a retrospective review of the documentation to verify that it was a medical emergency.

A provider should keep in mind that the thoroughness of his or her documentation is ultimately determined by the party paying for the medical procedure, not the provider. With this in mind, a provider should document that the proposed treatment satisfies the payer's minimum requirements for reimbursement, not merely what the provider feels is necessary to document. Failure to submit documentation that meets a payer's minimum requirements may result in needless delay in reimbursement for the service or a denial because there is not enough objective evidence to indicate that the patient needs the proposed intervention.

The following example illustrates this point: Dr. O was a skilled orthopedic surgeon with excellent training and experience. However, Dr. O spent much of his time talking with payer's reviewers who assessed his documentation and denied coverage for surgery because Dr. O's documentation did not show the trial of other alternatives to surgery, such as physical therapy. When Dr. O saw a patient for a sore knee, he would order an x-ray or MRI examination, and if there were an abnormality, major or minor, he would schedule surgery. However, best medical practices generally view surgery, which is invasive and carries the risk of infection and anesthesia, as a last resort, used only after failed conservative treatment alternatives. Payers who follow the principles of best medical practice will not approve surgery for a minor knee problem or an x-ray examination unless there is documentation that the patient has been on anti-inflammatory drugs and has completed the recommended course of physical therapy. Because Dr. O refused to follow these more conservative treatments before scheduling surgery, he often did not receive coverage for surgery from third party payers because the proposed procedure was not justified by the documentation submitted.

Requiring preauthorization and review of documentation before the performance of a service is a form of prospective utilization review performed by payers. Utilization review is generally a payer's review of a provider's use of resources in treating his or her patients. Utilization review may also take the form of *concurrent review*, a review of the utilization of health care services during a patient's hospital stay, or *retrospective review*, an audit of services that were previously provided. On a retrospective review, a payer may request patient charts and written documentation for support of services that were already performed, billed, and paid for by the payer, such as a review of medical emergency services that were already provided. Since a provider never knows what cases will be the subject of retrospective utilization review, it is important for the provider to consistently keep good documentation for all patient charts in a legible and organized manner. If the provider cannot justify a charge that was billed and paid, the payer may retract payment because the provider did not justify the medical necessity of the service or prove that the service was actually performed.

In performing utilization review, the payer will generally look for the documentation to support two elements: (1) that the treatment was indicated by the patient's condition and (2) that the treatment was actually performed. If the documentation shows that the patient's condition indicated that the proposed treatment was medically necessary but does not verify that the treatment was actually performed, the payer may deny or retract payment for that service. If the documentation shows that the service was performed but fails to show that the treatment was indicated by the patient's condition, payment may similarly be denied or retracted. Documentation that supports one without the other will not be sufficient. It must show that the treatment was indicated *and* that the treatment was performed.

Review of Documentation for Reasons Other than Payment

In the health care system today, there are competing and mounting pressures from patients and employer groups to keep health insurance premiums down. There are also pressures from physicians and other individual providers and from hospitals and other facilities to provide greater reimbursement for capital to improve equipment and facilities. This increase and competing pressure has resulted in increased scrutiny of provider billing, and the documentation that is submitted to support the billing, by insurance companies, HMOs, government health care programs, and other third party payers. Whereas in the 1970s it was rare that providers would be requested to submit their documentation, today it is a generally accepted business practice that third parties may request to review random charts for a variety of reasons. This possibility alone is incentive for a provider to ensure that his or her documentation is complete, accurate, and easy to retrieve.

Third party payers may request copies of your patient files for reasons other than claims payment and utilization review. HMOs, which approve the credentials of their network of participating providers, regularly monitor the quality of care their enrollees receive from these providers. An HMO may randomly request to review a number of patient records from one of its participating providers to verify that proper documentation was used and that quality standards were met. Payers will also review a provider's documentation to investigate and respond to patient complaints. For example, a patient may file a written complaint that he went to his primary care provider's office for a routine physical, and during the course of the physical, the provider also prescribed an allergy medication but billed the patient for two office visit copayments. In order to investigate the complaint, the HMO will request a copy of that patient's chart and billing ledger from the provider. If the documentation shows one visit and the collection of only one copayment, the complaint will not be substantiated. If, however, the documentation shows that the patient had visited the provider on consecutive days, once for a physical and once for his allergies and two office visit copayments were collected, HMO officials would want to talk to the provider and the patient to straighten out the facts. HMOs also request records from providers for a variety of other reasons, such as in order to respond to requests from government agencies for records or to help in the defense of lawsuits against the HMO. Often, the records may be requested on demand, so a provider will not have an opportunity to complete or correct his or her documentation prior to its being reviewed. Therefore, it is important to complete your documentation at the time services are performed.

Adopt a Global Documentation Method and Billing Strategy

It is important for the provider to be knowledgeable of how different insurance companies and government health care programs reimburse providers before performing a service. While billing requirements of third party payers are similar, they may differ in many ways. The most efficient way for you to approach these different billing requirements is to adopt one global billing strategy that will comply with the requirements of all third party payers with which you interact, not to adopt several different billing strategies, each unique to a particular payer.

Also, it is your duty to find the insurance coverage that will pay the bill for your services, not the patient's responsibility and not the insurance company's responsibility. For example, Medicaid has a two-year billing requirement for payment of a service. If you perform a service on a Medicaid patient that is covered by Medicaid and you fail to bill Medicaid within two years of the date of the service, you are forever forbidden from billing Medicaid and from billing the Medicaid patient, and you will take the loss on those services. Other insurance carriers and payers have shorter time requirements, such as a 90-day rule, to submit bills from the date of service. If the 90-day time frame is missed, you will not be reimbursed by the payer, and you will also be prohibited from billing the patient directly. There are other rules of coordination of benefits that you need to become familiar with to ensure that you will be paid for the services you render.

The following example illustrates how a provider's lack of understanding of billing requirements and reimbursement rules can result in denial of a claim.

Dr. S, a spine surgeon, evaluated a new patient in his office for severe back pain. In Dr. S's documentation, it is clear that the patient (P) told him that she was injured while she was working at a local restaurant. Although P was covered by her insurance company (IC), since this was an injury that occurred during work, it fell under the state's workers' compensation benefit program. This meant that workers' compensation was the sole remedy for the provider to be reimbursed for the proposed surgery. Under IC's insurance contract with P, workers' compensation claims for services provided by health care providers were excluded from coverage. Dr. S performed spinal surgery in the amount of $13,000 and billed IC for reimbursement. Dr. S failed to provide copies of his medical records and the bill for the spine surgery to the workers' compensation board. Simultaneously, IC denied the claim owing to workers' compensation exclusion in its contract with P. Around the same time, the workers' compensation board and P reached a settlement totaling $5,000 in full payment of all injuries, including all medical and surgical bills and claims. Because Dr. S neglected to provide his medical documentation and billings to the workers' compensation board, Dr. S's bills of $13,000 for the spine surgery were not included in the workers' compensation award of $5,000. P moved out of town within days of receiving the $5,000 workers' compensation settlement, leaving Dr. S. with an unpaid bill of $13,000. Dr. S had no recourse and had to write off the bill.

In this example, Dr. S was unaware that P had a workers' compensation claim. Had Dr. S sent the bill to the workers' compensation board, the board would have been aware that the medical bill alone was $13,000, and the settlement amount would have to take that bill into account. By failing to follow workers' compensation's reimbursement rules, Dr. S was stuck with a large unpaid bill.

While not receiving reimbursement for the health care services you provide is a severe consequence, you should also be mindful that there are numerous other consequences for failing to become familiar with payers' reimbursement requirements or for failing to maintain adequate documentation. As discussed earlier, inadequate documentation can result in a provider's having payments retracted by a payer on a retrospective review. In addition, if the retrospective review shows that the provider intentionally billed for a service that he or she knew should not have been billed, the payer may determine

that the provider committed fraud and may report the fraudulent billing to a state or federal licensing board. Furthermore, the payer may terminate the provider from its participating provider panel. While fraud in the health care delivery system has always been illegal for providers who treat Medicaid and Medicare patients, the government has recently enacted laws that require insurance companies and HMOs to establish fraud and recovery departments to monitor, investigate, and report all fraud or suspected fraud to the federal government. Payers now have an affirmative duty to conduct fraud investigations and report them to the government. This has increased the tension between providers and payers in the health care delivery system. If a provider is found guilty of billing fraud, he or she may be liable for fines and imprisonment. Now, more than ever, it is important for providers to maintain accurate and complete documentation for all of their services.

Legal Consequences of Inaccurate or Inappropriate Documentation

Under federal fraud and abuse laws, it is illegal for providers to knowingly and willfully make any false statement or representation of material fact in their application for payment under a federal health care program. While this is a simplified description of the Federal False Claims Act, the law provides severe criminal sanctions including a felony conviction and a fine of $25,000 or imprisonment for up to five years, or both, in the case of each such false statement. In addition, the provider may be limited, restricted, suspended, or forbidden to participate in federal health care programs, which include Medicaid and Medicare, an important source of payment for all providers. While these penalties may seem harsh, it is important to understand what the government considers a false statement and how it calculates such penalties. For example, if a provider bills Medicare or Medicaid (or any other federal health care program) for a certain CPT code that is not supported by adequate documentation to show that the diagnosis was indicated, that the treatment was documented and actually performed, this may be deemed by the government to be a false and fraudulent statement. The burden is on the provider, not the government, to have the necessary documentation to support billing codes, which are submitted to the government for payment.

A provider who regularly submits claims to the government without appropriate documentation may quickly find himself or herself potentially liable for millions of dollars in fines and subject to countless years in prison. The government considers each code that it receives to be a statement requesting payment, so that if a provider during the course of a year, for example, submits 5,000 claims on average to the government each year, and none of those claims have adequate documentation, the government may take the position that the provider made a false statement to the government 5,000 times during that year. After multiplying each false statement times the criminal penalties, the provider may be liable for up to $125,000,000 in fines and up to 25,000 years in prison, on top of the provider's being liable to repay the amounts he or she received from the government. While this is an extreme example, it should be enough to incite every health care provider to regularly maintain honest and accurate documentation and to regularly review their documentation and their billings to government entities and other third party payers to ensure that the claims are being submitted accurately. It is important to remember that the government still has the burden of proving that false claims were knowingly and willfully submitted in a false manner; however, providers who do not have any documentation to support the claims they submit will not be in a position to defend themselves. Conversely, a provider who maintains adequate and proper documentation will be able to show that documentation to the government and prove that if a billing code was improperly submitted, it was a clerical mistake or error and not an intentional and willful act to defraud the government. An example from case law may give a more realistic view of how a provider can stray from the law and how the government approaches cases of false claims:

In 1984, a grand jury indicted Dr. Larm, an allergist who treated Medicaid patients, and his wife, Mrs. Larm, who was his office manager and submitted bills to Medicaid on Dr. Larm's behalf. The Larms were indicted on 98 counts of Medicaid fraud. Counts 1 to 84 alleged that the Larms submitted claims to Medicaid for office visits, although Dr. Larm neither saw patients nor personally rendered the services. Counts 85 to 94 alleged that the Larms billed for giving injections to patients who actually administered the injections themselves. Counts 95 to 98 alleged that the Larms falsely submitted claims for allergy shots. The total of the excess charges was $882.21. For counts 1 to 94, the Larms' defense was that the claims were not false because each patient was given a routine allergy shot administered by a nurse, even though Dr. Larm was not in the office. The court noted, however, that the claim submitted for that service was billing code 90040, which is defined as a "brief examination, evaluation and/or treatment, same or new illness, including a brief or interval history, examination, discussion of finding and/or rendering of service." While the Larms argued that the treatment rendered fits within that definition, the Court held that the Larms falsely billed 90040 and should have billed code 90030, which defines the treatment as "minimal service: injection, minimal dressings, etc. not necessarily requiring the presence of a physician." Here, there was no dispute that patients were treated, but Dr. and Mrs. Larm were convicted because they submitted the wrong code, which was not supported by the documentation. As a result of the trial, the jury convicted Dr. Larm on 17 counts, which involved claim forms (documentation) that he signed, and acquitted him of all other charges. Mrs. Larm, who oversaw all the billing, was convicted on 94 counts (*United States v. Larm*, 824 F2d 780, 9th Cir. 1987).

It is important to note that although Mrs. Larm was not the health care provider and was merely the office manager, she was held equally responsible for the false claims submitted to the government and, in fact, was convicted on 70 counts more than her husband was. Because additional facts regarding the

Larms' practice are not readily available, it is difficult to ascertain the extent of the Larms' intent to defraud the government. However, this case illustrates the importance of proper documentation and billing for each and every service provided under a federal health program. Recall that the total excess charges billed to the government was $882.21, but, as a result of those false claims, the Larms were convicted on over 100 counts of defrauding the government. In addition, they may have been suspended or terminated from participating in federal health programs and most likely incurred hundreds of thousands of dollars in legal fees—all for $882.21.

Other providers have been found guilty of submitting false claims to the government by submitting claims for reimbursement for brand name drugs when generic or over-the-counter drugs had actually been dispensed to the patient. The government held that these claims submissions constituted misrepresentation of a material fact within the meaning of the Medicaid Fraud False Claims Statute.

If a provider has submitted incorrect claims to the government but did not do so with the intent to defraud or in bad faith, the provider may use his or her documentation to show that, although the billing code submitted may have been incorrect, the provider submitted the claims in good faith. Courts have held that good faith is an adequate defense to the charge of willfully and intentionally submitting a false claim. On the other hand, a physician was found guilty of submitting false claims to the government even though the physician submitted his claims to a private insurance company that had a contract with the government to receive payment for the services. In that case, the court held that since the physician was aware that the claims he submitted would ultimately be submitted to the government for payment, he had "caused" the carriers to submit the claims to the government. A physician was criminally liable on the false claims statute for submitting Medicare claims for services that were performed but which the physician knew were unnecessary or not therapeutic. This case illustrates the importance of documentation:

The service was performed, but the patient's condition was not indicated, the treatment was not medically necessary, and the treatment would not produce the required or desired result.

As a health care provider, you may be held ultimately responsible for false claims that are submitted by your office or your practice even though you did not personally submit the claims or sign the claims. In one case, the owner of a medical laboratory could not claim that he did not have knowledge of the claims or false statements because he authorized the signing and filing of claim forms by others in his office. It is therefore not enough for you as a health care provider to be aware of the Federal False Claims Act; it is important for each health care provider to regularly keep staff informed of the government's requirements as well as the requirements of other third party payers.

Exercise

DOCUMENTATION

Directions: Write a letter to a third party payer requesting reimbursement for services rendered and demonstrating your understanding of the need for documentation and legal ramifications involved. The patient, ailment, treatment plan, and results of treatment can be manufactured or based on a patient you have worked with in the past.

The payer requires that you explain how the patient came into your care, the patient's history and injury description, your evaluation, your plan of treatment, and the results to date. Reimbursement requires that you provide

- the rationale for treatment

- an explanation of your treatment that proves that it is medically necessary

- a description of your work in terms of the standards that apply (appropriateness of treatment)

- a document that educates the payer and the patient.

TYPES OF DOCUMENTATION

Notes

Much of a health professional's writing occurs in note form. In other words, writing an essay for publication is not always necessary if your goal is to chronicle evaluations or the progress of a patient. Although you may write notes frequently and not have much time to devote to writing glorious sentences, you should not feel licensed to break the basic rules of grammar or mechanics. Creating sloppy sentences or disorganized paragraphs can often bring about unintended results in your communication. Your license to practice may be damaged by incorrect or inaccurate representation of your work. Paying attention to precise and correct sentences and unifying your message will guarantee that your intended audience will receive your intended message.

Notes are usually brief bursts of information, presented in an organized format, that delineate your treatment procedures and the patient's evaluation and progress. Write your notes as close as possible to the time of communicating with the patient, to avoid information loss. However, do not write as the patient speaks. You will not be able to write word-for-word transcriptions of a patient's communication, and, furthermore, you should be focusing on the patient to read body language and to note other subtle clues the patient presents. Therefore, focus your attention on the patient while conversing, and then find a later time to write your assessments.

The process of writing notes also entails adopting a writing style that conflicts with the methods described in this text. To produce notes, you will most likely adopt an efficient method that is time saving. You may write elliptically, omitting certain words ("Patient complains of pain in stomach."), or you might adopt standard symbols and abbreviations that have precise meaning in your field. Be certain that such a writing style is not overused so that communication breaks down. Not all practitioners in the health care field will comprehend the meaning of all symbols or abbreviations used by others. Avoid creating confusion by understanding the limitations of your audience and by using standard abbreviations.

As with any form of documentation, basic patient information is required in a consistent place on the document: patient name, date of birth, and hospital or practice identification information or number. Always date progress notes, and use a consistent format for documenting allergies and medications. The form of the remainder of the note depends on the facility in which you are employed, but most health care facilities require either a SOAP note or a narrative.

SOAP Notes

The **SOAP note** is created by a consistent process of recording information that comprises four categories of data:

S: Subjective

O: Objective

A: Assessment

P: Plan

Use the SOAP note as a sketch of your methods. These headings allow your patient information to be presented in an orderly and organized fashion for easy reference by you, support staff, or colleagues. Such organized approaches allow others to assess your plan and any changes without sifting through a "wall of words" in essay form.

Narrative Method

However, the SOAP note does have a disadvantage in that comparative information is not readily available. If a patient's plan changes over time, those changes can be gathered only by reading the notes across an expanse of time. The SOAP note does not offer the flexibility to include such information. Instead of limiting yourself with a restrictive SOAP note, you could also write a narrative note. Narratives simply tell the story of the patient. Here, you re-create the patient's situation by writing in chronological order the events that transpire. This is advantageous in that that you can compare treatment plans, discuss changes that have occurred, or simply make necessary conclusions through strong and direct sentences.

Although the narrative may seem like the more effective means of chronicling your work, the narrative, because of the nature of its form, may require more time to write. Additionally, when given the time, many writers expand on the issues and write more than is necessary. Be aware of repetitiveness, wordiness, or rambling. Stay focused on events or changes that directly affect the plan or the patient's problem.

The notes that you write on a daily basis are the evidence of your work. Failure to document your work accurately can result in various problems, the least of which is a failure to be reimbursed for your work. Avoid complications by being thorough and accurate.

Initial Evaluation

The **initial evaluation** provides the blueprint for your rationale for treatment as you review the patient's condition. It provides your assessment of the patient's condition, your plan of treatment, and your short- and long-term goals for recovery. Use the following general guidelines for practical implementation of the first phase of documentation.

Initial Evaluation

1. Patient Identification Information
2. Referral Information
   Reason for Referral
   Referral Patient History
   Referral Diagnosis
   Requested Treatment
   Complicating Factors or Other Treatments Tried: Medical history, known allergens, other data.
3. Evaluation
   Assess Patient's Prior Condition: Include all pertinent physical and emotional conditions recorded by practitioner. Create a list with subheadings to define each. Exam-

ples: Ambulation, Cognition, Pain, Vital Signs, Vision, Hearing, Vascular, Diagnostic Tests, Lab Work.

4. Diagnosis
   Provide rationale for treatment.
5. Treatment Plan
   Prescribed medication, scheduled appointment for reevaluation, frequency and duration of treatment prescribed; short- and long-term goals.

Sample Narrative
INITIAL EVALUATION
Preliminary Assessment
REFERRAL

Barb Kowel, M.D., referred Michael Geigger to St. Nicole Hospital for physical therapy to decrease left shoulder pain, to improve mobility, and to return to work. His shoulder pain and decrease in mobility is a result of capsulitis in his left shoulder. The physician requested that patient's functional mobility be restored (to reach overhead with no difficulties).

Reason

Dr. Kowel referred patient to physical therapy to promote mobility and strength, as prior interventions, including wall-walking exercises to increase mobility, have been unsuccessful. The practical method of treatment is the properly supervised skilled care that is consistent with the payer's coverage guidelines. Without physical therapy, the decrease of mobility and strength will eventually result in the inability to return to work.

Specific Treatment Requested

The referring physician suggested three sessions of professional instruction per week for 4 weeks to increase the range of movement and to strengthen the patient's left shoulder. These exercises will be followed by an in-home exercise plan to ensure progressive strengthening and prevent future damage.

Data Accompanying Referral

General information regarding the patient about his past medical history and any complications was provided by the physician and discussed in the following.

Diagnosis/Onset Date

The patient is diagnosed with left shoulder capsulitis. The date of onset was November of 1999.

Secondary Diagnosis

March 22, 2000, was patient's first experience with a physical therapist. He previously attended appointments with his family physician regarding left shoulder complications. The patient used a sling for a period of 2 weeks, immediately following the accident; the sling is no longer being used. Patient received injections of cortisone to minimize pain in shoulder. He currently takes an anti-inflammatory and tries a home program of wall-walking exercises for mobility.

Medical History

His past medical history states that he had cancer (CA) in his right kidney approximately 10 years ago with no reoccurrence. In July of 1990, he had surgery for the CA in his kidney. At this point, patient has only his left kidney and sees his physician on a yearly basis. The loss of his right kidney has no relevance to his shoulder pain, but when medications are prescribed, the loss should be taken into consideration. Due to his shoulder injury, he is currently not working as a mason but intends to return to work when instructed by physician.

Medications

Patient is currently taking Decadron to reduce inflammation in his left shoulder. Patient reports that Advil reduces the amount of pain in his shoulder, and he takes these when necessary.

Comorbid Conditions

No complications will directly affect or influence his progress in physical therapy.

PHYSICAL THERAPY INTAKE HISTORY

Michael Geigger is a 50-year-old male who was born on November 21, 1949. He is alert and physically active. He defined "physically active" as briskly walking two miles per day.

Start of Care

March 22, 2000, was the start of physical therapy care for this patient. The delay in initiation of physical therapy was a result of the examinations and x-ray studies required by the physician before referral.

Primary Complaint

The patient is suffering from severe pain when he reaches for or lifts objects over 5 pounds. He has difficulties getting dressed in the morning, getting items out of the kitchen cupboards, and reaching for objects behind his back. Both pain and lack of motion continue in his shoulder. The first two injections helped decrease the amount of pain, but he did not notice a difference after subsequent injections. Restoring his range of motion (ROM), strength,

and functional use of his shoulder will allow him to return to everyday activities without complications.

Referral Diagnosis

The patient was referred to physical therapy to aid in the strengthening of his left shoulder and to enable him to return to work.

Mechanism of Injury

This patient reports that he has experienced sharp pain in his shoulder since November of 1999. He was helping to build a home and was working on the roof. He does feel that his shoulder may have started bothering him after that time. On March 18, 2000, the patient received an injection in his shoulder to reduce the pain. He states that when his arm is at rest, he has minimal pain to no pain. When he tries to lift an object heavier than 5 pounds or reach higher than his shoulder, the pain is acute and severe; on a scale of 1 to 10, 10 being the worst, he rates his pain level to be a 10. Patient reports that he has mild (3 on a pain scale) aching into his left upper arm when he lifts or reaches.

Prior Diagnostic Imaging

The patient's family physician previously diagnosed patient with a fractured left shoulder. With further testing and an x-ray examination on December 3, 1999, the physician determined that the patient's shoulder was not fractured, but the shoulder joint was irritated. The physician proceeded with this diagnosis and injected pain relievers and instructed him to perform specific home exercises.

EVALUATION
Baseline Evaluation Data

Information establishing objective and functional deficits is determined and documented in the following. Evaluation components include areas that may be pertinent to the patient's rehabilitation.

Vascular Signs

The patient's skin color and temperature appear normal. His skin circulation is intact. On palpation, the patient has no focal pain or tenderness.

Sensation

Patient denies any numbness or irregularities in the lower arm or hand. He states he has acute aching in the shoulder. He senses a sharp pain in the shoulder itself when he reaches back, up above his shoulder, or to the right and left sides.

Posture

The therapist did not note any irregularities in the patient's posture when he was standing or sitting.

When he raises his left arm above the shoulder, his spine curves to the right. Verbal cues improve his posture but do not allow him to reach any higher or farther.

AROM/PROM

Patient's left shoulder does appear limited in his movement, on general observation. In the supine position the following readings were recorded:

- Flexion was 116°, active
- Flexion was 130°, passive
- Abduction was 70°, active
- Abduction was 72°, passive
- Internal rotation was 45°
- External rotation was 20°, active
- Muscle guarding noted at end range

Strength

Patient demonstrates functional strength within his available range. When muscle testing was performed by the physical therapist, he received a 2 of a possible 5 because of an inability to go through the full ROM. On this scale of 1 to 5, 5 is the greatest range of motion and 1 is the least. He is able to lift a 4-pound weight without straining himself, recording the level of pain as a 2 on a scale of 1 to 5. The lack of motion range and inability to lift excessive weight (greater than 20 pounds) cause him to be incapable of performing his necessary work duties.

Pain

On a scale of 1 to 10, 10 being the most painful, patient stated his pain level was a 3 at any given time. He defined "at any given time" as the time when he was not lifting, reaching, pulling, or moving his shoulder in any manner. When asked to demonstrate the highest point he could reach, the pain level was an 8/10. This decreased mobility affects his everyday living: his inability to get dressed, to get dishes out of the cupboard, and to brush his teeth with his left hand.

Activity Tolerance

The evaluation indicated that pain decreased following 15 minutes of rest and that pain is more severe during work and after activity, including getting dressed and reaching. Activity tolerance needs to be addressed, as it will influence the patient's ability to return to work.

Special Tests

Joint mobilization of anterior and posterior glides appears limited as well as inferior glide. The drop arm test was performed and was negative.

Requirements to Return to Work

Patient must minimize lifting objects heavier than 10 pounds above his waist to 25 times a day. He must lift the object using his arms and not his back, as this will result in more complicated problems, such as back and neck injuries.

Prior Level of Function

Mobility (home)

Prior to the accident, the patient was able to retrieve objects from a cupboard, dress himself, and brush his teeth using his left shoulder, arm, and hand. He was also capable of mowing the lawn with a push mower. These activities were accomplished without pain and with a full range of motion, at least 170°.

Employment

Michael is employed by BB's Bricks as a mason but is currently on medical leave owing to shoulder complications. The patient was previously able to stack and lift bricks up to 30 pounds approximately 200 times per day. Presently, the patient reports the inability to lift any object more than 4 pounds of weight 15 times per day.

FINAL PLAN OF TREATMENT

Following are methods that the physical therapist will act upon to increase the mobility and use of the patient's left shoulder.

Treatment Diagnosis

Patient had decreased functional abilities, loss of range of motion, increased pain, and lack of strength in left shoulder.

Assessment

Patient presents a decreased range of motion and strength of the left upper extremity resulting in decreased functional activity.

Reason for Skilled Care

Patient would benefit from three physical therapy sessions per week. Frequency and repetition are important in strengthening muscles and joints, and improving their ROM. Three sessions per week would ensure that the patient is receiving the utmost assistance in improving strength, ROM, and functional use. Without this professional assistance from a therapist, he will continue to lose his ROM and functional use. With treatment provided in a controlled setting by the physical therapist, the patient will be able to gain up to 95% of his initial range of motion and 100% of his functional use. In a controlled setting, the physical therapist is able to supervise the activity performed by the patient and assist him when necessary. The care offered by the therapist will ensure that the strengthening and training are completed properly. Supervised training will provide a transition to the exercises he will be instructed to perform at home.

Problems

The patient's problems have affected his life at home and at his place of employment. His current problems are as follows:

- Decreased mobility
- Decreased strength
- Decreased functional use.

Plan of Care

The final elements needed for a successful functioning outcome for the patient, and methods that will be used, are declared in the following.

Specific Treatment Strategies

The patient will apply moist heat and phonophoresis for 10 minutes at 0.4 watt per centimeter squared. Additionally, the patient will follow the heat application by joint mobilization and active and passive range of motion exercises. Finally, he will proceed in the plan of treatment by using clinical equipment to strengthen the upper body, and overhead pulleys to strengthen and increase the functional use of his left shoulder.

Frequency and Duration

Three physical therapy sessions per week are required to aid this patient in increased mobility, strength, and functional use. These sessions must continue for 4 straight weeks to ensure complete recovery from the accident. Exercises guided by physical therapists are necessary and must be repeated three times per week. The exercises assigned by the therapist and performed by the patient must be supervised to guarantee that the tasks are done correctly and to the patient's fullest potential. This thorough supervision will ensure proper healing in the shortest time period possible.

Patient Instruction/Home Program

After intensive therapy in the controlled facility, the patient is instructed to do arm lifts at home, initially with no weights and gradually increasing to 10 pounds. Patient will begin by performing unweighted arm lifts and gradually increase their size by 2 pounds every 5 days, until the left arm can be lifted parallel to the floor. The second exercise, arm circles, should be performed just as for the arm lifts, increasing the weights and the size of the circles gradually, 2 pounds every 5 days. Exercise according to these explicit instructions

will increase the patient's range of motion and strength of the left shoulder.

Short-Term Goals

The short-term goals of the patient are to improve mobility by at least 10–15° in his ROM. After 4 weeks of supervised physical therapy, he should be well versed in a home exercise program and be able to correctly demonstrate the exercises back to the therapist. The pain in his shoulder will be decreased by 75% in 2 weeks to enable patient to improve lifting ability at work. The patient will be able to do overhead reaching in low cupboards by April 1, 2000.

Long-Term Goals

The patient will be restored to functional mobility of at least 155–165° of flexion and abduction allowing the patient to reach over his head with no pain by June 1, 2000. The patient will be able to return to work by April 30, 2000.

Rehabilitation Potential

Patient has the potential to gain 95% of his original range of motion back after his completion of the 4 weeks of physical therapy sessions. He will be able to return to work and perform everyday tasks such as dressing himself and brushing his teeth without pain. His rehabilitation potential is excellent.

Progress Report

A **progress report** documents the continuity of care provided over a specified period of time. This amount of time may be a few days, a week, a month, or longer, depending on the patient. Additionally, the progress report supports the practitioner's need to carry on further treatment. As with any document listed in this section, format depends on the work environment (progress reports are often in the SOAP note format), but the purpose of all progress reports should be clear: to establish the medical necessity of continued care.

When creating this or any other document, one of your first tasks is to build unity throughout the document to carry forward a singular purpose or thought. That same consistency should be applied here, first to the internal workings of the document, and again to build continuity between this and any previous documents written about or for this patient. For example, if a patient suffers from head wounds, and the initial evaluation addresses the lacerations that you have treated, the progress report should address the same lacerations. In many cases, patients develop further complications, which may distract the practitioner from the original purpose. These further complications can be addressed, but they should appear as a secondary finding in the document. Use the following general formula as an outline to address the progress of a patient.

Progress Report   (Date)

1. Patient Information

2. Current Evaluation

3. Diagnosis

   Review the original diagnosis and address the new one.

4. Treatment Provided

   Describe what was accomplished to treat the patient and events occurring during or since last treatment.

5. Assessment

   Describe the reaction the patient has to treatment.

6. Complications or Further Developments

   Discuss the problems that arise out of treatment. Patients may have reactions to a prescription drug, they may fail to take their medication, physicians may change orders, or the patient may develop new complications from related events. Be precise about assessments, as you will not want any information misinterpreted.

   At this point, you may consider offering information in chart form to provide an easy comparison of findings for other practitioners who treat the patient or who may make changes to the orders.

7. Recommendations, Changes to Treatment, and Goals

   Offer suggestions or make changes to treatment, and set both long- and short-term goals in response to the goals set in the initial evaluation.

   Establish a follow-up schedule.

Sample Narrative
PROGRESS REPORT

Michael Geigger was seen three days a week as recommended by the physical therapist. He attended physical therapy from March 22, 2000, to April 17, 2000, for a total of twelve sessions, and he missed zero appointments. His consistent attendance assisted in the exceptional rehabilitation of his left shoulder. The girth measurement of the patient's shoulder, at the time of initial evaluation, was 46 cm, and his present girth measurement is 49 cm. The skilled care provided by the physical therapist influenced the increase in the patient's girth measurement; the strengthening exercises increased the muscle capacity of the patient's shoulder. The strengthening of the patient's shoulder diminished the acute aching in his shoulder. In the initial evaluation, the patient sensed acute pain when he reached back, up above his shoulder, or to the right and left side with weight over 15 pounds; currently, he can reach above his head with a maximum of 20 pounds without pain. The continuation of skilled care will continue to reduce the acute pain and increase the girth measurement in his left shoulder.

The controlled exercises assigned by the therapist facilitated improvements in the patient's posture and resulted in an increase in the range of motion (ROM) of his left shoulder. On March 22, 2000, the physical therapist recorded the ROM of the patient in the supine position, as listed in the table:

Measurements of patient's left shoulder	Measurements at the March 22, 2000, session	Measurements at the April 17, 2000, session
Flexion, active	116°	150°
Flexion, passive	130°	160°
Abduction, active	70°	71°
Abduction, passive	72°	78°
Internal rotation	45°	48°
External rotation	20°	26°

The patient reports that he continues to sense a dull pain in his deltoid muscle, resulting in an inability to complete the exercises assigned by the physical therapist. The patient's active and passive ROM has not improved as stated in the goals established in the initial evaluation; therefore, the continuation of physical therapy in a controlled setting is necessary to assist in complete rehabilitation of his left shoulder.

The patient demonstrates functional strength within his available range. The strengthening of his muscles also assisted in the improvement of his ROM. The therapist instructed the patient to use the upper body exercise machine (UBE) for 10 slow repetitions, to perform 25 repetitions of pulleys, to complete 10 repetitions of wall ladders, and to perform upper body rows for 10 minutes. Initially, the patient received a 2 out of a possible 5 on the strength examination because of his inability to move actively through his full range of motion; currently, he receives a 4/5. Previously, he was unable to lift a 4-pound weight, recording the level of pain as a 2/5. The patient demonstrates the ability to lift 15 pounds with his left shoulder; the pain level is a 1/5. The increase in motion range and the ability to lift an increasing amount of weight, when compared with findings on the initial evaluation, enable him to perform his necessary activities of daily living (ADL). With the professional assistance from a physical therapist, the patient will continue to regain his ROM, strength, and functional use.

The mobility and strength of the patient has increased; therefore, he is able to return to work lifting objects with a maximum weight of 15 pounds above his waist no more than 40 times a day. The continuation of skilled care will enable the patient to remain at work and to continue to increase the amount of weight he is capable of lifting. The persistence of skilled care will improve the functional abilities, the ROM, the level of pain, and the strength of the patient's left shoulder. With continued treatment provided by the physical therapist, the patient will gain up to 95% of his initial ROM and 100% of his functional use. In a controlled setting, the skilled physical therapist supervises the activities performed by the patient to ensure that the strengthening and training are completed properly and to assist him when necessary. Such supervised training also provides instruction that aids the patient in the performance of exercises at home.

The physical therapist performs the following actions to aid in the rehabilitation of the patient's left shoulder. I apply moist heat and phonophoresis for 10 minutes at 0.4 watt per centimeter squared; these modalities relax the deltoid muscle, resulting in a reduction of pain and an increase of the ROM. The patient proceeds in the plan of treatment by making use of clinical equipment to strengthen the upper body. The patient utilizes overhead pulleys to strengthen and increase the functional use of his left shoulder. The supervision of skilled care during this plan of treatment

ensures that the tasks are properly acted out, which will reduce the risk of further injury.

The current problems of the patient, which have affected his life at home and at work, are the same as stated in the initial evaluation but less severe. The following are the patient's problems that continue to require attention:

• Decreased mobility in the left shoulder
• Decreased strength of left shoulder
• Decreased functional use of left shoulder

Controlled care, three times per week, will aid the patient in increasing mobility, strength, and functional use. The sessions must continue for 2 additional weeks to ensure the complete recovery from his previous accident. The patient must repeat the sessions, which the physical therapist instructs, three times per week to ensure proper healing. The physical therapist supervises the assigned exercises to guarantee that tasks are done correctly and to the patient's fullest potential. Thorough supervision by the therapist and dedication by the patient ensure proper healing in the shortest possible time period.

With the previous standard for care established by the physical therapist, I have developed a plan for future treatment. After intensive therapy in the controlled facility, the physical therapist will instruct the patient to perform arm lifts at home, initially with no weight and gradually increasing the weight to 10 pounds. The patient will perform small unweighted arm lifts, gradually increasing by 2 pounds every 5 days, until he has the ability to lift his arm parallel to the floor. The patient will complete the second exercise, arm circles, just as for the arm lifts, increasing the weights by 2 pounds and the size of the circles every 5 days. The physical therapist will encourage the patient to visit a local gym and/or aquatic facility to receive the maximum benefit from rehabilitation. The explicit instructions stated above will increase the patient's ROM and strength of the left shoulder.

The patient's improved functional use depends on the continuation of skilled care to assist in the strengthening the left shoulder. The therapist instructs the patient, as well as the family of the patient, to perform the instructed exercises, which continuously strengthen the left shoulder and prevent future injury.

The short-term goals of the patient, as stated in the initial evaluation, were to improve his mobility by at least 10° in his ROM; this goal was met on April 7, 2000. The new goal is to improve his ROM by an additional 15° by April 30, 2000.

The pain in his shoulder has been reduced by 75% within the 2-week time period. Consequently, with this progress, the patient's functional mobility will return to the minimum of 160° of flexion and abduction allowing the patient to reach over his head with no pain by May 15, 2000, instead of the original goal of June 1, 2000. The patient has the potential to regain 95% of his original range of motion after the completion of the three remaining physical therapy sessions. He will return to work by May 1, 2000, with no restrictions, and perform everyday tasks such as dressing himself and brushing his teeth without pain. His rehabilitation potential is exceptional.

Discharge Report

The **discharge report** describes the success of the treatment provided and clears the patient to return to living, and in some cases, with limitations or restrictions. The discharge report has a secondary purpose in that it explains the interactivity between and among providers. It chronicles, in brief, the patient's path to success from the initial evaluation (or from the practitioner's first intervention or evaluation) and releases the patient from the care of the practitioner.

In form, the discharge report should reflect the same categories of discussion presented in the progress report, but it should also reflect final outcomes and assessments. Following is a sample outline of categories.

Discharge Report (Date)

1. Patient Information
2. Final Evaluation
3. Diagnosis
   Review the original diagnosis, or identify any changes.
4. Treatment Provided
   Describe what was accomplished to treat the patient.
5. Assessment
   Describe the patient's successful response to treatment.
6. Complications or Further Developments
   Discuss the problems that may arise out of treatment.

At this point, you may consider offering information in chart form to provide an easy comparison of findings for other practitioners who handle the patient or who may make changes to the orders.

7. Recommendations and Goals
   Provide restrictions and set both long- and short-term goals (if necessary) in response to the goals set in the initial evaluation and progress report.

   List medications and establish a follow-up schedule.

Sample Narrative
DISCHARGE REPORT

After Benjamin Christopher Lewis tore his anterior cruciate ligament (ACL) while skiing at the Peak 'n Peek Ski Resort on December 17, 2001, he underwent ACL reconstructive surgery by Dr. Phillip C. Carnes at St. Vincent's Hospital in Erie, Pennsylvania. Following his surgery, Mr. Lewis implemented a home rehabilitation treatment program, which not only hindered his recovery time due to his lack of motivation in the program but also resulted in the formation of excess scar tissue within the knee joint capsule. At this time, Dr. Timothy N. Banks performed surgery to remove the scar tissue and referred him to Erie Rehabilitation. On January 8, 2002, I admitted Mr. Lewis into my care.

Most patients who have undergone ACL reconstruction demonstrate full extension and a flexion of 140° at the 3-week post-ACL surgery period; however, Mr. Lewis displayed only a 170° extension and a 120° flexion during his first visit. These impediments resulted from both the unsuccessful home treatment program and his second surgery to remove scar tissue. Despite these initial shortcomings, Mr. Lewis displayed full flexion and extension by the end of his 6-month treatment, and consequently, I am discharging Mr. Lewis at this time.

At the beginning of each therapy visit, I applied a moist hot pack to Mr. Lewis' knee for approximately 20 minutes prior to his exercise program and ended with 15 minutes of icing. During the first week, the patient concentrated on regaining some of his lost flexion by performing three sets of heel, shuttle, and wall slides for 15 repetitions each. To aid in his full extension efforts, Mr. Lewis completed the same amount of heel props, prone hangs, and towel stretches during this first week. At the end of his first week with me, Mr. Lewis made significant progress and increased his flexion to 124°. At the start of the second week of treatment, I established a plan to help Mr. Lewis regain patellar tendon strength to better support his knee joint, which was done by adding step-down exercises, leg presses, and knee extensions. Mr. Lewis executed 3 sets of 12 repetitions for each of these exercises. By the end of the third week, Mr. Lewis had reached full extension and a flexion of 135°. After almost a month of treatment, the patient not only enhanced his strength and conditioning by utilizing the Stairmaster and bicycle for 20 minutes each day but also increased his sport-specific agility by adding forward and backward running, lateral slides, and jumping rope. At this point in his recovery, I reduced his weekly visits to the clinic from the original four to five times a week to only twice a week. In addition to the exercises that Mr. Lewis performed within our clinic, he also completed several in-home exercises to help regain strength in his quadricep and calf muscles by performing 3 sets of 10 repetitions of both partial squats on the involved leg and calf raises to better stabilize his knee.

At this time, which is 6 months from the first time I met with Mr. Lewis, he has achieved a full recovery. Even though Mr. Lewis underwent a full functional progression back to activity to include near-normal strength, decreased swelling, full motion, excellent stability, and complete running program, I still urge him to continue his strengthening exercises while returning to his normal activities at home. In addition, I also created a specific knee-strengthening program for Mr. Lewis to decrease the possibility of further knee injuries. The patient will stand on one leg, bending the other leg behind his body, concentrating on a single-stance one-third knee bend. Continuing the exercise at a steady rate for three minutes, working up to 5 minutes on each leg, Mr. Lewis will complete a series of flexions and extensions from approximately 30° to 80°. I also recommended to Mr. Lewis that he add specific hamstring and side-to-side exercises as a preseason and intra-season workout. This 20-minute-a-day program, concentrating on the knee musculature, will improve performance, increase strength, and diminish injuries for Mr. Lewis during ski season.

Due to Mr. Lewis' full recovery from his ACL tear, I am discharging him from my care at Erie Rehabilitation. He may return to all of his normal activities, including skiing, and wear his sports brace when participating in activities, if needed.

Exercise

EDITING FOR CONTINUITY AND FLOW

Directions: Examine the following paper, submitted by a student as a rough draft, and consider the italicized text, which indicates problems, and correct. Then look at the paragraphs throughout the paper and find the ones that read like lists. Consider how you might draw transitions between these paragraphs to build continuity and coherence.

Christopher Adams, a seventeen-year-old high school student, started attending physical therapy on September 29, 2000. Dr. Matthew Myers referred Christopher to therapy after he underwent reconstructive surgery on his left patellofemoral joint (knee). Christopher entered physical therapy with pain and stiffness in his knee, which he was unable to flex or extend with ease. Since he first attended physical therapy a *(one?)* month ago, he has made significant progress and will be able to finish therapy at an earlier date than originally anticipated, if *there are* no complications. He will need to continue therapy for at least three more months for supervised exercising and strengthening to ensure that he does not further injure his knee. *Chris (appropriate?)* has been attending therapy regularly three times a week for the past month, *and* has only missed one visit due to lack of transportation.

When Chris started physical therapy, he was confined *(is this the right word? I don't think HE himself was confined to the brace)* to a knee brace that limited his movement. He no longer needs the brace and has *progressed nicely (vague)* without it. Chris has made *excellent (vague)* progress on both active and passive range of motion for his patellofemoral joint. With active range of motion, he has increased in extension from 140 degrees to 165 degrees and in flexion from 90 degrees to 100 degrees. With passive range of motion, he has increased in extension from 160 degrees to 175 degrees and in flexion from 95 degrees to 110 degrees. This is an above *(hyphenate)* average increase considering he has been attending therapy for only one month.

Christopher also showed improvement in the manual muscle test for strength. For extension, he *progresses (past tense?)* from a two out of five to a four out of five. For flexion, he *progressed* from a three out of five to a four and a half out of five. *(Since you are using a numerical scoring method, you can use numbers here. Example: 4 1/2.)*

Chris reports decreased pain in his leg using the same scale of one out of ten with ten being the worst pain. When walking, his pain has decreased from a seven out of ten to a four out of ten. During excessive movement, he now experiences a five out of ten instead of a nine out of ten, which is still his worst pain. He now sleeps much better since his pain has diminished from a five and a half out of ten to a two out of ten. *(Relevance? Was sleep an issue?)*

Christopher's ability to perform his exercises has *enhanced (word choice)* to a level close to his previous capability of performance. He has now moved beyond simple stretching to more intense stretching along with leg presses and squat exercises on the Total Gym. While warming up, he continues to alternate between the bicycle and the treadmill. He also performs exercises at home two to three times a day. Even though he is progressing smoothly and effectively, his mother has reported that he is not performing the exercises on a regular schedule. I have talked with Christopher about *doing (word choice)* his exercises at home and explained to him the importance of them. *(Transition)* He will not receive therapy for an extended period of time and needs to continue his exercises in order to keep up his strength and mobility. The exercises are also important for him to reduce scar tissue, which can *immensely slow down (awkward and vague—find a single word as a substitute for these)* his recovery process.

(Transition) Chris has progressed on the platform system for balancing. He now has the capability to bear full unilateral weight on his left leg and balance on his leg without the assistance of a therapist or a wall. A therapist does, however, stand by in case he loses his balance.

(Transition) Chris has electrical stimulation with cold packs applied to his left leg by a therapist to provide increased input to the quadriceps and hamstrings. This technique will alleviate pain and stiffness to the patellofemoral joint making it easier for Chris to perform his exercises.

Physical therapy may not be required for the full six months, but *it is* in Christopher's best interest to continue therapy three times a week for at least two more months, after which he will be reevaluated on his progress. Chris needs to continue attending physical therapy for supervision while performing his rehabilitation program to alleviate any possibility of re-injury to his knee.

My short-term goals for Christopher's rehabilitation include a continuation of better range of motion of his patellofemoral joint and increase

(increased?) strength of his lower extremity muscles. I would like to increase his range of motion two to three degrees for both flexion and extension within the next week. The pain in Chris's knee should be alleviated within the next month.

Christopher desires to play football again along with other sports, *so* in long-term, I would like to return Chris's range of motion and strength to normal *so* he is capable of playing sports again. In relation to Chris's right knee, his left knee should possess full range of motion and full strength by the time therapy *is completed (passive)*.

Exercise

EDITING FOR WORD CHOICE AND DICTION

Directions: Examine the following paper, which a student submitted as a rough draft, and consider the words and phrases highlighted in italics. Review each mark and determine why these comments are made.

Preliminary Assessment

Christopher Adams tore the anterior cruciate ligament (ACL) of his left knee at a high school football game, which required reconstructive surgery. *It is* essential for Chris to attend physical therapy to repair his range of motion of the patellofemoral joint (knee) and *to strengthen his* . . . strength of the quadriceps and hamstring muscles.

REFERRAL

An orthopedic surgeon, Dr. Matthew Myers, referred Chris to the Physical Therapy Department at St. Joseph's Hospital in order to advance with the recovery process following a weekend of rest.

Data Accompanying Referral

Dr. Myers diagnosed Chris on September 8, 2000 *(comma)* with a torn ACL *(comma)* and on the 15th of September, reconstructive surgery was performed *(who performed? = passive voice. Dr. M performed . . .)* on Chris's knee. Dr. Myers prescribed ibuprofen for any pain and/or inflammation accompanying the surgery. Crutches and a functional knee brace will also be needed after surgery. For the first two to three weeks after surgery, the brace needs to be set with limitations of the final 20-degree extension and flexion to 90 degrees or greater. Following those initial weeks after surgery, the brace is adjusted so *there is* unlimited flexion with some limitations on extension that progressively decrease until full extension is possible.

Patient History

- Name: Christopher Adams
- Date of birth: June 30, 1983
- Age: 17
- Gender: Male
- Start of care: September 29, 2000
- Primary complaint: stiffness and soreness in the knee and weakness in the muscles of the left leg

Referral Diagnosis

Christopher tore his ACL in a football game when he was tackled on a play. He was sent to the hospital for x-ray and MRI examinations to diagnose the injury. *These tests showed how serious the tear was (awkward)* and what type of treatment would be necessary.

Prior Therapy History

Chris has not undergone physical therapy prior to our first session.

EVALUATION

While performing the evaluation and tests, the following data were collected about the patient's injury.

Baseline Evaluation Data

Christopher is *very (omit)* cooperative and follows direction well. He is anxious to get his rehabilitation program started so he can get back to his everyday activities, including football.

Posture

Chris's posture is excellent, which will *greatly (omit)* benefit his progress with rehabilitation. Good posture is essential for him because it will help with his aerobic capacity for sports, and it will benefit treatment because posture affects joint integrity and mobility *(comma)* which *is what we are trying to get the most out of (awkward and wordy)*.

AROM/PROM

Chris *demonstrates* normal range of motion for his injury with his active range of motion (AROM) at 140° for extension and for flexion, he *demonstrated (verb tense problem—is he currently demonstrating this or did he demonstrate in his tests at a previous date/time? Answer this question and you have your answer. However, be sure to stay consistent with verb tense throughout each section)* his AROM to be 90°. When testing passive

range of motion (PROM), he demonstrated 160° for extension and 79° for flexion.

Before his injury of his left knee and with his right knee, Chris had full range of motion, which included 180° for extension and 70° for flexion.

Strength

During the manual muscle test for strength, Chris showed that his muscle strength of extension is a 2/5 and for flexion his strength is a 3/5. Normally, Chris shows full strength of 5/5 for both extension and flexion.

Pain

When asked about pain, Chris stated that he notices pain in his knee when walking or with excessive movement *(comma)* and when he is sleeping, it wakes him up when he rolls onto his left side. Based on a scale from 1 to 10, with 10 being the worst amount of pain, he describes his pain when walking to be a 7/10 *(comma)* and with excessive movement, *his pain is the worst being at a (awkward)* 9/10. When Chris sleeps, his pain is not unbearable, but it *is enough to* wake him up being at about a 5.5/10.

Activity Tolerance

Chris performs the exercises well and has a high *tolerance to the activities (what does this mean?).* He complains of pain and discomfort when his knee is stretched beyond his ability, making us aware of what he can handle and how fast we can progress his rehabilitation. He is able to walk upstairs and perform daily activities with a small level of difficulty and few complaints.

Wound Description

Chris does not possess *and* open wounds and shows good progress in the appearance of his scars. The scars do not show any signs of discoloration. The main scar is about three inches long and two centimeters wide. The smaller scar is a one-centimeter diameter circle *(relevance?).*

Requirements to Return to Home, School, and/or Job

Christopher needs to be taken out of gym class and school and also needs to limit the number of stairs he climbs. At home, he needs to rest as much as possible and also *perform his exercises he is given to do by himself (wordy).*

DIAGNOSIS

In evaluating the information obtained during the examination (this phrase must modify the next word: "it"?), it can be organized and interpreted in the following way.

Treatment Diagnosis

The patient has undergone reconstructive surgery of his ACL, which has caused some movement and strength limitations. Through the process of physical therapy, Chris will be able to increase his movement and strength ability back to *it's* original status.

Reason for Skilled Care

It is necessary for Chris to attend physical therapy because he needs to be watched and guided carefully. *It is* essential for Chris's rehabilitation to be gradual because if the process occurs too fast, his injury could regress. If he is not monitored closely during his program, he could develop effusion, laxity, and joint surface irritation.

PLAN OF CARE

It is important to have early motion because it decreases effusion, pain, and inhibition. Weights should also be used early, but in small amounts *and little by little*. Isometric, concentric, and eccentric techniques are needed where the patient is most deficient in the range of motion. In the early stages, flexion-adduction and flexion-abduction diagonal patterns are used so the knee can maintain flexion from 30 degrees or greater. Extension-adduction external rotation with knee extension is also needed in order to decrease the stress placed on the ACL.

When Chris gets his ROM at a better standing, he will progress to strength and endurance exercises. Using the leg press and squat exercises on the Total Gym offers a wide range of help to the patient with various degrees of incline and the ability to add weight resistance. Stationary bicycling will also be used when Chris has adequate ROM.

Balancing on the injured leg can be assisted through training on a platform system. He will begin with partial body weight on his injured leg and slowly progress to full unilateral weight bearing.

Electrical stimulation will be used to provide increased input to the quadriceps and hamstrings.

As Chris's strength increases, more exercises, including toe raises, squats, step-ups, resisted gait, reciprocal lower extremity extension, treadmill walking/running, and stair climbing, will be added to his program.

Frequency/Duration

Christopher needs to attend physical therapy 2–3 times a week for approximately six months. He will be reevaluated in six months to see how well he has progressed *(comma)* and if he has not progressed to the right standards *(comma)* then therapy will continue.

Patient Instruction

The patient will be instructed on how to perform all the exercises assigned to him in each of his sessions. He will be encouraged to continue those exercises when he is not in the clinic *(comma)* and he will also be given some additional exercises that can be done strictly at home and do not need a therapist's supervision to perform.

Short-Term Goals

The therapists in this department are going to work with Christopher to get his ROM and strength back to *where it needs to be* to function properly in everyday activities.

Long-Term Goals

Christopher would like to be able to play football and other sports again, so as therapists, we will perform at the best of our abilities to get Chris's ROM and strength *where it needs to be* in order for him to play sports again.

Rehabilitation Potential

The patient has a high potential for a full recovery from his injury. He is anxious to get started and willing to cooperate and work to return his knee to where it started.

12

The Business
of Writing

Key Terms

Asynchronous Not occurring at the same time

Cover letter Business letter introducing a longer, more descriptive document

Curriculum vitae A lengthy description of qualifications usually emphasizing educational experiences relevant to job

Electronic communication Writing in asynchronous environments using computer technology

Executive summary A description of a proposed business program—the introduction

Grant proposal A document seeking funding for support of research

Investment potential The type of investment offered and rates of return

Market The product or service in terms of the competition

Mission statement Language stating the overall direction of the organization; also called *vision statement*

Overhead The facilities needed to be operational and the personnel associated with operations

Projected revenues Estimated growth and development in relation to capital expenditures

Request for proposal (RFP) A document prepared by a company or grant-offering institution advertising for a project to be completed

Request for qualifications (RFQ) A document prepared by a supporting institution that ensures that the right organization has been targeted for a project

Resume A brief description of qualifications usually emphasizing employment experience

chapter objectives

On completion of this chapter, the reader should be able to

1. Develop a letter meeting business standards.

2. Develop cover letters that serve to enhance the documents they introduce.

3. Understand that electronic forms of communication should be treated like any other form of professional communication.

4. Design a resume or curriculum vitae using standard practices of presentation.

5. Develop business plans that meet industry standards.

6. Develop a scheme to approach proposal writing using standard categories for presentation.

Once you are employed, you are a functional element of a profession, and professions are businesses, whether their administrators like to admit it or not. Businesses operate under a set of standards, and meeting those standards is often the difference between merely surviving and succeeding.

Although this is not a text about business writing, this chapter does serve that function, to some extent. Clear communication is as important as communication protocol in business. Therefore, these chapters discuss the modes of communication and the forms under which they operate.

Additionally, communicating with patients is another element of being a good or successful business person. This chapter helps the reader gather an understanding of how to prepare information for a less educated audience.

WRITING LETTERS

Some allied health care providers operate under the direction of a supervising physician. In such cases, a simple discharge report (or progress report) is not completely useful unless additional information is provided. A **cover letter** summarizing treatment and results should supplement the discharge report to the supervising physician and should act as a conduit to the report.

A letter should ultimately serve to educate its audience. Consequently, be sure that it makes clear and direct points, instead of using vague and imprecise language that fails to communicate. Many allied health professionals complain that they are not considered equals to others in the health professions or that they do not receive the respect that, for instance, physicians do. Earn the respect of your colleagues by writing clearly and acting like a professional should.

Consider the following points to avoid the pitfalls of bland and vague communication.

- When introducing a patient to the audience (physician or another allied health professional), provide detailed information about the patient and the patient's condition. Without specific details, the recipient of the letter may be forced to produce a file to review the patient's condition. Make your reader's job easy ("easy reading comes from hard writing") by offering the necessary details to make clear connections. You may also be just as specific when writing about the patient's history. Give a clear explanation of the condition(s) and treatment(s) in a brief but complete form.

- Provide a clear rationale for treatment. Many letters fail to explain why treatments were followed or why a plan was initiated. Be sure to illuminate the reader by offering the details.

- Give full explanations of the results of treatment. Be sure to address issues that have not been resolved or limitations that the patient may experience as the result of treatment, temporarily or long term.

- Follow sound practices of writing business letters, such as attention to format, addresses, closings, signatures, and general writing concerns.

- Do not assume that all health care professionals will understand the jargon of your specific niche. Stop using abbreviations or shortened versions of terms that may be acceptable only within an informal office setting. In other words, make sure your audience understands your directives or explanations and gets your message. Do not allow your reader to lose focus because of mental shortcuts you have deployed.

- Understand your position as a professional in the field. You want to send the message that you belong, and writing as if you worship the practitioners with whom you work will send the message that you are uncertain of your space in the profession. Be polite and direct, but do not ask permission unnecessarily, ask for forgiveness for your incompetence, or assume that your work needs outside approval (unless you have been directed to seek approval from an overseeing professional).

You are a professional, and your competence in the way you act, write, and present yourself will send the message to others that you belong in your position.

Sample Student Essay
COVER LETTER

Directions: With your knowledge of documen-tation procedures, examine the discharge letter presented in Figure 12-1. Then review the comments following the letter.

Department of Physical Therapy
January 4, 2002

Dr. Kelsch
Director of Orthopedic Medicine
Buffalo General Hospital
Buffalo, NY 14202
RE: Joe Marshall

Dear Dr. Kelsch,

Thank you for referring this man with knee pain, who we first saw in the PT department three weeks ago. He presented with pain effecting his sleep and limitation of movement in the knee and hip, which has since responded to ice, ES, and clavical traction.

Mr. Marshall has reported symptomatic relief for his Osteoarthritis. If you are agreeable, I will see him once more and then discontinue Physical Therapy.

Yours truly,

Megan Clarke

Figure 12-1 Sample Discharge Letter

COMMENTS

- The overall message is weak: Specifics are lost. The patient history cannot be re-created here, as the writer of the letter expects the physician to pull the chart or notes. More problematic is the fact that the writer does not specify which shoulder received treatment and the duration and frequency of that treatment. The writer provides no personal details about the patient and his condition.

- The writer provides a vague discussion of patient treatment in that the rationale for treatment and medical necessity is not evident. What is ES? Do all medical professionals use this term? Also, why was the clavicle in traction? Is this appropriate treatment? The outcome of treatment is not evident, and no specific data regarding pain relief or clinical improvement are supplied. *(Allied health professionals complain that they do not receive the respect of their colleagues in a medical setting. This letter demonstrates how respect can easily be lost.)*

- Closing: The patient discharge depends on the response of the director. If the director fails to reply, what is the course of action to take? The therapist is trying to be respectful here, but she does not need approval to perform her job. Again, act like a professional and receive professional treatment from colleagues.

- Letter format: The general appearance of the letter is unprofessional in that paragraph indentation is not consistent; punctuation problems are ignored; the return address, salutation, and closing do not meet standard business letter formats; and the spacing of the elements of the letter is inconsistent.

- Writing concerns:

  Word choice: The writer fails to distinguish between *affect* (to influence) and *effect* (to bring about).

  The meaning of the word *agreeable* is pleasant or pleasing. This is not the appropriate term for this sentence.

  The terms *I* and *we* are used interchangeably, which creates confusion for the reader.

  Verb tense shifts: The letter makes unnecessary verb tense shifts, which can create confusion and inaccuracies.

  Mechanics: The writer demonstrates inconsistent capitalization of the title *Physical Therapy*. The name of the profession need not be capitalized, nor does the term *physical therapist*.

  The name of a condition, such as "osteoarthritis," does not require capitalization, unless it contains a proper noun, such as in *Parkinson's disease*.

  In the first paragraph, *who* should be *whom*. In sentence 2, *pain* and *limitation* are the words that *which* refers to, so *has* should be *have*.

E-MAIL ETIQUETTE

E-mail, **electronic communication** in **asynchronous** form, is unique to the world of professional writing and standards because it is a hybrid of several types of writing. For example, the forms you fill in that contain the recipient's E-mail address, subject, CC, and RE are set up as if the message is in "memo" format. However, since E-mail is primarily for communicating or exchanging documents, most people write as if they are composing a letter. In view of these format issues, E-mail has an identity problem. Furthermore, some people use E-mail as a means to write notes or messages to another person; consequently, writers use a style that is imprecise, unprofessional, and grammatically incorrect, or they may eliminate salutations or closings under the assumption that a quick note should carry less formality than a business letter. Such an assumption is made in error.

Consider all E-mail messages to be representations of your academic abilities. Use a style that is professional when you communicate with others on a professional basis. As a result, you should lead with a formal greeting, and the body paragraphs of your message should be organized, the content should be clear, and you should provide a conclusion to your message. Close appropriately, and then proofread for any errors. Many people assume that the informal nature of E-mail allows for inconsistencies and errors. This is not true. Any reader who knows the rules of writing will be offended by mistakes and blatant disregard for the rules. Your writing should be a representation of you, in any format.

You should always think that what you write is not secure. Most E-mail services are secure, but you should write as if your work could possibly be reviewed at any time by anyone in your organization. You would not want to represent yourself in one way to a colleague and then represent yourself in another to your employer.

Likewise, you should never forward anyone's comments or E-mail letters to someone else unless you have received permission first. Confidential information should not be transferred via E-mail, but in the case that some confidential information is provided, you do not want to take the chance of abusing privacy privileges.

Finally, check your E-mail frequently and respond promptly. People depend on E-mail messaging services for a quick and absolute means of communicating. Do not let your "In box" be the "vacuous hole" of E-mail that never is answered. You are provided with E-mail in your workplace to increase efficiency in communicating. Use it to promote such efficiency by being constantly aware of your role in the communication network.

E-mail can also be used for nonproductive purposes or for nonbusiness purposes. Use the following guidelines to ensure professionalism in the workplace:

- Answer personal E-mail messages on your own time using your own home computer.

- Never forward or send messages that are not work related.

- Never participate in promoting or sending pornography or lewd messages and jokes.

- Never become part of the network of complainers on E-mail. Be careful that lists and mail groups are used for appropriate purposes and not to humiliate or unfairly criticize others in the workplace, especially employers.

If you receive E-mail that asks you to engage in any of these practices, simply send the message to your "Trash" or "Recycle Bin," or ask the sender to remove you from the group or list.

COVER LETTERS AND RESUMES

Cover Letters

When you are applying for a job, writing a proposal, or producing a report, a cover letter may be necessary to introduce you or your credentials—typically presented in a **resume** or a more detailed document called a **curriculum vitae**—to the audience. For writing reports or applying for grants, the cover letter serves as an introduction that leads the audience into the actual proposal. For applying for jobs, the cover letter is often the only piece of evidence that future employers have to gauge the applicant's written communication skills. This is important to remember because many people think that prospective employers do not consider the cover letter when reviewing applicants' credentials; they think that the resume or curriculum vitae is the most important element of the application process. This is not true.

When I worked for a large institution, I had the interesting experience of sifting through piles of resumes and cover letters looking for qualified applicants. Most of the applicants had the minimum qualifications for the job. Those who did not meet the minimum were immediately moved to the "Unlikely" pile. The other two piles were the "A" pile, of applications from those likely to get an interview, and the "B" pile, of applications from those whose credentials were competitive but who showed some kind of weakness in communicating their position. The resumes that were discarded into the "B" pile got there mostly because of inconsistencies in format or writing problems, such as in clarity, organization, style, grammar, and mechanics. With the huge number of qualified applicants hunting for jobs, employers must have a way of weeding out the weak so that they can deal with a reasonable number of applicants. The only piece of evidence that represents you is your cover letter.

The cover letter should conform to standard business letter format: heading (your address and the date of the letter), inside address (the recipient's address), salutation ending with a colon ("Dear _____ :"), body (the paragraphs that make up your message), closing ("Sincerely," "Respectfully,"), and signature with your name in type beneath it.

Helpful Tips

Alignment: How you align the elements of the letter on your paper is your choice. Some people like to align the heading and the closing/signature in the middle of the page. Others like to skip spaces between paragraphs, and thus align all the paragraphs and sections of the letter with the left margin. Be consistent in the style you choose. Any inconsistency in format is considered a disorganization problem.

Purpose of letter and resume: Always keep in mind that the cover letter should elaborate on specific qualifications that are listed in the resume or curriculum vitae. It should never repeat what is listed on the resume. Many people find that they have little to say in the cover letter; accordingly, they rewrite the resume in the cover letter. Be aware, however, that the cover letter serves an entirely different purpose from that of the resume. Know the difference, and prove that you know it.

Introductory paragraph: State what you want. Ask for consideration for the job. Many people unfamiliar with cover letters simply assume that by submitting a letter, they qualify themselves for a position. Be sure to clarify what position you seek, since the company may offer several different types at once, and then ask to be considered for the position. Simply sending a letter that says that you have an interest does

not qualify you for the job. You are writing for a purpose: to be considered for the job. Be sure to ask for it, because asking will indicate that you are clear in your intent as you write.

Body paragraphs: Elaborate on experiences that you offer in your resume or curriculum vitae. Your resume should be specific in listing your qualifications and experiences, but a bulleted list should not be sufficient to describe all that you have experienced or learned. Give yourself the opportunity to expand on your learning experiences in the body paragraphs, and relate them to the job requirements. Remember to write for the purpose of qualifying yourself for the job. Make clear connections between your work experiences and the qualifications your prospective employer seeks.

Concluding paragraph: You do not need to thank anyone who reads your letter for his or her time. This is a mistake made by many unprepared job seekers. Simply reinforce the fact that your qualifications meet the expectations of the employer. Finally, you can offer to make yourself available for interviews. In doing so, recognize that your schedule is not the important one here. You should not dictate which days or dates you are available. If you want the job, you will do what is necessary to be available.

Do not offend: You do not want to tell employers what they already know. Telling a prospective employer that the company is "a quality place" or "the standard in the profession" has no relevance to your qualifications. Furthermore, companies that represent the industry standard are already aware of their favored status—they do not need you to tell them.

Closing and signature: Your closing can often make an impact if you are serious about searching for the right word. Often, the average letter will close with "Sincerely." Although "Sincerely" is appropriate for personal correspondences, it does not feel appropriate for business correspondences. Find the term that fits the mood and tone of your letter. Try different words and experiment with their effectiveness. "Respectfully" and "Cordially" are appropriate. Think of others that will fit your purpose.

Below your signature, you should type your name. If you have a title, you should include it after your printed name and separate the name from the title with a comma. Do not tack on unnecessary or inappropriate titles for the sake of adding one. You do not want to risk sounding immodest.

Resume or Curriculum Vitae

A resume provides a brief description of your preparation, qualifications, and experiences. The standard format of the resume helps the reader gather and process information quickly and efficiently.

The curriculum vitae offers similar experiences, but it allows for inclusion of published materials or listings of academic preparation. It follows a format similar to that of the resume.

Organizational Structure

Personal information: At the top of your resume or curriculum vitae, present your name, address, telephone numbers, and E-mail address. You can experiment with the design of this section. If you have a variety of information to include here, divide the information into columns and separate it at the top of the page. If you have the minimum information, center this section (see Figure 12-2). In either case, make your name stand out, through the use of either a bold font or another typeface.

Body: In the remainder of the resume or curriculum vitae, you should include specific information about your training, education, work experiences, and other information that qualifies you for the job you seek.

Each section is presented on the page in descending order of importance. If you have just completed an educational program and have no full-time employment experience, then education is your most valuable attribute. Start your list of qualifications with this heading and, as always, provide the information in reverse chronological order (meaning most recent degrees first).

Consider the following categories for inclusion in your resume or curriculum vitae:

Education

Relevant work experience

Related work experience

Volunteering

Relevant course work—such as independent studies or upper division courses (do not include standard course descriptions here; provide information that will allow your work to be recognized as unique)

Academic or professional awards and achievements

Publications and conference presentations

Skills and certifications

References—state that these are available on request, or include them on a separate sheet

Notice that the category "Objective," which appeared in many standard forms in the past, has been eliminated.

Design

As you design your resume or curriculum vitae, you should consider your audience and how a prospective employer will react to the information you present. The content is controlled by your experiences, but the design of the resume is not. Your presentation should incorporate the following standard design principles.

Headings: Be consistent with heading locations and purpose. Allow your text beneath the headings to feed from them in consistent and logical ways. As always, like elements, such as headings, should be parallel in structure.

General layout of headings: Placement of headings, either centered or justified on the left margin, is a matter of personal preference. Be consistent with headings and the text that flows under it. Most resumes use a hanging indentation format. The heading appears on the left margin, and the information placed under it is indented. More specific information is indented further.

Details in headings: When presenting information such as about a job experience or a degree, consider what is important to the reader. The reader, or prospective employer, wants to know

YOUR NAME, RPA-C
123 Maple St. Anywhere, NY 10000
(555) 123-4567
yname@e-mail.com

EDUCATION
BA/MA **Daemen College**, 2001 *(magna cum laude, Honors)*
Physician Assistant (3.8 GPA)
Honors Thesis: "The Effect of Stretching on Arthritis Patients"

PROFESSIONAL/BUSINESS EXPERIENCE
Medical Transcriptionist—Buffalo Medical Services, Buffalo, NY. 1999—present
- Performed general office duties
- Provided transcription services for the three partners in the company

Phlebotomist—Millard Fillmore Hospital, Amherst, NY. 2000—present
- Extracted blood from patients
- Ran centrifuge and conducted tests

RELEVANT COURSE WORK
Independent Study: Arthritis and Its Causes and Treatments
Advanced Studies: PA 447: Orthopedic Rehabilitation
PA 420: Musculoskeletal Disease
PA 414: Degenerative Neuromuscular Disorders

PUBLICATIONS AND CONFERENCE PRESENTATIONS
"The Effect of Stretching on Arthritis Patients." Daemen College Academic Festival
Presentation, 2001.
Arthritic Patients and the Impact of Nonsteroidal Anti-Inflammatory Drugs. Research Assistant
under author Professor Timothy Bankwell.

VOLUNTEER WORK
Office Assistant—Sister's Hospital. Buffalo, NY. Summers: 1999–2001
Clinical Orderly—Buffalo Medical Facilities. 1997–1998

ACADEMIC HONORS AND PROFESSIONAL AWARDS
Daemen College: Honors Program, 1999–2001; Academic All-American, 2000
Albert's Academic Scholarship, Daemen College, 1999–2001
New York State Regents Scholarship, 1997–2001

PROFESSIONAL ACTIVITIES, MEMBERSHIPS, AND CIVIC INVOLVEMENT
Buffalo Society for Physician Assistants; APAA
Member, Scottish Rite #342 F&AM
Officer, Daemen Rugby Club

REFERENCES AVAILABLE UPON REQUEST

Figure 12-2 Sample Curriculum Vitae

first, what position you held or the degree you hold; then, which institution employed or graduated you; and finally, how much time you spent there. Consequently, in your heading, include information that fills this need in that order. You can manipulate the text with bold or italic fonts to highlight categories, but the main purpose is to present this information in a logical form. Under the heading, you can now delineate your experiences, accomplishments, or responsibilities.

Use space to your advantage: Readers may become intimidated by long paragraphs of information. Move information farther down the page and condense. Create space in your document, sometimes through headings, that allows for easy access to information.

Issues of consistency: If you use one heading type, use it for all others that are of equal weight or importance. This also applies to typefaces, italic and bold fonts, underlining, and capitalization. Additionally, use parallel structure (consistency) for phrasing and verb tense. Another important issue of consistency is in punctuation. You are using language in an abbreviated form throughout your resume or curriculum vitae, and this technique often allows for manipulations of punctuation rules. The manipulations are acceptable; just be consistent in their use, whether it is standard or a variant.

Style: Instead of writing full sentences that take up valuable space, trim your entries by offering the text in lists or in bulleted formats. To do so, you will present your information in sentence fragments or even as short bursts of language. These are acceptable in the resume, but you should make the entries parallel and be consistent with punctuation.

Length: A resume intended for an entry-level position should not exceed one page in length. Upper management, academic, or professional positions can and should exceed the one-page limit to accommodate necessary information.

Jargon, abbreviations, and symbols: Do not assume that your readers will understand the language shortcuts that you use in your area of experience. Spell out terms and explain to be thorough.

Grammar and usage: Make no mistakes. Presence of typographical errors or other evidence of failure to proofread sends an ominous message about your commitment to your job prospect or your interest in the position. Send the right message about you by being accurate, precise, and correct.

BUSINESS PLANS

Business plans are similar to proposals in that they offer to start a business or expand an existing one. However, the focus of a business plan usually is to get approval from a bank or lending institution for a loan to support the business. Other types of business plans may be directed to company executives to propose plans and details of those plans to make changes in an existing business. For example, consider the possibility that you work for a well-established practice that has room for growth. While working there, you discover that the practice could benefit from offering additional services. Your expertise fits this niche, and you are the logical one to head this new development. To do so, your partners will want to weigh options and project costs and revenues to determine if expansion is possible or logical.

Content and Headings

The headings for your proposed business plan will reflect certain key business concepts, including **market**, **overhead**, **projected revenues**, and **investment potential**. The following list presents possible headings with definitions of the categories and terms used.

Sample Business Plan

Introduction: Describes the new business idea and explains the product or service.

Market: Describes the product or service in terms of the competition. Also explains how your product or service will be successful or different.

Production Process: Describes how the product will be made or the service will be offered.

Overhead: Describes the facilities needed to be operational and the personnel associated with operations.

Projected Revenues: Estimates growth and development in relation to capital expenditures. The bank or any investor will want to predict the rate of return. Estimate, but do not be overzealous. Be realistic in your approach, which may suggest that you will lose money for a few years until the operation is functional.

Funding: Defines the amount of money to get started as well as operational costs. You may consider presenting this information in a chart or spreadsheet.

Legal: Highlights any and all regulations that are imposed from government legislation and how they will affect the business.

Qualifications: Describes your experiences and education to assure bankers and investors that you will make the business a success.

Investment Potential: Defines the type of investment you are offering, if applicable.

Standard Business Plan

The standard business plan is based on similar categories. Additional terms used in such plans include **executive summary** and **mission statement** (or *vision statement*). The following list is an outline of the standard business plan:

Introduction or Executive Summary: Provides a description of the program or service and key capabilities or impact.

Mission Statement: Defines the link to the overall direction of the organization; also called *vision statement.*

   Environmental Assessment
      Internal Analysis
      External Analysis: Industry and Competitor
      Analysis
   Assumptions and Implications
   SWOT Analysis (Strengths, Weaknesses, Opportunities, Threats)
   Critical Success Factors
   Performance Metrics and Objectives (measurable targets)
   Implementation Plan

Communications Plan (Marketing, Public Relations, Creative Services)

Financial Analysis (revenue projections, income statements, balance sheets, cash flow statements, and capital requirements)

Organizational Structure

Appendices

Add or delete headings and information as appropriate to meet the demands of your audience.

Format

The design of your plan, as for any other document targeted to a business audience, should make the plan easy to read and allow easy and quick access to information. Obviously, you will want to include a cover letter, which should outline your rationale, but the remainder of the plan must be logical and follow a reasonable sequence of thinking.

If your plan contains a large section that comprises more than five pages of text, move this information to an appendix. An appendix serves to accommodate these larger parts of the plan or proposal that would normally interrupt the flow and consistency of the main document. Appendices also house charts and graphs if the author finds that they too disrupt the flow or are too large to fit neatly into the main document.

PROPOSAL WRITING

Much of the writing you do in your professional environment will be persuasive, convincing others to support your research projects with money, administrative and/or technical support, or professional collaboration. To pull people and resources together, you need a standard format for explaining your ideas and listing the pertinent information that your readers seek. This format is the *proposal.* Although different types of proposals exist, most follow the general categories or scheme described in this section.

A proposal is the springboard into implementation of the project. In research, it provides the blueprint for further research to be performed in the field. Note that in research proposals, much of the research has already been established in order for the writer to form a clear and strong hypothesis. You would not propose to prove something with research without knowing if your project will be successful. You will provide a research proposal for any thesis or dissertation you plan to write because your advisors will want a firm understanding of your methods before you embark on a lengthy journey into research and writing.

Other proposals are generated from the needs of organizations such as private research institutes or foundations, business institutions such as drug companies, or government agencies that have an interest in solving medical dilemmas. Allied health professionals often write **grant proposals** to these institutions to fund their projects. For example, the National Institutes of Health may offer grant support for anyone who can find treatments for hand tremors affecting patients with Parkinson's disease. Such institutions will advertise their interests, and researchers and other professionals will compete for these grant dollars. The best proposals usually win the contract. The same pattern can be seen in business. Often, governments, businesses, or funding agencies will call for submissions to complete a project. Other companies or private entrepreneurs will submit proposals outlining their plan, and the best and most cost-effective or competitive plan wins the contract.

When a company or grant-offering institution advertises for a project to be completed, they write a **request for proposal** (RFP), and this document has clear and restrictive guidelines to follow. Some grant-offering institutions may target specific researchers or companies to complete the project. Often, to assure themselves that the right organization has been targeted, they will submit a **request for qualifications** (RFQ), which asks the writer to delineate recent research completed, listing the companies and the work completed in a detailed format.

In any of these request forms, the company seeking information will ask for specific information in a specific format. The wise and successful writer will follow these recommendations and produce a proposal meeting the exact specifications of the document. You will want to be innovative in your methods and procedures, but you should not take liberties with the proposal guidelines. Stay within the page limit, submit charts and graphs if requested, meet the deadlines, write clearly and concisely, and—most important—proofread. A document that fails to meet the standards provided can and should be rejected because of participant negligence. A document that contains grammatical and mechanical errors will be rejected because it reflects the attitude of the writer. If the document is carelessly constructed, it sends the message to the reviewers that the author too is careless. No one wants to work with a person who is careless or nonprofessional.

The proposal, then, competes for grant dollars or other support mechanisms, and it does so through a simple formula: identify a problem, explain how the research will solve it, and show how you plan to proceed with the research. The following categories can be used as headings or subheadings to outline the proposal.

Summary of Problem

The summary of the problem section introduces the issue to be studied. The summary itself describes the issue by providing background information and clarifying the necessity of the research proposed. In total, the summary section is a microcosm of the entire proposal in that it describes the need for the proposed research and convinces the reader to support the writer's cause.

Proposed Plan

The section on the proposed plan can address several issues at once. First, you should outline the various methods that can be used to solve the problem, to allow your reader to understand that you fully comprehend the magnitude of the issue to be solved. You should then dictate which of these methods is most effective and your rationale for choosing one method over the others.

The plan will also make clear to the reader what will be studied and what will be omitted from the course of action. In this section, you may want to outline the specifics of the plan by setting goals and describing how they will be met and in what sequence. This section calls for you to define the scope of your project, which will set the boundaries.

The methods you will use to accomplish your goals should appear next in the proposal. Methods are determined by the study. Some studies call for research only, and you will outline your sources of information in a literature review of pertinent research. Other studies will require subjects to be tested, and you will provide descriptions fully explaining how subjects are acquired and complications or biases present in this group. Other projects may require statistical analysis, and you will explain which methods of analysis will be used to provide the best quality of results. This section allows you some latitude in your subject matter to discuss other problems that may arise in your analysis of data, research, or subjects. Be sure to explain the fallible aspects of your project if these conditions arise.

Schedule and Facilities

Providing a list of the proposed schedule of events helps your supporters gauge time to be spent on the project. As always, you should schedule your project to fit the demands and deadlines outlined in the requests. In your schedule, begin with the date the proposal is submitted and continue, in list form, with dates and clear headings that signal the accomplishment of the components of the project. Finish with the date you will submit the final report.

List all facilities and equipment to be used in the study, to demonstrate that you have the hardware, software, and physical capabilities to perform the research proposed. This step also provides a rationale for you to include in your budget the purchase of equipment that you do not have.

Personnel

List all the personnel involved with the study and their qualifications. Be as specific as possible, because your supporting institution wants to be certain that its money is being spent on the efforts of professionals in the field. Avoid any delay in confirming the personnel involved (do not designate any personnel as "TBA"—to be announced), as your uncertainties may be perceived as poor planning. You should also indicate who is the principal investigator (PI) for the project, who are coinvestigators, and who are support staff. The credentials of the PI are most important to the reviewers. If appropriate, define the PI's philosophical stances on pertinent issues related to the project's outcome or to the methods used to obtain results.

Budget

Outline in list form the costs of the project and the research. Unfortunately, the budget is often an important factor in determining support. If a project is too costly, it may be rejected. Stay within the proposed limits, if they are listed, and do not pad your budget to meet costs that you cannot foresee. Padding the budget produces unrealistic costs that are easily identified by reviewers. Be realistic and be precise. Think through the costs carefully, and include direct and indirect costs.

Conclusion

Reaffirm your position in the conclusion by stating your expertise, your reasons for being the person best suited to complete the project, and your ability to get the results that you propose.

Other Concerns

You may want to provide other information that will help solidify your standing with the reviewing committee. These may include letters of reference, appendices (charts, graphs, and other documents, if appropriate), titles that fully explain your qualifications and intentions, bibliographic information, and forms to be used in the process of gathering data from test subjects.

Reasons for Rejection

Most often, proposals are rejected because of a flawed method. The design of the study should fit within standard practice and reveal that the researcher is performing "good science." A flawed methodology may also result from poor management and recruitment of test subjects or faulty analysis of data. Proposals are also rejected on the basis of their main hypothesis or overall goal. In other cases, the information that a researcher claims as the result of the study may not be appropriate at this time or will not add to the field's scholarly dialogue, and these proposals will be rejected as well. Finally, proposals are rejected, with less frequency, if the PI's credentials are weak or if the preliminary research presented is inadequate. The PI must also be certain to list the facilities that will be used, because proposals may be rejected on the basis of poor environment.

Other Considerations for Proposals

Not all proposals that professionals write are grant proposals. Some may target business plans, while others may simply offer a service or a means to perform a job. Consider including the following topics, depending on the type of proposal you plan to produce.

Introduction: Gives overview of proposal and encourages the reader to act.

Background: Provides a discussion of issues that have raised interest in implementing changes.

Benefits/Feasibility: Provides the reader with the advantages of the proposal and the likelihood of its success.

Description and Results: Describes the finished product, which includes outlines, graphics, facts, and figures.

Method/Theoretical Framework: Explains how the proposal will be completed by including a detailed discussion of the methodology. Proves the author is using good reasoning principles.

Schedule: Outlines important dates and major sections of the proposed project.

Qualifications: Demonstrates that the author of the proposal is the best person for the job. If others are included in the project, their credentials are listed too. Although this section is not calling for a resume, it does call for highlights of the author's career and education.

Costs/Budget: Describes the purpose of dollars to be spent. Estimating costs may be the most difficult section to write because unforeseeable variables exist in every project. The proposal writer should try to plan for the unforeseeable and create a budget that clearly describes the purpose of each dollar spent.

Conclusions: Reinforces the need for the proposal and the advantages/benefits. This section, like all conclusions, should establish that the purpose will be met and the method for achieving that purpose is sound.

Organization

Notice that the proposal sections follow a logical progression of thoughts and ideas that your reader may encounter. Consider that the proposal introduces the subject, provides background information, provides a solution to the problem discussed in the background and its benefits, describes the details of the project and the methods behind it, outlines a schedule and budget, proves that the author is capable and qualified, and then reinforces the need and benefits in the conclusion. This format considers the audience's needs and anticipates the questions the reader will ask. If other issues arise that are project specific, include these in a separate category or find a way to blend the issues raised into information under an established heading.

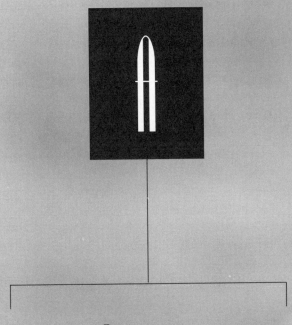

Answers

to

Exercises

CHAPTER 1

PAGE 27
EXERCISES: COHERENCE AND UNITY
RECOGNIZING COHERENCE BREAKS

Directions: Following are examples of incoherent paragraphs. Study each one and determine various means to solve incoherence: organization, development of ideas, or transitions. In all cases, the reader's expectations have not been met.

1. Tom and Jim crouched in the old shed, waiting for someone to discover them. He *(which one?)* thought that the farmer had passed by. He felt safe in the silence, but he looked at Jim's foot and he knew he couldn't go on. *(At this point, the paragraph shifts to Tom's emotional attachment to Jim, which doesn't help the reader understand the reason they cannot continue.)* He was happy to be there with Jim. *(Is he happy to be there with Jim because they were a long way from home? The passage does not help answer this question.)* They were a long way from home.

2. The Rocky Mountain summer was hot and dry. Steve wanted to go trail riding. His friend, Tom, wanted to go rock climbing. Tom was a great rock climber because he had a low center of gravity. The summer days were long, and the boys were free to roam the countryside. *(A major concern in this paragraph is the choppiness created by the sentence openers. Every sentence begins with a noun, and the sentences are short and choppy. Consider adding transitional phrases and sentences to connect ideas.)*

3. When the doors of the stadium opened, thousands of fans rushed in. The seats were the last to fill up as the mass of people flooded the floor. The stage extended across the field, and *(Here, the issue of time creates a problem. The reader assumes that the sound of the siren is associated with the start of the concert, but the stadium has just opened. The logical connection of time is lost.)* the sound of sirens could be heard. *(The previous sentences are describing the scene, while this last sentence attends to the emotional connection of the writer without alerting the*

reader to the change in perspective.) This will be the best show of the year.

4. The Eastern coyote hunts mainly for mice and rabbits. *(Although the connection between coyotes and Jones is not available here, the shift in verb tense, from present to past, compounds the coherence break.)* Jones was deep in the Adirondack Mountains, and the noise of the village and the highways could not be heard. Many hunters had seen the coyotes, and a few had been shot. Their carcasses were hanged on the fence rows to warn others of their fate. Jones' mission was to rid the neighbors of these rascals that have been trading rabbits and mice for the neighbors' small dogs and cats.

5. Prince Edward Island is busy during the summer. *(The connection between the Island and the house is not clear. Is the house on the Island?)* The grasses have grown tall over the season, and weeds surrounded the old house. Some of the windows needed painting. Shutters were hanging loosely from their frames. *(At this point, the writer has been moving from a broad landscape description to a narrowly focused description of the windows. To return to a description of the fields disrupts the logic that the reader expects.)* Soon, the fields will be plowed under and the preparations for winter will begin.

PAGE 28
BUILDING UNITY AND COHERENCE

Directions: Find the breaks in the line of reasoning. Fix all coherence problems by considering a thesis, connecting ideas clearly, and offering mechanisms to help guide the reader to that singular purpose.

Mrs. Jones, a female born on November 1, 1970 has five primary complaints. She has pain when showering, brushing her hair, washing dishes, dressing and driving. The patient suffers extreme stiffness in her right shoulder and has low strength. She complains of pain when moving her shoulder and arm with limited coordination. *(Did the patient stop work because of her pain? If so, lead into the next sentence with a clarifying phrase.)* Mrs. Jones stopped work.

(This sentence should be developed to include the plan of treatment, since it is vague.) The problems of strength, reduced mobility, and pain need to be improved. *(Sentences are short and choppy, and most begin with a subject-verb combination that becomes monotonous. Consider transitional elements for sentence openers, and combine short sentences that have similar purposes.)*

Mrs. Jones will be shown how to use an elastic band for her home exercises. The band will improve her mobility and stiffness. She will be doing weight lifting. The patient will have two short-term goals. She will return to her previous functioning and her discharge date is set for three months. The patient does not need long-term goals because the duration of treatment is short. *(Shift in verb tense)* Mrs. Jones completed physical therapy three times with the same complaint. When discharged, she improved her status, but her condition deteriorated over time. No home exercises were prescribed on the time of discharge.

(The first paragraph alerts the reader to Mrs Jones' five complaints; however, the second paragraph describes the plan of action to heal her. At no time in the introductory paragraph is the treatment alluded to.)

PAGE 28
IDENTIFYING UNITY AND COHERENCE PROBLEMS

Directions: The following sample is a student's essay before it was revised. This was the first attempt at putting words to paper.

Coherence breaks are identified with the following symbol: ^. Notice that the sentences before the indicator carry forward a particular subject. The sentence following the indicator starts a new idea but fails to carry the reader from the previous point to the present.

Problems in unity are identified using this symbol: ~ . Notice that the sentences following the indicator suggest a topic or an idea that is not on task. The essay contains a thesis, and the information provided in the paper should support that thesis. If you provide information that is related to your thesis, explain that tangential connection to your reader. Do not ask your reader to make such connections.

Punishing a child teaches children what is right and what is wrong. Many parents punish their children by talking to them or by reward and punishment. ^ Child abuse consists of hurting a child physically, mentally, or emotionally. *(Notice that the first two sentences discuss the issue of punishment. The sentence after the indicator defines child abuse. These two ideas are not connected in any way. Any reader could make the connection, given the time to do so, but this task is not the reader's job. It is the job of the writer.)* ~ There have been parents beating their children for hundreds of years. *(In this example, the borrowed information suggests that parents have been beating their children over time. How does this information support the thesis? It does not, and consequently, this error leads to a mistake in unity.)* Some punishments do consider spanking but do not hurt the children. Spanking a child is considered a soft slap to show the children that they did something wrong. Beating a child leaves bruises and psychological problems. ~ Unfortunately, there are parents all over the world who deliberately hurt their children. Child abuse causes many unresolved issues that usually do not get explored. Discipline can often be used in different ways. In case a child does not relate to a certain way, the parent can approach them in different ways to teach them morals.

As hard as it is to punish children, it needs to be done. ~ Our society focuses on parent-child relationships and specializes in natural parenting. Punishment gives children a sense of what proper behavior is. Children need to learn the difference between right and wrong. Punishing children can be done in many different ways. One example to discipline a child is isolation. When a child is left alone they get bored easily. When they are forced to pursue something they do not get motivated unless they want to do it. Then they realize what they did was wrong. Another way to discipline children is by reward and punishment. When children are young, they react well to this. They realize that when you take something that they want away, they did something wrong, but when they do well or if they do something that you ask them to do, they get a reward. People believe that reward and punishment works well with children. This creates problems because every time they do something right, they expect to get something in return. If they know that they are not going to get something in return, they may not do what you ask them to do. If this happens, you may have to approach the situation in a different way. ^ Lastly, talking to children begins a great relationship and tells them what is right and what is wrong. In this case, punishment may not be the answer, but explaining to them what is wrong can create an image of what is right. Speaking to your children can be a powerful tool for explaining morals. ^ ~ A theme is created from experiments and it shows the relations between a parent who wants to raise their children properly and the society in which they live. If you talk to children, it teaches them to trust you and to respect you and the decisions you make. The examples you set for your children also teach them what is wrong and right by your actions.

Many parents do not understand the concept of talking to your children like they are human. This is when spanking gets too far. ^ Child abuse creates mental, physical, and emotional problems. Children who are hurt constantly deal with numerous problems and side affects. Some examples include becoming sensitive to pain, destructive, and depressed. The child becomes unlovable and is likely that they will not be loved by anyone because of their behavior. ^ Usually when there seems to be child abuse in a family, the parent is usually the one with the problem and they hit the child to blame someone else. ~ As a society we project problems of child abuse and try to concentrate on helping the parents. They are usually dealing with mental health issues or they have expectations of their children to do unrealistic things. In many cases, the child gets stressed out and needs to take his or her aggression out on someone who won't fight back. ~ Child abuse is used as a form of control but sometimes the child is left with destructive organs or even death.

PAGE 29

Directions: Now read the remainder of this essay and use the given symbols to identify the problems in coherence (^) and unity (~).

Child abuse stems from stress or the parents' childhood. ^ Changes have occurred by giving the parent therapy and treatments. *(This next sentence should connect with first sentence of this paragraph.)* The parent may think that beating a child is normal if they were hit as a child. The parents need to recognize what they are doing to their children and realize the relationship that they could have with them. *(Vary sentence openers. Also, consider a new paragraph here, creating one paragraph for one reason and a second for another reason.)* It has been shown that the link between economic and social atmospheres affect families that are involved in child abuse. ^ Physical abuse normally occurs with low-income families because they have too much stress keeping control in their life and to support their families. Evidence proves that there is a relationship between child abuse and low-income families. They get stressed easily because of poverty and become likely that they are unable to support their families. ^ Emotion becomes very natural to a human being in how they respond to certain situations. ~ In the past, it has been shown that people are embarrassed to deal with the poor. Emotional abuse usually takes place within a high income-tax family, because they don't seem to spend enough time with their children and they search for attention. Rich families create a life worth living but do not create time to spend with their children. Parents involved in this need to realize that they need to care for their children and give them guidance.

~ Children who are in an abused situation usually need psychological help. *(Is this paper prepared to define abuse and then offer treatments? This is too much information for a short paper.)* After a child is abused they suffer many side effects. These side effects include that they cannot trust, they have shame and doubt in anything they do, and they become destructive with people and property. It *(unclear pronoun reference creates coherence problem)* strains their brain and creates an image so they perceive themselves as not being good enough. ^ Many abusive parents have low self-esteem and some do not even know who they are. *(Move the following sentences to paragraph above. The subject of this paragraph is* treatment*; the previous paragraph discussed* reasons.*)* Hitting a child is wrong and often enough parents who do this need mental and emotional help as well as the children. For some reason, the parents believe beating someone satisfies their urge to control something and forces them to believe that it is right. Child abusers form discipline into an extreme level. The parent's attention should be on the child and what they can do to help them, not what they can do to help themselves. ^ *(Can this sentence be connected with this paragraph after moving the previous sentences?)* Discipline creates morals and behavior, so telling them to do something right by doing something wrong and hurtful is not the right approach. ^ Sadly, child abuse is done in many ways. They may not be hitting them, but child abuse can also be from not taking care of them. Some examples are leaving a baby in a hot car for hours, not cleaning up after the children, or even not feeding them. ~ If these parents can't take care of themselves then they should not be taking care of children. *(This sounds more like moralizing instead of being objective.)*

~ Control is an issue that needs to be resolved before the children are born. Control helps life and releases some stress. Control leads to a natural relationship between parents and their children. They *(unclear pronoun reference creates coherence break)* can learn how to discipline them by finding out what their children react to and how they can learn. If a parent is stressed, they should seek help if they cannot control it. Control seems to be one of the main problems because if they can't control something in their life, they need to control something else. Lack of self-control usually leads to child abuse. Punishment deals with a child's behavior and teaches them what they did wrong. It does not physically harm them. Child abuse is not discipline. It controls the way a parent reacts to certain situations. When trying to discipline children, hurting them is not the point, teaching them a lesson is. Parents need to understand that and if they don't, they need psychological help. This will help parents

deal with their problems and create new relationships with their children.

(A concluding paragraph should reinforce the issues covered in the paper and demonstrate that the thesis has been proved. This paragraph opens new avenues for discussion that have not been raised in the paper. Consequently, the reader does not expect this paragraph to serve as a concluding paragraph and leads to a disruption of logical progression.)

PAGE 30
EXERCISE: IDENTIFYING AND CORRECTING COHERENCE AND UNITY PROBLEMS

Directions: Examine the following sample student essay and find coherence breaks and problems with unity. Provide possible transitions to solve some of these problems.

A New York study found that most people would support a restriction on the use of cell phones (Holsendolph, 2002*), (This run-on sentence should be separated with a semicolon. As a transition word,* then *is weak because the date does not correspond with a previous date)* then on November 1st, 2001, New York State introduced a "hands free" law for all automobile drivers to follow while driving. *(The next two sentences interfere with the continuation of the sentence previous. Continue the thought about the law, or move the definition to a separate paragraph.)* "Hands free" implies that all drivers must have both hands on the wheel at all times while driving. The driver must be clear of interference, ensuring that he has complete control of his car. When implemented, the law focused on the increasing number of drivers talking on cell phones while driving. *(What is thesis? Do you support the law?)*

(This sentence does not begin the paragraph well since reckless driving *and thinking* are not connected clearly. The paragraph could use a more organized approach that identifies the purpose with a topic sentence that continues the thought from the thesis.)* When asked about talking on cell phones while driving, Chuck Hurley, of the Illinois-based National Safety Council claimed "It's not where the hands are, but where the head is" (as quoted in Hands-free . . . , 2001,

p. 19). When used in certain circumstances, hand-held cell phones can lead to reckless driving (Copquin, 2002).

(This sentence, again, begins the paragraph poorly. Who is Holsendolph? Is he an expert of some kind or just a casual observer of people's driving habits? Why should the reader be inclined to hear his testimony?) Ernest Holsendolph (2002) tells of a situation that he encountered while driving on the Atlanta Interstate that has attracted attention from safety experts. He observed a white Ford Bronco that drifted toward the right lane, then back into the original lane. Then, the driver of the SUV spotted a car she was about to crash into, she then turned to the right lane, again. Gradually, the SUV then drifted back to the center lane. Ernest then pulled up next to the SUV to observe the driver holding a cell phone in her right hand, distorting her view of the righthand lane (Holsendolph, 2002). *(How does this episode relate to the thesis? Explain.)*

Once implemented, "hands free" *(the law?)* tried to decrease the number of automobile accidents caused by drivers being distracted while driving. The law specified the use of cell phones while driving and not other distractions that occur every day: applying makeup, eating fast food, shaving, changing the radio or station, and smoking cigarettes. Any of these distractions impairs the driver from having complete control of their car, yet, none are illegal except for the use of cell phones. The law does not state that eating a cheeseburger while driving is equivalent to talking on a cell phone. Still, one hand is needed to hold the cheeseburger, which would be the same hand that would be holding a cell phone while you were talking on it. The same argument could be presented for shaving, applying makeup, smoking, or adjusting the controls of your vehicle. Tom Wheeler, president and CEO of the Cellular Telecommunications and Internet Association concludes, "Any activity a driver engages in, besides the task of driving, has the potential to distract" (as quoted in Hands-free . . . , 2001, p. 19). Driver distractions lead to 20–30 percent of all crashes as estimated by the National Highway Traffic Safety Administration (Hands-free . . . , 2001,

p. 19). *(Are you supporting the law or showing its weaknesses?)*

Since the introduction of the law, companies have introduced "hands free" kits for talking on cell phones while driving. Earpieces that connect to the phone, and then attach to your ear, are most common. These earpieces must connect to the phone once it rings, causing attention to drift from the road to the preparation of the device. *(Coherence break: This quote does not adequately represent an attention drift, as mentioned in the previous sentence.)* Claudia Copquin of *The New York Times*, said "I don't know what to do first: insert the ear jack or press the talk button?" She also admits that she struggles to keep her eyes on the road when her phone rings, as her head drifts from the road to the phone itself (as quoted in Copquin, 2002). *(Does this next sentence support the previous? If so, connect them by demonstrating their relatedness.)* One study showed that hands-free devices do not actually reduce driver distraction (Hands-free . . . , 2001, p. 19). Even with the use of these "hands free" kits, distraction still exists while talking on the phone.

(The word one *was used to describe a test in previous paragraph. Is this the same test being referred to here in* **bold***?)* In **one** test, it was found that there was no significant difference between drivers using hands-free devices and those using hand-held phones (Hands-free . . . , 2001, p. 19). The law states that the driver is to have complete control of their car. The focus of the driver even while being "hands free" is still on the phone call. *(Does this mean that the driver does not have control of the car? What is the significance of this sentence in terms of the thesis?)* The drivers' hands may be on the wheel now, but their attention still drifts to the person on the other end of the conversation. David Stayer, a University of Utah psychologist, found that listening and talking on a phone while driving were both distractions (as quoted in Holsendolph, 2002). The person talking to the driver doesn't know what types of conditions the driver is occurring *(experiencing?)* (weather, road work, and hazards) and doesn't realize the distractions that the driver occurs. *(In this*

previous sentence, would the person on the other end of the line change communication style? Again, what is relevance of this statement to thesis?) Stayer further concluded:

> There is a different quality of communication between two people in a car and people on phones. The people in a car share the awareness of how demanding the driving may be, and they tailor their conversation accordingly, getting quiet if the driver had to do certain maneuvers in busy traffic, and talking more relaxed if they are traveling on a quiet street. (Holsendolph, 2002, p. 1)

"Hands free" was originally implemented to allow a driver to have complete control of his car and to be free of distractions. *(Connect this sentence and the next.)* Free of distractions would imply that nothing interferes with the driver. Stayer says that using cell phones can be dangerous, because talking makes drivers "sluggish" (as quoted in Holsendolph, 2002). University of Utah researchers concluded that the distraction with cell phones is caused by the concentration on the conversation, and not by dialing or holding the phone (Hands-free . . . , 2001, p. 19). If a driver's attention is focused on a phone call, their attention is diverted, endangering not only themselves but other drivers on the road as well. Also, Stayer claims, "When you're talking, you're impaired" (as quoted in Holsendolph 2002). *(Verb tense shift between the previous sentence and the next.)* The goal of the "hands free" law was to decrease the number of accidents caused by distractive driving: car crashes, pedestrians and animals being hit, and speeding. Yet, all of these accidents still occur due to the drivers' attention still not being focused on the road. *(Should the information in the following sentence be included in a paragraph in the early stages of this paper? This is a classic coherence break in that the sentence does not connect to the paragraph surrounding it.)* A study involving nearly 6,000 Canadians proved that a driver using a cell phone "quadrupled the risk of a collision" (Holsendolph, 2002). The law has managed to ensure that both hands are on the steering wheel at all times, but it has done noth-ing to ensure that the attention of the driver is on the road at all times.

The mistake that was made when introducing the "hands free" law was the extent to what was considered a distraction while driving. Anything that distracts a driver while driving should be included under the law, not just the banning of talking on a cell phone while driving. The number of car accidents caused due to cell phone use while driving increase daily. Studies have also proven that the use of hands-free phones has made no difference in crash risk compared to the use of hand-held phones. Now, the law must state clearer what is considered distractive, and what should take a "hands free" approach.

References

Copquin, C. G. (2002, September 1). I can't talk now. Call me back! *The New York Times*, p. 17.

Hands-free cell phones distracting: Study finds device no boon to safety. (2001, August 17). *Houston Chronicle*, p. 19.

Holsendolph, E. (2002, January 13). Hand-held? Hands-free? Critics say it doesn't matter—cell phones are not safe to use while driving. *The Atlanta Journal*, p. 1.

CHAPTER 2

PAGE 37
EXERCISES: PRONOUNS
CHOOSING THE APPROPRIATE PRONOUN

Directions: From the options in parentheses, choose the appropriate pronoun in each sentence.

1. All of the employees on the unit believed that (his or her) actions were medically necessary.

2. Both the charge nurse and the nurse manager found (their) schedule too busy to attend to all of the needs of their patients.

3. In the event of an emergency, the therapists understand the procedures to care for (their) patients.

4. The patients insisted that the technician make copies of the CT scan films and send (them) to his doctor.

5. The results of the study provoked debate because of (their) controversial nature.

6. Although ovaries produce estrogen, the anterior pituitary gland regulates (their) activity.

7. The anterior pituitary produces hormones, and (they) effect various biological processes.

8. After discovering that they both had the same disease, the patients discussed (their) treatment methods, and neither patient could determine the appropriate course of action for (his or her) disease.

9. Neither of the doctors decided on (his or her) position on the embryonic stem cell issue.

10. Both the doctor and the nurse documented (their) actions during the surgical procedure.

PAGE 37
CORRECTING PRONOUN INCONSISTENCIES

Directions: Find and correct any pronoun inconsistencies in the following sentences.

The correct pronoun is in **bold** *type.*

1. The doctor informed his patient that his test results were negative and that **the patient** could be discharged from the hospital immediately.

2. The surgical resident was pleased with **the operation's** outcome and had a positive ending to his day.

3. I injected the patient with a 2-ml bolus of lidocaine, and **this drug** relaxed the patient.

4. If the results returned insufficient, **I** would be forced to repeat the procedure.

5. The doctor, a successful cardiologist, discussed **the case** openly with his neighbors.

6. I informed the patient's daughter of her grave condition and inquired into **the daughter's** wishes for end-of-life care.

7. The chest x-ray films provided by the radiology department demonstrated **the department's** role in the diagnosis.

8. The paper reported the results of the new drug, and it discussed many positives to **the new drug's** use.

PAGE 38
EXERCISES: DANGLING MODIFIERS
EXERCISE SET 1

Directions: Use the example provided to revise the following sample sentences.

EXAMPLE: Believing what the labels and advertisements say, their minds believe it to be true and trick their body into thinking the same.

The writer should ask himself or herself the following: Whose mind believes?

For correct revision of the sentence, the implicit and explicit subjects must be identical.

REVISION: As people believe what the labels and advertisement say, they believe the information on the label or in the advertisements to be true and trick their bodies into thinking the same.

1. The results of the test underwent extensive reviews, thus finding the cause of the flaw.

   The results of the test underwent extensive reviews; consequently, the doctor found the cause of the flaw.

2. Having finished the chores, the television was turned on.

   Having finished the chores, she turned on the television.

3. Realizing the need for more time, the agency delayed its decision.

   Realizing the need for more time, the agents delayed their decision.

4. Further comparative studies were conducted, hoping to find the most efficient method.

   Hoping to find the most efficient method, the doctors conducted further comparative studies.

5. Upon the achievement of higher degrees in Physical Therapy, direct access is being considered.

   On the achievement of higher degrees in physical therapy, accreditation agencies will consider direct access for therapists.

6. Realizing the need for more practice, week-end schedules were implemented.

   Realizing the need for more practice, the administrator implemented weekend schedules.

7. After reading the study, the article remains unconvincing.

   After reading the study, I found the article unconvincing.

8. By receiving intercessory prayer, their minds believe they will achieve healthiness.

   By receiving intercessory prayer, patients believe they will achieve healthiness.

Other Possible Revisions

1. We revised the results of the test extensively, thus finding the cause of the flaw.

2. Having finished her chores, Kate turned on the television.

3. Realizing the need for more time, we delayed the decision.

4. We conducted further comparative studies to find the most efficient method.

5. Since physical therapy students are now able to achieve a doctorate in physical therapy, New York State is now considering making direct access available to physical therapy clinics.

6. Realizing the need for more practice, the coach scheduled weekend practices.

7. After reading the study, I find the article unconvincing.

8. By receiving intercessory prayer, the ill believe prayer alone will aid them in overcoming their illness.

PAGE 38
EXERCISE SET 2

Directions: Correct all sentences containing dangling modifiers.

1. The patient's left leg measured 2 inches larger than the right, caused by the accident.

2. Having declared an emergency situation, the charge nurse ordered the removal of the patients from the unit.

3. To easily remove the dressing, sterile water was poured onto the wound.

4. Discovered in the closet, the nurse used the Kelly clamps to secure the drainage tube and stabilize the patient.

5. On the IV pole that I had found on the floor upstairs, I hung the saline solution.

6. During manual muscle tests, the patient's right shoulder demonstrated less strength than the left, resulting from the trauma.

7. After reading the chart, the patient was put on strict "npo" status by the physician.

8. Due to his progress in therapy, the therapist recommended Mr. Smythe's discharge.

9. Following an insulin injection, the nurse recorded a low blood glucose reading on the patient.

10. Resulting from prolonged exposure to secondhand smoke, the doctor diagnosed the patient with lung cancer.

11. Due to an increased dosage of anesthesia, the nurse believed the patient felt better.

12. During the surgery, the anesthesiologist nearly administered 3 units of O positive blood.

13. I instructed the patient to do only 10 repetitions of each exercise prescribed by the therapist.

14. After running multiple tests, the laboratory reported the patient's blood pH at 7.5 almost.

15. While preparing the settings on the ventilator, the respiratory therapist only set the VIO_2 at 80%.

16. The heart monitor nearly registered the patient in bradycardia for 5 minutes.

17. Following examination by the doctor on call, the patient was admitted almost with a 3-inch-diameter wound.

18. The patient swiftly attempted to rehabilitate from the surgery and, as a result, aggravated the injury.

19. Admitted to the emergency room for dehydration, the patient received an IV saline solution that the nurse hung for over 3 hours.

20. The patient bravely and willingly accepted the diagnosis and treatment options.

21. The wound indicated the extent of the accident, obviously beyond repair.

Possible Revisions

1. The patient's left leg measured 2 inches larger than the right, an abnormality caused by the accident.

2. Having declared an emergency situation, the hospital official directed the charge nurse to order the removal of the patients from the unit.

3. To easily remove the dressing, the attendant poured sterile water onto the wound.

4. Discovered in the closet, the Kelly clamps were used to secure the drainage tube and stabilize the patient.

5. I hung the saline solution on the IV pole that I had found on the floor upstairs.

6. During manual muscle tests, the patient's right shoulder demonstrated less strength than the left, as a result of the trauma.

7. After reading the chart, the physician restricted the patient to "npo" status.

8. Due to his progress in therapy, Mr. Smythe was recommended for discharge by the therapist.

9. Following an insulin injection, the patient registered a low blood glucose reading.

10. Resulting from prolonged exposure to secondhand smoke, the patient was diagnosed with lung cancer.

11. The nurse believed the patient felt better after an increased dosage of anesthesia.

12. The anesthesiologist administered nearly 3 units of O positive blood while the patient was in surgery.

13. The therapist instructed the patient to do only 10 repetitions of each prescribed exercise.

14. After running multiple tests, the laboratory technician reported the patient's blood pH at 7.5 almost.

15. While preparing the settings on the ventilator, the respiratory therapist only set the VIO_2 at 80%. *(Correct)*

16. The heart monitor reading nearly registered the patient in bradycardia for 5 minutes.

17. Following examination by the doctor on call, the patient was admitted with a wound approximately 3 inches in diameter.

18. The patient aggravated the injury by attempting to rehabilitate from the surgery. *(More information needed)*

19. Admitted to the emergency room for dehydration, the patient received an IV saline solution for 3 hours.

20. The patient bravely and willingly accepted the diagnosis and treatment options. *(Correct)*

21. The wound, obviously beyond repair, indicated the extent of the accident.

PAGE 39
EXERCISE: PARALLEL STRUCTURE

Directions: Examine the following sentences and correct the problems in parallel structure.

1. I have an apple and pear.

2. In the group were a carpenter, locksmith, a painter, and plumber.

3. I am hot, tired, and I wish I had something cool to drink.

4. She hoped to fly to Buffalo and that she could rent a car there.

5. My friend can tutor students who need help in English and lead orientation sessions.

6. Some examples include becoming sensitive to pain, destructive, and depressed.

7. Towards females, the media portray Barbie doll-like women as successful in life and can achieve anything.

8. The methods help you achieve a state of mind, not cure illnesses.

9. Treatment will include the use of a hot pack, various stretching techniques, aerobic activity on a stationary bike, and conclude with ice on the back of his neck.

10. The exercises will help him keep the muscles loose, flexible, and eventually recover full range of motion.

Possible Revisions

1. I have an apple and a pear.

2. In the group were a carpenter, a locksmith, a painter, and a plumber.

3. I am hot, tired, and thirsty for something cool to drink.

4. She hoped to fly to Buffalo and rent a car there.

5. My friend can tutor students who need help in English and lead orientation sessions. *(Correct)*

6. Some examples include becoming sensitive to pain, destructive, and depressed. *(Correct)*

7. The media portray Barbie doll-like women as successful in life and as achievers.

8. The methods help you achieve a state of mind, not cure illnesses. *(Correct)*

9. Treatment will include a hot pack, various stretching techniques, aerobic activity on a stationary bike, and ice on the back of his neck.

10. The exercises will help him keep the muscles loose and flexible, and this treatment will help him eventually recover full range of motion.

PAGE 41
EXERCISE: VERB TENSE SHIFTS

Directions: In the following sample essay, mark the unnecessary shifts in verb tense.

Instances of inconsistent verb tense are in **bold** *type.*

Throughout the course of reading the short story, "The Story of An Hour," the reader begins to wonder what traits make up the character of Mrs. Mallard. Her character is mysterious and peculiar. She **experienced** several emotions that can be interpreted differently by different people. The author **wrote** in such a manner that leaves the reader asking questions about Mrs. Mallard's character.

The story begins with an element of foreshadowing. The reader is told that Mrs. Mallard has heart trouble. This statement leads the reader to believe that, later in the story, Mrs. Mallard's physical ailment will be a factor. When Mrs. Mallard hears the news of her husband's death, she cries uncontrollably in the arms of her sister and **retreated** to her bedroom. Then,

a look of intelligent thought **came** over her face. She **reflected** on life without her husband and **thought** about the possibilities of her new freedoms. Such ambiguity in this situation forces the reader to interpret the relationship between her husband and she. Later, a force **came** and "takes over" Mrs. Mallard. She could have been feeling guilt for feeling freedom.

PAGE 46
EXERCISE: THE FOUR MAJOR ERRORS

Directions: For each of the following sentences or groups of words, make sure each is grammatically correct.

Revisions are in **bold** *type.*

1. Every one of the professional golfers **donates his or her** time to charity.

2. When I watch television, **a desire** to look like the actresses **fills** my mind.

3. The young viewers never see behind the scenes; they only witness the final product.

4. Although he had been well recommended by his former employer, **he still did not get the job**.

5. The mission is dedicated to serving the following countries: China and Guatemala.

6. The driver spotted the car; therefore, she avoided the crash.

7. Some of the collection **were** not sold.

8. Acquiring alcohol as a teen is easy. **T**hey have someone buy it for them.

9. The officer, climbing out of his check-station, **took** out his pencil and book.

10. The more things change, inevitably, the more they stay the same.

11. In the group **were** science, English, foreign language, and the health professions professors.

PAGE 47
EXERCISE: THAT VERSUS WHICH; ESSENTIAL VERSUS NONESSENTIAL

Directions: Insert the appropriate word, *that* or *which*, into the following examples using the information provided earlier.

1. Please help me with my duffle bag **that** is third in line.

2. The stewardess helped me stow my duffle bag, **which** I had brought with me on the trip.

3. After much searching, we found a store **that** sells authentic Scottish kilts.

4. After much searching, we found the liquor store, **which** was selling gin at a discount. *(Could be "that" if the store we seek is one that sells gin at a discount.)*

5. I am walking because I own only one car **that** is now being repaired.

PAGE 49
EXERCISES: COMMAS
COMMAS WITH NONESSENTIAL ELEMENTS

Directions: Consider the use of commas with nonessential words, phrases, or clauses to make any necessary changes in the following sentences.

Added commas are in **bold** *type.*

1. Slee Hall, the recently completed fine arts building, is acoustically perfect.

2. The toy that I wanted to buy is no longer available. *(Correct)*

3. Dr. Jones decided, however, that this procedure was best.

4. The Genesee River, which flows north into Lake Ontario, flows through the city of Rochester and is used to make beer.

5. Watching the mouse intently, the cat crouched in the grass.

6. Mark Twain, one of America's greatest storytellers, worked as editor of the *Courier Express*. *(Correct)*

PAGE 49
COMMAS WITH INTRODUCTORY ELEMENTS

Directions: Identify the introductory element in each sentence and apply the appropriate mark of punctuation.

Introductory elements are in italics; added commas are in **Bold**.

1. *As my fishing line tightened,* the reel began to scream.

2. *Having changed her major,* Kara had to enroll in biochemistry.

3. *Consequently,* she now has time to meet me for lunch.

4. *Changing her major* has been a positive experience for her.

5. *When she was in high school,* she did not know what career path she should choose.

6. *To gain a full understanding of the program,* Kara met with faculty members.

7. *To make a lot of money* has been his goal.

PAGE 50
COMMAS IN A SAMPLE STUDENT ESSAY

Directions: Read the following student essay. Then identify the problems in punctuation and offer suggestions for revision.

Revisions are in **bold** *type.*

One of the most common neurological disorders, Parkinson's disease, affects both men and women, and the disease most often develops after the age of 50. A cause of Parkinson's disease **includes** *(word choice:* is?*)* the progressive deterioration of the nerve cells of the portion of the brain that controls muscle movement. The brain normally produces dopamine, a substance used by cells to transmit impulses. The degeneration of the brain reduces the amount of dopamine available to the body. An insufficient amount of dopamine disturbs the balance between this substance and other transmitters such as acetylcholine. Resulting from the insufficient amount of dopamine, a loss of muscle function creates an inability of the nerve cells to properly transmit messages. The reason for deterioration of these cells remains unknown. The disorder may affect one or both sides of the body, *(comma creates nonessential element)* with varying degrees of loss of function. To help minimize the degree of functional loss for a patient without Parkinson's, the stretching and manipulating of muscles can be helpful; consequently, this research aims to determine whether physical therapy can assist Parkinson's patients in maintaining their current muscle strength. A physical therapist can aid the patient in maintaining the muscle that she possesses.

Physical therapy undertakes a significant role in the muscle maintenance of a Parkinson's patient, and it uses active and passive exercise, gait training, practice in normal activities, hot or cold treatments, water therapy, and electrical stimulation. To stretch and manipulate the patient's muscles, the therapist uses passive exercises, and the range of motion [ROM], coordination, and speed of the patient improve by active exercises. In order to maintain ROM and lessen abnormal posture, physical therapists should teach Parkinson's patients useful relaxation techniques. Preliminary research regarding Parkinson's patients indicates that physical therapy intervention is unlikely to permanently reverse the rigidity, which is directly affected by the nervous system.

Physical therapy plays a significant role in patient education. During physical therapy, the therapist must emphasize the importance of self-relaxation to reduce rigidity and to apply the patient's remaining postural response methods by encouraging the patient to subconsciously practice correct posture ~~voluntarily~~ *(Can you perform something voluntarily if it is subconscious?)*. Physical therapy would be a practical way to teach patients methods in which they can compensate for the physical weaknesses associated with the disease, and the therapists demonstrate methods that reduce the potential for the impairments to return. When relaxation techniques and strengthening exercises are assigned by the physical therapist, the patient reduces rigidity and maintains a stable ROM, and he decreases atypical posture and encourages musculoskeletal change. Using relaxation methods first allows the therapist to develop the intervention to active mobility and stretching once the patient becomes facile with self-relaxation.

To achieve mobility throughout each segment of the spine, the therapist encourages exercises. The following experiment presents an explanation for physical therapy in identifying the provisions that eventually result in disability and immobility. Our team of researchers, Jones, Davies and Scott, conducted an experiment with 20 out-patients *(no comma)* affected with the Parkinson's disease to determine the importance of strengthening exercises and to conclude the degree of ease that the exercises provided the patients to help change their body position. The test group consisted of 12 males and 8 females ranging from ~~the age of~~ *(repeats)* 64 to 83 years of age. Motor training for the **patient's** various exercises repeated 5-10 times, twice a week for 5 consecutive weeks, included mobilization exercises for the trunk, upper and lower limbs, and the individual divisions of the spine. To rectify movement and rid the patient of atypical posture, the therapist practiced the previously listed exercises. The results of the study showed a general improvement in all exercises performed in all but four patients; the reason 4 of the original 20 *(no comma)* patients failed to improve has not been determined.

New research addressing musculoskeletal detriments, by the therapist, **allows** *(the research allows?)* the patient to gain sufficient ROM for automatic movements, which permits the therapist to focus on balance impairments. A Parkinson's patient's ability to successfully survive everyday activities of reaching, dressing, and being jostled in a crowd centers on the patient's capability to weight shift and to balance. Patients with gait impediments demonstrated significant improvement when performing exercises of standing balance and weight shifting. Implicated in essential activities, gait patterns require the ability to move in a continuous and slow motion, **to compose** weight shifts, and **to change** in the direction of movement.

A recent article presented two case studies **that** were conducted according to the intervention described above depicting the early treatment of patient's with Parkinson's disease. One of the two cases involved one man not taking medication for Parkinson's disease and a second man receiving medication for the disease. In case one, a man, **aged** 67 **years**, experienced impaired balance and difficulty with functional movements. He was referred to physical therapy for the necessary exercises to delay the intervention of pharmacology. Treating the individual for 1 month, **three sessions each week,** for approximately 1 hour each time *(no comma)* made **it** *(unclear pronoun reference)* possible for the ROM of his limb to nearly return to its original measurement. The second case involved a man, **aged 68, who** experienced a tremor in his right hand and gait complications. He chose to receive a medication that reduces rigidity and assists him in contending with the disease. His symptoms at the time of physical therapy intervention *(no comma)* included balance complications and poor functional difficulties. Case two patient attended physical therapy for 6 weeks**,** three sessions per week**,** and 1 hour per session**;** these treatments concentrated on gait and functional activities. When 6 weeks of physical therapy were completed**,** his everyday functional activities and his gait improved.

In light of the literature that was previously reviewed**,** we can assume that this disease needs to continue to be studied**,** and researchers must determine the necessity of physical therapy for Parkinson's patients. The experiments conducted by researchers demonstrated the importance of physical therapy in maintaining the muscle that she possesses**,** and they prove that strengthening and manipulating muscles can help to minimize the degree of loss of function for the patient.

PAGE 51
PUNCTUATION READING FOR RULES OF COMMA USAGE

Directions: The following passage abides by the rules of comma usage listed in this chapter. Read the writing sample and identify the rules governing each comma insertion.

Note that nonessential elements contain two commas when used internally.

In light of the research, *(introductory prepositional phrase)* physical therapy helps Parkinson's patients maintain the muscle that he possesses, *(independent clauses joined by a coordinating conjunction)* and this can be proved in the following discussion.

Parkinson's disease (PD) affects movements; therefore, *(introductory word)* exercising may assist patients to improve their mobility. Some doctors prescribe physical therapy or muscle-strengthening exercises to tone muscles and to develop underused and rigid muscles through a full range of motion. Exercises will not prevent disease progression, *(independent clauses joined*

by a coordinating conjunction) but they may improve body strength. Schenkman's conclusion supports the previously stated ideas: Exercise does not have the ability to end disease progression, *(independent clauses joined by a coordinating conjunction)* but it can develop the patient's body strength:

> "Physical therapy may not be very effective in remediating the direct effects of pathology of Parkinson's [disease] on the integrative mechanisms for balance. Physical therapy, however, *(nonessential phrase or word)* could be effective in reducing contributions of other impairments, *(nonessential phrase or word)* such as loss of trunk and pelvic mobility, in remediating balance impairments" (Schenkman et. al., 1989, pp. 544–545).

Also, *(introductory word)* exercises improve balance, *(nonessential word or phrase)* helping people overcome gait problems, *(independent clauses joined by a coordinating conjunction)* and they strengthen certain muscles that allow people to speak, swallow, walk, *(items in series)* and function better.

Physical therapy, *(nonessential element)* extremely important for the Parkinson's patient, usually follows an approach that uses active and passive exercise, gait-training, practice in normal activities, and if needed, hot or cold treatments, water therapy, and electrical stimulation *(items in series)*. Giving particular emphasis to upright posture, gait training, and extension exercises for the neck, trunk, and legs *(items in series)* stabilizes the patient. Passive exercise, *(nonessential appositive phrase)* mainly stretching and manipulating muscles by a physical therapist, aim at preventing muscles from shortening. An active exercise program, *(nonessential participial phrase)* used to help ROM, coordination, and speed, *(items in series)* that begins with slow and gentle exercises and becomes progressively more intense, may improve mobility in patients with early and mid-stage Parkinson's disease (WebMDHealth). Relaxation techniques that the patient is capable of using *(no comma)* should be taught to the patient in order to reduce rigidity, *(independent clauses joined by a coordinating conjunction)* and these will maintain ROM and lessen abnormal posture. Essentially, *(introductory word)* physical therapy encourages the well-being of patients; it acts as a common denominator in patients who are able to maintain productive years.

Responsibility for teaching the Parkinson's patient a formal home exercise program that will guarantee continued effective intervention and will provide the patient with some control over the disease depends on the physical therapist. According to Schenkman in *Physical Therapy* (1989), *(introductory participial phrase)* on the intervention that consists of teaching the patient self-relaxation of rigidity, *(introductory prepositional)* assisting the patient in maintaining flexibility and ROM, *(nonessential element)* and restoring the patient's automated movement patterns through repetition, the patient should continue in a home exercise program that continues to maintain flexibility, *(items in series)* ROM, and movement; once the patient has achieved maximum therapeutic gains, *(introductory prepositional phrase)* the patient must continue to maintain those gains through self-exercise. Postural reeducation, *(nonessential appositive)* an important aspect of the home exercise program, incorporates the flexibility acquired in therapy into appropriate postural alignment throughout the day.

Physical therapy intervention reduces disabilities by improving the patient's ability to function. Schenkman and Butler state that *(no comma, as quote runs into sentence grammatically)* " . . . functional activities should be incorporated into mobility exercises" (1989, p. 948). Any form of exercise is beneficial, *(nonessential clause)* although task-specific exercises are the most effective; this concept supports the notion that physical therapists are necessary to assist the patient in performing the exercise effectively. Once the physical therapist establishes exercises, *(introductory prepositional)* the patient's role revolves around efforts to practice movements, *(parenthetical element)* even simple ones, such as marching in place, making circular arm movements, and raising the legs up and down while sitting *(items in series)*. Therefore, the

template exercises established by the physical therapist enable the patient's physical activity.

Muscular and articular restrictions, *(nonessential element beginning with* which*)* which are ultimately caused by Parkinson's disease, contribute to reducing muscle content. Exercise, *(nonessential dependent clause)* when coupled with sensory reinforcements, proves efficacious for Parkinson's patients. An experiment reported in *Disability and Rehabilitation* (1999) presents an explanation for the physical therapist to encourage exercise to achieve mobility. The results in this study supported " . . . the rationale that physical therapy intervention is to identify the underlying and composite mechanisms which gradually lead to disability and immobility." This case study supports the demand for continuing study on the effect of physical therapy on patients suffering from Parkinson's disease; the results confirm that "the degree of disability in PD can be reduced by adding a simple physical therapy programme to the [patient's] pharmacological treatment" (Viliani et al., 1999, p. 73).

The studies suggest that the disability of Parkinson's disease can be reduced with early physical therapy intercession as gains are made in musculoskeletal flexibility, alignment, and overall functional movement *(items in series)*. Schenkman and colleagues (1989) demonstrate the necessity of physical therapy, *(independent clauses joined by a coordinating conjunction)* and the two case studies exemplified the changes that occurred in two Parkinson's individuals who received physical therapy early in disease. The study concluded that " . . . physical therapy intervention contributed to [the] changes, *(nonessential dependent clause)* although further study will be necessary to establish [a] relationship" between the changes in the patients and physical therapy treatment (p. 925).

Physical therapy successfully combats the rigidity and the ROM losses in Parkinson's patients. Preliminary assessment of physical therapy reveals beneficial results for Parkinson's disease patients, *(independent clauses joined by a coordinating conjunction)* but continued research regarding these effects on patients remains necessary. Gait training, posture, mobility, and functional activities *(items in series)* will improve with the assistance of physical therapy.

References

Parkinson's disease. Retrieved from http://my.webmed.com/content/dmk/dmk_article_40066

Schenkman, M., & Butler, R. A. (1989). A model for multisystem evaluation treatment of individuals with Parkinson's Disease. *Physical Therapy, 69*, 932–940.

—. (July 1989). A model for multisystem evaluation, interpretation, and treatment of individuals with neurologic dysfunction. *Physical Therapy, 69*, 538–547.

Schenkman, M., Donovan, J., Tsubota, J., Kluss, M., Stebbins, P., & Butler, R. B. (1989). Management of individuals with Parkinson's disease: Rationale and case studies. *Physical Therapy, 69*, 944–955.

Viliani, T., Pasquetti, P., Magnolfi, S., Lundardelli, M. L., Giorgi, C., Serra, P., & Taiti, P. G. (February 1999). Effects of physical training on straightening-up processes in patients with Parkinson's disease. *Disability and Rehabilitation, 21*, 68–73.

Young, R. (1999). Update on Parkinson's disease. *American Family Physician.* Retrieved from http://www.aafp.org/afp/990415ap/2155.htm

PAGE 54
EXERCISES: GRAMMAR, MECHANICS, AND PUNCTUATION
PUNCTUATION AND THE FOUR MAJOR ERRORS

Directions: Correct the following sentences with punctuation or identify the error as a comma splice (CS), run-on (RO), sentence fragment (SF), or subject-verb disagreement (SV). After identifying the error, correct the mistake. A sentence may have more than one error.

*Revisions are in **bold** type.*

1. The patient complained of angina**,** and the doctor administered nitroglycerin to make the patient more comfortable.

2. A list of the patient's allergies **was** posted in the chart that the nurse referenced. **SV**

3. The patient's current health, family history, and lifestyle **suggest** an increased risk of heart disease. **SV**

4. Blood tests revealed high clotting factor in the patient's blood **after** I administered a heparin IV bolus. **SF**

5. Following the procedure, the doctor prepared the patient for recovery**;** it became evident that the patient needed further care. **RO**

6. I changed the dressings on the abdominal wound**;** I found the dressings saturated with and the area irritated. **CS**

7. Although I found the patient had clear sputum, good breath sounds, and normal temperature**, the** patient's differential white blood cell count tested high. **SF**

8. I assigned the patient therapeutic exercises to aid in her discomfort**;** she benefited from the therapy. **CS**

9. The nurse practitioner prescribed a sulfa antibiotic for the patient's infection but the bacteria **were** resistant to the drug**. The** NP then prescribed Cipro to cure the infection. **CS**

10. Due to the severity of the trauma, the patient could not breath on his own**;** therefore, the physician **inserted** an endotracheal (ET) tube **that** was attached to a ventilator**, which** the respiratory therapist maintained throughout the patient's stay in the hospital. **CS**

11. As a result of the surgery, the patient's right knee **exhibits** decreased range of motion in flexion and extension. **SV**

12. The woman began labor contractions in her seventh month of pregnancy**;** because of the early labor**,** the obstetrician performed a cesarean section to ensure the safety of the mother and child. **CS**

13. The patient's blood tests reveals a high count of cancerous white blood cells, which **led** his doctor to the diagnosis of leukemia. **SV**

14. Chest x-ray films of the patient demonstrated an accumulation of fluid within her pleural spaces**,** and the doctor ordered a thoracentesis to relieve the pressure on her lungs and to enable **the** patient to **breathe** with ease.

15. The patient, Mr. Smith, **sustained** an infection in his right foot for 2 months. **SF** The undetected infection spread and induced secondary inguinal lymphadenopathy.

16. After **Mrs. Whitman complained** of bilateral knee pain, **her** physician performed **an** arthroscopy and determined that she had decreased cartilage in her knees and hypertrophy of her femur**. For** the pain and discomfort the doctor recommended aspirin, glucosamine, and chondroitin**; he then** recommended that she have total knee replacement if these treatments proved insufficient. **RO**

17. The radiologist performed an ultrasound examination of the patient and identified two cysts in her breast**, although** the mammogram revealed no abnormalities. **SF**

18. Mrs. Banks, a 37-year-old office assistant, complained of wrist pain and a tingling sensation in her fingers**;** Dr. Sanki diagnosed her with carpal tunnel syndrome. **CS**

19. Although other dermatologists diagnosed Mary with eczema, Dr. Horn **determined** her problem to be psoriasis**,** and the physician provided a prescription for a topical cream.

20. Hank **suffered** from noticeable anisocoria due to a massive head trauma, and the ophthalmologist offered no solution to improve his physical appearance. **SF**

PAGE 55
PUNCTUATION

Directions: Insert semicolons, colons, dashes, quotation marks, and italics as needed in the following sentences.

1. The players on the Wall of Fame—Jim Kelly, Kent Hull, and Cookie Gilchrist—deserve awards.

2. Several cities participated in the clean-up effort: Buffalo, Rochester, Syracuse, and Binghamton.

3. "Give me liberty" is one of my favorite quotes. I cannot remember who said it, though.

4. In last week's *New York Times*, Larry Felser was quoted from his most recent book entitled, *The Glory Years*.

5. He left us with one choice: swim for the shore.

6. The word *is* is often considered weak in verb-based writing strategies.

PAGE 55
GRAMMAR RULES AND WORD CHOICE

Directions: Correctly rewrite any sentences containing mistakes in mechanics, punctuation, or grammar or informality of language.

*Revisions are in **bold** type.*

1. After her surgery, Mrs. Sanders complained of **overheating, fatigue, and thirst**.

2. Dr. Francis intends either to operate on the patient *(no comma)* or **to** instruct her to attend physical therapy.

3. After stocking all the rooms, weighing all the patients, and recording all the vital signs, Susie, the nurse's aid**e**, then distributed all the lunches, supplied the phlebotomy kit, and cleaned all the medical equipment.

4. The patient complained that his ankle was painful and swollen, and he experienced **problems** *(unclear:* dyscoordination? weakness?*)* while walking.

5. The therapist demonstrated appropriate exercises, answered the patient's questions**,** and **documented** the patient's history.

6. For the procedure, the nurse prepared a multitude of sterile gauze **and** a suture kit, and **she** anesthetized the area.

7. For a primary diagnosis, Dr. Davis believed the **patient's** problem could be Crohn's disease, irritable bowel syndrome**,** or a duodenal ulcer, but to solidify a diagnosis**,** the physician requested a barium swallow, a barium enema, and **possible** exploratory surgery.

8. When the nurse answered the call bell, the patient asked the nurse to help him to the chair and **find** his glasses.

9. Months of occupational therapy enabled Mr. Appolito to walk**,** dress, and **eat** independently.

10. While bathing the patient, the nurse noticed redness **and** poor capillary refill, and **the patient complained of** numbing to his coccygeal region.

PAGE 56
PUNCTUATION, GRAMMAR, AND MECHANICS IN AN ESSAY SAMPLE

Directions: Correct any mistakes in grammar, punctuation, or mechanics within the following paragraph.

Revisions are in **bold** *type.*

Admitted to the ER on Thursday, January 26, the patient complained of angina. A **60-year-old** man, he has an extensive history of heart problems. At the age of **51,** the patient, Mr Rouge, suffered from a minor heart attack. **Congestive heart failure (CHF)** developed, presumably, as a result of this myocardial infarction**;** however, Mr. Rouge sustains a healthy lifestyle including *(no punctuation)* walking, gardening, and cross-country skiing. The **patient's** family reports that he is a **pillar of strength** *(cliché)*. Throughout his ER visit, the physician's monitor**ed** his pulse, heart rate, and ~~taking his~~ temperature. A blood test revealed high troponin levels indicating that the patient, again, suffered from a myocardial infarction. Following his diagnosis, the patient was transported to the cardiac unit on the 3rd floor. While on the cardiac unit, Mr Rouge will remain on a cardiac monitor, which will allow the nurses 24-hour monitoring of his heart.

▌CHAPTER THREE

PAGE 69
EXERCISES: ADOPTING A VERB-BASED WRITING STYLE

Directions: Rewrite the following sentences into a verb-based writing style by reducing nominalization, eliminating weak verbs, eliminating "it" and "there" as subjects, eliminating passive voice, and limiting the use of "to be" verbs.

EXERCISE SET 1

1. There were many patients waiting to see the doctor.

   Many patients waited for treatment from the doctor.

2. The patient was feeling uncomfortable due to high temperatures and a pain in her arm.

   The patient felt uncomfortable due to high temperatures and a pain in her arm.

3. The paramedic was providing oxygen to first the child and then to the mother in order to help them breath after the car accident.

   The paramedic provided oxygen first to the child and then to the mother to assist their breathing after the accident.

4. There are many reasons why this 43-year-old patient could have suffered from a stroke including; his diet, the amount of exercise he did, his stress levels at work and home, and others.

   Many reasons exist for this 43-year-old patient's stroke, including diet, amount of exercise, and high stress levels at home and at work.

5. After the nurse administered chest compressions, the doctor injected some dopamine which helped the situation because the patient's heart beat came back.

   After the nurse administered chest compressions, the doctor injected dopamine, which helped the patient to recover her heartbeat.

6. It became evident that the patient would need surgery to fix the damages from his skiing accident, so the nurse was preparing for the procedure.

   The patient needed surgery to repair damages from his skiing accident; the nurse prepared for the procedure.

7. No one was sure about the protocol for evacuation in the case of a bomb threat. It seemed that the problem had never before been faced.

   The protocol for evacuation in the case of a bomb threat was never established; no one had ever faced the problem before. *Note: Passive voice is acceptable in first independent clause because the doer of the action is unknown.*

8. Later the patients will be given their dinner trays and then the nurses will need to record the amount of food and liquids they had eaten.

   Later, the nurses will provide the patients with their dinner trays and then record the amount of food and liquids the patients had eaten.

9. Because of the fact that the nurses were very busy, the patients complained that they were not receiving the care that they deserved.

   Because other responsibilities demanded the attention of the nurses, the patients complained about neglect.

10. The physician became troubled over the patients status because the patient was looking jaundice and was recording a high temperature.

   The physician struggled with the patient's status because the patient appeared jaundiced and recorded a high temperature.

EXERCISE SET 2

1. Recently the recordings from John Doe's blood pressure has provided the nurses with reason to believe his days are numbered.

   Recently, the recordings from John Doe's blood pressure indicated his certain and imminent death.

2. The patient is going to radiology, and he is receiving a CT scan to verify his doctor's diagnosis.

   The patient will transfer to radiology where he will undergo a CT scan to verify his doctor's diagnosis.

3. It seems that the doctor's are agreeing on the appropriate billing procedures regarding this procedure of a localized biopsy.

   The doctors agree on the appropriate billing procedures for a localized biopsy procedure.

4. The nurse said to the aide to call for the doctor because it was an emergency.

   The nurse instructed the aide to contact the doctor for an emergent situation.

5. The patient was examined in order to determine the problem that was causing her abdominal pain, and it was found to be from a weakness of the pyloric sphincter.

   The patient was examined, and her condition was diagnosed; a weakness of her pyloric sphincter caused her abdominal pain. *Note: Passive voice can be acceptable here if the actor performing the diagnosis is not known.*

6. The patient is returning today for his final and third hepatitis B vaccine booster shot.

   The nurse will administer the third and final hepatitis B vaccine booster for the patient today.

7. Following her stroke, Dr. Metting gave the indication to Mrs. Hinman that an EEG should be done to determine if any brain damage had occurred.

   Dr. Metting indicated to Mrs. Hinman that an EEG would help determine if any brain damage has occurred after her stroke.

8. After piecing together the patient's history obtained from family and friends, it seemed that the patient may well have forgotten to take his insulin shot and was suffering from ketoacidosis.

   After reconstructing the patient's history, the physician determined that the patient may have failed to administer his insulin shot and currently suffers from ketoacidosis.

9. The psychiatrist came to believe that Megan suffered from bipolar disease as indicated by her rapid mood changes.

   The psychiatrist concluded that Megan suffered from bipolar disease, using her rapid mood swings as evidence.

10. The patient has presented with complaints of fatigue, sore throat, and swollen axillary lymph nodes, and the preliminary blood tests give an indication of mononucleosis.

The patient complains of fatigue, sore throat, and swollen axillary lymph nodes, and the preliminary blood tests indicate mononucleosis.

PAGE 70
EXERCISE: REVISING A SAMPLE STUDENT ESSAY

Directions: In this sample student essay, the overuse of the verb "to be," dependence on passive voice, use of weak verbs, unnecessary nominalization, and *It* and *There* used as subjects limit the effectiveness of the writing. The weak and ineffective verbs are *italicized*. Find ways to revise these sentences to create a more effective message. In some circumstances, the use of the "to be" verb forms is necessary, such as in the exceptions to the rules of passive voice and in describing a state of being. In most cases, however, the "to be" verb forms can be eliminated by revising the sentences or subordinating "to be" constructions in phrases or nonessential elements.

Within the field of medicine, many treatments *are being found* from ancient remedies. Many remedies used in ancient societies *are* now being studied to *see* if *there is* any validity in using them as a treatment. A major area of the world *being sought after* is Asia. In many of the oriental cultures there, acupuncture *has been used* for thousands of years. Acupuncture *has been implemented* to aid in medical problems such as arthritis, pain management, addictions, and cancer. *There are* many reasons for using it.

Acupuncture *is* simply the insertion of extremely small needles into specific points in the body. Generally, moxibustion *is used* in association with acupuncture. Moxibustion *is* burning specific herbs while acupuncture is performed. Varying types of acupuncture *are used* depending on ailments. Electroacupuncture *is* a new technique in which small electrical impulses *are sent* through the needle. Electroacupuncture *is generally used* as a pain reliever. Another type

of method *is* sonopuncture. Sonopuncture *is* the use of sound waves within the ear to reach other parts of the body. Ailments such as obesity *have been treated* with sonopuncture. Another treatment that is synonymous with acupuncture *would be* acupressure. The only difference between the two *is* that one *is based* on using needles while the other uses pressure.

Possible Revision

Within the field of medicine, many scientists have rediscovered ancient remedies and plan to study their efficacy for modern illnesses. In many of the oriental cultures in Asia, acupuncture *has been used* for thousands of years. Acupuncturists have implemented strategies to aid in medical problems such as arthritis, pain management, addictions, and cancer, and have many reasons for using accupuncture.

Acupuncture *is* simply the insertion of extremely small needles into specific points in the body. Generally, acupuncturists employ a method called moxibustion, burning specific herbs while acupuncture is performed, in association with acupuncture. Additionally, acupuncturists use a variety of other treatments depending on ailments. For example, electroacupuncture, a new technique in which small electrical impulses *are sent* through the needle, relieves pain. Sonopuncture, the use of sound waves within the ear, reaches other parts of the body, and ailments such as obesity *have been treated* with sonopuncture. Acupressure, another treatment that is similar to acupuncture, uses pressure instead of needles and results in similar success.

PAGE 71
EXERCISE: WEAK VERBS

Directions: Examine the following sample student essay and identify the problems with weak verbs. This essay was used in an earlier chapter to represent coherence breaks and problems with unifying the essay. Consider how a strong use of verbs might help alleviate some of these problems as sentences are revised.

Revisions can vary. Target areas are in **bold** *type.*

Punishing a child teaches children **what is right and what is wrong**. Many parents punish their children by **talking to them** or by reward and punishment. Child abuse consists of hurting a child physically, mentally, or emotionally. **There have been** parents beating their children for hundreds of years. Some punishments **do** consider spanking but do not hurt the children. Spanking a child **is considered** a soft slap to show the children that they did **something** wrong. Beating a child leaves bruises and psychological problems. Unfortunately, **there are** parents **all over the world** that deliberately hurt their children. Child abuse causes many unresolved issues that usually **do not get** explored. Discipline can often **be used** in different ways. In case a child does not **relate to a certain way**, the parent can approach them in a different ways to teach them morals.

As hard as it is to punish children, **it needs to be done**. Our society focuses on parent-child relationships and specializes in natural parenting. Punishment gives children a sense of what proper behavior **is**. Children need to learn the difference between right and wrong. Punishing children **can be done** in many different ways. One example to discipline a child is isolation. When a child is **left alone** they get bored **easily**. When they are forced to pursue something they **do not get motivated** unless they **want to do it**. Then they realize **what they did** was wrong. Another way to discipline children is by reward and punishment. When children are young, they react well to this. They realize that when **you** take something that they want away, they did **something** wrong, but when they do well or if they do **something** that you ask them to do, they get a reward. People believe that reward and punishment works well with children. **This** creates problems because **every time they do something** right, they expect to **get something** in return. If they know that they **are not going to get something** in return, they may not **do** what you ask them to do. If this happens, you may have to approach the situation in a different way. Lastly, talking to children begins a **great** relationship and **tells** them what is right and what is wrong. In this case, punishment may not be the answer, but explaining to them **what is wrong**

can create an image of **what is right**. Speaking to your children can **be** a powerful tool for explaining morals. A theme **is created** from experiments and it shows the relations between a parent who wants to raise their children properly and the society in which they live. If you talk to children, **it** teaches them to trust you and to respect you and the decisions you make. The examples you set for your children also teach them what is wrong and right by your actions.

Many parents do not understand the concept of talking to **your** children like they are human. This **is when** spanking **gets too far**. Child abuse creates mental, physical, and emotional problems. Children who **are hurt constantly deal with** numerous problems and side **effects**. Some examples include becoming sensitive to pain, destructive, and depressed. The child becomes unlovable and **is** likely **that they will not be loved by anyone** because of **their** behavior. Usually when **there seems to be** child abuse in a family, the parent **is** usually **the one with the problem** and they hit the child to blame someone else. As a society we project problems of child abuse and try to concentrate on helping the parents. They are usually **dealing with** mental health issues or they have expectations of their children to do unrealistic **things**. In many cases, the child **gets stressed out** and needs to **take his or her aggression out** on someone who won't **fight back**. Child abuse is used as a form of control but sometimes the child is left with destructive organs or even death.

Child abuse stems from stress or the parents' childhood. Changes have occurred by **giving** the parent therapy and treatments. The parent may think that beating a child **is** normal if they **were** hit as a child. The parents need to recognize **what they are doing** to their children and realize the relationship that they could have with them. **It has been shown** that the link between economic and social atmospheres affect families that are involved in child abuse. Physical abuse normally occurs with low-income families because they have **too much stress keeping control** in their life and to support their families. Evidence proves that **there is** a relationship between child abuse and low-income families. They **get stressed easily** because of poverty and become likely that they are unable to support their families. Emotion becomes **very natural** to a human being in how they respond to certain situations. In the past, **it has been shown** that people are embarrassed to **deal with** the poor. Emotional abuse usually takes place within a high income-tax family, because they don't seem to spend enough time with their children and **they** search for attention. Rich families **create a life worth living** but do not create time to spend with their children. Parents involved in **this** need to realize that they need to care for their children and **give** them guidance.

Children who **are in an abused situation** usually need psychological help. After a child **is abused** they suffer many side effects. These side effects include **that** they cannot trust, they have shame and doubt in **anything** they do, and they become destructive with people and property. **It** strains their brain and creates an image **so** they perceive themselves as **not being good enough**. Many abusive parents have low self-esteem and some do not even know who they are. Hitting a child is wrong and often enough parents who do **this** need mental and emotional help as well as the children. For some reason, the parents believe beating someone satisfies their urge to control **something** and forces them to believe **that it is right**. Child abusers form discipline into an extreme level. The parent's attention **should be on** the child and **what they can do** to help them, not **what they can do** to help themselves. Discipline creates morals and behavior, **so** telling them to **do something right by doing something wrong** and hurtful is not the **right** approach. Sadly, child abuse **is done** in many ways. They may not be hitting them, but child abuse can also **be** from not taking care of them. Some examples are leaving a baby in a hot car for hours, not cleaning up after the children, or even not feeding them. If these parents can't **take care** of themselves then they should not be **taking care** of children.

Control **is** an issue that needs to be resolved before the children are born. Control helps life and releases some stress. Control leads to a nat-

ural relationship between parents and their children. **They** can learn how to discipline them by **finding out** what their **children react to** and how they can learn. If a parent **is stressed**, they should seek help if they cannot control it. Control **seems to be** one of the main problems because if they can't control something in their life, they need to control something else. Lack of self-control usually leads to child abuse. Punishment **deals with** a child's behavior and teaches them **what they did wrong**. It does not physically harm them. Child abuse is not discipline. It controls the way a parent reacts to certain situations. When trying to discipline children, hurting them **is not the point**, teaching them a lesson is. Parents need to understand that and if they don't, they need psychological help. This will help parents **deal with** their problems and create new relationships with their children.

PAGE 78
EXERCISE: REVISING SENTENCES TO ELIMINATE WORDINESS

Directions: Revise these sentences to state their meaning in fewer words. Avoid passive voice, needless repetition, and wordy phrases and clauses. The first sentence has been completed as an example.

1. There are many nurses in the area who are planning to attend the meeting which is scheduled for next Friday.
   Many area nurses plan to attend next Friday's meeting.

2. Although Smithery Hall is regularly populated by the medical students, close study of the building as a structure is seldom undertaken by them.

3. He dropped out of nursing school on account of the fact that it was necessary for him to help support his family.

4. It is expected that the new dress code for the therapists will be announced by the hospital administrators within the next few days.

5. There are many ways in which a graduate student of physical therapy who is interested in meeting other physical therapists may come to know one.

6. It is very unusual to find a health professional who has never told a deliberate lie on purpose.

7. Trouble is caused when patients disobey rules that have been established for the safety of all.

8. A recent rally in front of a hospital was attended by more than a thousand nurses and residents of the local area. Six residents were arrested by hospital guards for disorderly conduct, while several other nurses are charged by hospital administrators with organizing a public meeting without being issued a permit to do so.

9. The courses that are considered most important by students pursuing a career in health science are those that have been shown to be useful to them after graduation.

10. Upon graduation, occupational therapists who have recently graduated from college must all become aware of the fact that there is a need for them to make contact with other health professionals in other health fields concerning the matter of a patient.

11. In our clinic there are wide-open opportunities for professional growth with a clinic that enjoys an enviable record for allowing our patients to get rid of walking problems as soon as possible.

12. Some people believe in direct access, while other people are against it; there are many opinions on this subject.

Possible Revisions

1. Many area nurses plan to attend next Friday's meeting.

2. Medical students seldom recognize Smithery Hall's structure upon entering.

3. He withdrew from nursing school to support his family.

4. Hospital administrators will announce the therapists' new dress code soon.

5. A physical therapy graduate student may meet other physical therapists at many different places.

6. Most health professionals have lied.

7. People who disobey rules jeopardize the safety of others.

8. Hospital guards arrested six area residents for disorderly conduct at the hospital rally, while hospital administrators charged several other nurses for meeting without a permit.

9. Health science students have found the course information used after graduation most important.

10. Occupational therapists must closely associate with other health professionals when treating a patient.

11. Our clinic, which prides itself in quick ambulation rehabilitation, provides wide-open opportunities for professional growth.

12. Many opinions exist on the direct access subject.

PAGE 80
EXERCISES: ELIMINATING WORDINESS
REWRITING SENTENCES TO CORRECT IMPROPER USAGE, DICTION, AND WORDINESS

Directions: Rewrite the following sentences, correcting any improper word usage, wordiness, or informality.

1. As a physician, I, personally, believe Mrs. Strom's health problems relate to her drinking.

   In my medical opinion, I believe Mrs. Strom's drinking contrributes to her health problems.

2. After prescribing the antibiotic, the nurse practitioner was not aware of the fact that the patient was allergic to sulfa drugs.

   The nurse practitioner who prescribed the antibiotic did not realize that the patient was allergic to sulfa drugs.

3. On one hand, the patient required physical therapy after the intense surgery, but, on the other hand, he required rest.

   The patient required physical therapy after the intense surgery; however, he also required rest.

4. Discussing the diagnosis, Mr. Fuller excepted the necessary treatment course and the risks involved.

   After discussing the diagnosis with his physician, Mr. Fuller accepted the necessary treatment course and weighed the risks involved.

5. Following the examination, Dr. Schlay determined the patient was in alright condition to continue participation on the basketball team.

   Following the examination, Dr. Schlay released the patient to full physical activity.

6. Repeatedly, the nurse keeps talking the patient's temperature and checking my blood glucose to ensure that he doesn't go into diabetic shock.

   The nurse regularly measures the patient's temperature and blood glucose to avoid or anticipate diabetic shock.

7. For her stroke rehabilitation, Mrs. Adams believed that physical therapy was equally as important as speech therapy and that all the people she worked with were a fine bunch of fellows.

   For her stroke rehabilitation, Mrs. Adams believed that physical therapy and speech therapy would complement each other and that her coworkers would support her.

8. When choosing her physician's assistant, Dr. Knowles couldn't decide which candidate was more preferable.

   When choosing her physician's assistant, Dr. Knowles could not decide between the two candidates.

9. The unproductive nature of the contract talks with the nurses' union made Carrie's blood boil.

   The unproductive nature of the contract talks with the nurses' union made Carrie furious.

10. With the advancement in research, Mrs. Collins explored lots of different treatment options.

    Considering recent advances in research, Mrs. Collins explored various treatment options.

PAGE 80
ELIMINATING WORDINESS USING VERB-BASED WRITING

Directions: Rewrite the following sentences into a verb-based writing style by reducing wordiness, replacing weak verbs, and replacing passive voice with active voice construction. Correct any other errors within the sentence.

1. There were many patients waiting to see the doctor.
   Many patients waited for the doctor.

2. The patient was feeling uncomfortable due to high temperatures and a pain in her arm.
   The patient's fever and pain in the left arm caused her discomfort.

3. The paramedic was providing oxygen to first the child and then to the mother in order to help them breath after the car accident.
   After the accident, the paramedic provided oxygen first to the child and then to the mother.

4. There are many reasons why this 43-year-old patient could have suffered from a stroke including; his diet, the amount of exercise he did, his stress levels at work and home, and others.
   Diet, lack of exercise, and stress could have caused the 43-year-old patient's stroke.

5. After the nurse administered chest compressions, the doctor injected some dopamine which helped the situation because the patient's heart beat came back.
   After the nurse administered chest compressions, the doctor injected dopamine to recover a normal heartbeat.

6. It became evident that the patient would need surgery to fix the damages from his skiing accident, so the nurse was preparing for the procedure.

The nurse prepared for the surgical procedure to treat the patient's injury from his skiing accident.

7. No one was sure about the protocol for evacuation in the case of a bomb threat. It seemed that the problem had never before been faced.

   Because of the infrequency of an event such as a bomb threat, no one knew the protocol for evacuation.

8. Later the patients will be given their dinner trays and then the nurses will need to record the amount of food and liquids they had eaten.

   The staff will deliver dinner trays to the patients, and the nurses will then record amount ingested.

9. Because of the fact that the nurses were very busy, the patients complained that they were not receiving the care that they deserved.

   Because the nurses were occupied with administrative duties, the patients complained about neglect.

10. The physician became troubled over the patients status because the patient was looking jaundice and was recording a high temperature.

    The patient's high fever and jaundiced appearance caused concern for the physician.

11. Recently the recordings from John Doe's blood pressure has provided the nurses with reason to believe his days are numbered.

    John Doe's recent blood pressure readings signaled certain and imminent death.

12. The patient is going to radiology, and he is receiving a CT scan to verify his doctor's diagnosis.

    X-ray films and a CT scan will verify the doctor's diagnosis.

13. It seems that the doctor's are agreeing on the appropriate billing procedures regarding this procedure of a localized biopsy.

    The doctors agree on the proposed procedures for localized biopsy billing.

14. The nurse said to the aide to call for the doctor because it was an emergency.

    The nurse declared an emergency and ordered the aide to call for the doctor.

15. The patient was examined in order to determine the problem that was causing her abdominal pain, and it was found to be from a weakness of the pyloric sphincter.

    The physician examined the patient and found that her abdominal pain resulted from a weakness of the pyloric sphincter.

16. The patient is returning today for his final and third hepatitis B vaccine booster shot.

    The patient will receive his third and final hepatitis B vaccine booster today.

17. Following her stroke, Dr. Metting gave the indication to Mrs. Hinman that an EEG should be done to determine if any brain damage had occurred.

    Dr. Metting recommended to Mrs. Hinman an EEG to determine the extent of brain damage post stoke.

18. After piecing together the patient's history obtained from family and friends, it seemed that the patient may well have forgotten to take his insulin shot and was suffering from ketoacidosis.

    A reconstructing of the patient's history revealed insulin non-compliance that triggered ketoacidosis.

19. The psychiatrist came to believe that Megan suffered from bipolar disease as indicated by her rapid mood changes.

    Megan's mood swings indicated bipolar disease.

20. The patient has presented with complaints of fatigue, sore throat, and swollen axillary lymph nodes, and the preliminary blood tests give an indication of mononucleosis.

    The patient presents with fatigue, sore throat, and swollen axillary lymph nodes, and the preliminary blood tests indicate mononucleosis.

PAGE 81
SAMPLE STUDENT ESSAY: WORD CHOICE AND DICTION

Directions: In the following sample student paper, identify the word choice problems and offer suggestions for change. Eliminate wordiness and vague constructions as well, replacing them with precise and accurate terms or language.

Revisions will vary. Target areas are in **bold** *type.*

Anorexia is an eating disorder that could be life-threatening and cause **seriously problematic health problems**. A **major** symptom of the disease consists of a fear of becoming **too heavy and gaining weight**. Sufferers of the disease will count calories, exercise excessively, and eat **little amounts** of food. An increase in pressures from family members can result in a **really** unhealthy outcome. The media, and other forms of radio and television, **send out** negative and false **images and messages about body images**. A perfect body, defined as tall, thin, and beautiful in all ways, **remains** an impossible **appearance to accomplish** within today's society and **leads to the idea of an unhealthy being**. The reality of reaching such a body state or such **a dream coming to life remains** unreal.

Parents, especially mothers, add to the pressures of young adult life. Many mothers, unhappy with their own appearances and who suffer from eating disorders themselves, **pass the grief onto** their daughters. Recent studies **fit** well with **this idea** of eating disorders. Mothers who constantly influence daughters to lose weight and **to become thin** can lower self-esteem and lead a child to feel **bad** about herself, ultimately resulting in anorexia in order to **halt the nasty comments**. Words **remain** more powerful **when compared to a mother simply loses** a dramatic amount of weight and the daughter witnesses the success story. **In the long run, the idea** of negative comments from a parent can **destroy someone internally** and **make one feel like less of a person**. People desire to feel loved and accepted, but if others view a person as unattractive, especially parents' views **on** their children, the out-

come may result in an eating disorder. Two people in a child's life are most important: mother and father, **the parents**. If parents criticize their children too much, a child may starve in order to feel **beautiful** in **their** parents' eyes. Teens are especially **unstable** about personal perceptions of self during adolescent years, **so** parents who comment **negatively** about the child can emotionally destroy **a teen**.

The researchers raise **a good point** because **a lot** of **girls I associated** with fear becoming heavy; overweight **means** a person **is shunned from her surroundings**. In society, fat **associates** with ugly and isolation, and thinness connects with beautiful and and popular. **Personally**, I am terrified of weight gain **because it people** may not like me or reject me from the **work place** in the future. Dieting **consumes** my mind and **literally drives me crazy** because I can never lose enough weight.

CHAPTER 4

PAGE 92
EXERCISES: USING PHRASES FOR SENTENCE VARIETY
COMBINING SENTENCES USING PHRASES

Directions: Work through these monotonous, simple sentences and rewrite each one five times using all of the five commonly used phrases.

1. Alabama was organized as a territory in 1817. It was admitted to the union in 1819.

   Appositive: Alabama, a territory organized in 1817, was admitted to the union in 1819.

   Prepositional: In 1817, Alabama was organized as a territory; it was admitted to the union in 1819.

   Infinitive: To admit Alabama to the union in 1819, it was organized as a territory in 1817.

   Gerund: Organizing Alabama as a territory in 1817 cleared the path for admittance to the union in 1819.

   Participial: Admitted to the union in 1819, Alabama was organized as a territory in 1817.

2. Virginia is nicknamed "The Old Dominion." It was the oldest of the English colonies. It remained loyal to the king during the English Civil War.

   Appositive: Virginia, "The Old Dominion," was the oldest of the English colonies, and it remained loyal to the king during the English Civil War.

   Prepositional: During the English Civil War, Virginia, nicknamed "The Old Dominion" and the oldest of the English colonies, remained loyal to the king.

   Infinitive: To earn the nickname "The Old Dominion," Virginia, the oldest of the English colonies, remained loyal to the king during the English Civil War.

   Gerund: Remaining loyal to the king during the English Civil War allowed Virginia, the oldest of the English colonies, to be nicknamed "The Old Dominion."

   Participial: Nicknamed "The Old Dominion," Virginia was the oldest of the English colonies, and it remained loyal to the king during the English Civil War.

3. Rhode Island is the smallest state in the union. It has played a great part in American history. It was a haven for individuals seeking religious freedom.

   Appositive: Rhode Island, the smallest state in the union, has played a great part in American history as it was a haven for individuals seeking religious freedom.

   Prepositional: As a haven for individuals seeking religious freedom, Rhode Island, the smallest state in the union, played a great part in American history.

   Infinitive: To play a great part in American history, Rhode Island, the smallest state in the union, was a haven for individuals seeking religious freedom.

   Gerund: Being a haven for individuals seeking religious freedom allowed Rhode Island, the smallest state in the union, to play a great part in American history.

   Participial: Playing a great part in American history, Rhode Island was a haven for individuals seeking religious freedom, and it is the smallest state in the union.

4. Dr. Jones is a professor of comparative literature. He believes that Wordsworth is the founder of modern literary criticism.

   Appositive: Dr. Jones, a professor of comparative literature, believes that Wordsworth is the founder of modern literary criticism.

   Prepositional: In his view, Dr. Jones, a professor of comparative literature, believes that Wordsworth is the founder of modern literary criticism.

   Infinitive: To understand Dr. Jones' perspective, you must understand that he is a professor of comparative literature, and he believes that Wordsworth is the founder of modern literary criticism.

   Gerund: Believing that Wordsworth is the founder of modern literary criticism has lead Dr. Jones, a professor of comparative literature, to further study on the subject.

   Participial: Believing that Wordsworth is the founder of modern literary criticism, Dr. Jones is a professor of comparative literature.

5. Professor Holland is our soccer coach. She also teaches American literature.

   Appositive: Professor Holland, our soccer coach, also teaches American literature.

   Prepositional: For the sake of the soccer team, Professor Holland agreed to teach American literature.

   Infinitive: To coach our soccer team, Professor Holland sometimes applied lessons from American literature.

   Gerund: Teaching American literature allowed Professor Holland to coach our soccer team.

   Participial: Teaching American literature, Professor Holland is also our soccer coach.

6. My father graduated from USC. He is now a professor at Tufts.

   Appositive: My father, a graduate from USC, is now a professor at Tufts.

Prepositional: At Tufts, my father, a graduate of USC, is a professor.

Infinitive: To earn a professorship at Tufts, my father graduated from USC.

Gerund: Graduating from USC led my father to teach at Tufts.

Participial: Graduating from USC, my father teaches at Tufts.

PAGE 93
REVISING FOR SENTENCE VARIETY

Directions: Revise the following paragraph using phrases to create variation.

Many rivers flow out to sea. They take the most direct route. They flow quickly down the sides of mountains. They flow more slowly on flat terrain. Rapidly moving water wears away the land. The wearing-away process is called erosion. The planting of trees, shrubs, and grasses can prevent erosion.

Possible Revision

*Revisions are in **bold** type.*

Taking the most direct route (*participial*), many rivers flow out to sea. **Down the sides of mountains** (*prepositional*), they flow quickly, and **on flat terrain** (*prepositional*), they flow more slowly. **Wearing away the land** (*gerund*), **a process called erosion** (*appositive*), is the result of rapidly moving water. **To prevent erosion** (*infinitive*), plant trees, shrubs, and grasses.

PAGE 95
EXERCISES: USING THE FOUR TYPES OF SENTENCES
COMBINING SENTENCES USING DIFFERENT SENTENCE TYPES

Directions: These are the same sentences that appeared in the section about phrases. Work through these monotonous, simple sentences and rewrite each one four times using all four types of sentences.

1. Alabama was organized as a territory in 1817. It was admitted to the union in 1819.

   Simple: Alabama, organized as a territory in 1817, was admitted to the union in 1819.

   Compound: Alabama was organized as a territory in 1817, and it was admitted to the union in 1819.

   Complex: Since Alabama was organized as a territory in 1817, it could be admitted to the union in 1819.

   Compound-Complex: Although other states would follow its lead, Alabama was organized as a territory in 1817, and it was admitted to the union in 1819.

2. Virginia is nicknamed "The Old Dominion." It was the oldest of the English colonies. It remained loyal to the king during the English Civil War.

   Simple: Virginia, nicknamed "The Old Dominion," was the oldest of the English colonies and remained loyal to the king during the English Civil War.

   Compound: Virginia, nicknamed "The Old Dominion," was the oldest of the English colonies, and it remained loyal to the king during the English Civil War.

   Complex: Since it remained loyal to the king during the English Civil War, Virginia, the oldest of the English colonies, was nicknamed "The Old Dominion."

   Compound-Complex: Since it was the oldest of the English colonies, Virginia remained loyal to the king during the English Civil War, and it was nicknamed "The Old Dominion."

3. Rhode Island is the smallest state in the union. It has played a great part in American history. It was a haven for individuals seeking religious freedom.

   Simple: Rhode Island, the smallest state in the union and a haven for individuals seeking religious freedom, played a great part in American history.

   Compound: Rhode Island, the smallest state in the union, has played a great part in American history, and it was a haven for individuals seeking religious freedom.

   Complex: Although Rhode Island is the smallest state in the union, it has played a great part in American history as a haven for individuals seeking religious freedom.

Compound-Complex: Although Rhode Island is the smallest state in the union, it has played a great part in American history, and it was a haven for individuals seeking religious freedom.

4. Dr. Jones is a professor of comparative literature. He believes that Wordsworth is the founder of modern literary criticism.

   Simple: Dr. Jones, a professor of comparative literature, believes that Wordsworth is the founder of modern literary criticism.

   Compound: Dr. Jones is a professor of comparative literature, and he believes that Wordsworth is the founder of modern literary criticism.

   Complex: Since Dr. Jones is a traditional professor of comparative literature, he believes that Wordsworth is the founder of modern literary criticism.

   Compound-Complex: Since Dr. Jones is a traditional professor of comparative literature, he believes that Wordsworth is the founder of modern literary criticism, and Coleridge was his pupil.

5. Professor Holland is our soccer coach. She also teaches American literature.

   Simple: Professor Holland, our soccer coach, also teaches American literature.

   Compound: Professor Holland is our soccer coach, and she also teaches American literature.

   Complex: While Professor Holland is our soccer coach, she also teaches American literature.

   Compound-Complex: Professor Holland is our soccer coach, and she also teaches American literature, although she prefers to British literature.

6. My father graduated from USC. He is now a professor at Tufts.

   Simple: My father, a graduate from USC, is now a professor at Tufts.

   Compound: My father graduated from USC, and he is now a professor at Tufts.

   Complex: Although my father graduated from USC, he is now a professor at Tufts.

Compound-Complex: Although my father graduated from USC, he is now a professor at Tufts, but he was not considered at other universities.

PAGE 95
REVISING FOR SENTENCE VARIATION

Directions: Revise this entire passage using sentence variation techniques. When finished, rewrite it again using combinations of the four types of sentences and the five commonly used types of phrases:

Many rivers flow out to sea. They take the most direct route. They flow quickly down the sides of mountains. They flow more slowly on flat terrain. Rapidly moving water wears away the land. The wearing-away process is called erosion. The planting of trees, shrubs, and grasses can prevent erosion.

Sentence Types

As many rivers flow out to sea, they take the most direct route. **CX** They flow quickly down the sides of mountains, and they flow more slowly on flat terrain. **CP** Although rapidly moving water wears away the land, this wearing-away process, called erosion, can be prevented by the planting of trees, shrubs, and grasses. **CX**

Sentences and Phrases Combined

As many rivers flow out to sea, they take the most direct route. **CX** They flow quickly down the sides of mountains, and they flow more slowly on flat terrain. **CP** Wearing away the land *(participial)*, rapidly moving water carries soil to flat terrain. **S** This wearing-away process, erosion *(appositive)*, helps enrich the farmland in these flat areas. **S** Planting trees, shrubs, and grasses *(gerund)* can prevent erosion. **S**

PAGE 96
EXERCISE: SUBORDINATION AND COORDINATION

Directions: Combine the following sentences using the four types of sentences and appropriately subordinating relevant parts of the original in your reconstruction.

1. Professor Jones teaches English. She is also our rugby coach. Her coaching duties are part of her job.

Although Professor Jones teaches English, she is also our rugby coach, and her coaching duties are part of her job.

2. Many colleges in New York are private. Most students attend the public colleges and universities. Many of these students do not live in New York State.

While most students attend the public colleges and universities, many in New York are private, and many of the students attending private colleges do not live in New York State.

3. My English professor for composition was good. He taught me how to formulate coherent essays. He also taught me how to recognize grammatical problems.

My English professor for composition taught me how to formulate coherent essays and how to recognize grammatical problems.

4. The buildings on campus are old. Some are still useful and have character. Others are outdated and need to be demolished.

Although the buildings on campus are old, some are still useful and have character, while others are outdated and need to be demolished.

PAGE 97
EXERCISES: SENTENCE VARIATION
COMBINING SIMPLE SENTENCES FOR SENTENCE VARIETY

Directions: Combine the following groups of sentences into one effective simple or complex sentence.

1. The nurse prepared the sterile tray. The physician intended to perform a lumbar puncture.

As the nurse prepared the sterile tray, the physician intended to perform a spinal tap.

2. A woman went into labor. Her family waited nervously. They were to be informed of any new details.

As her family waited nervously to be informed of any new details, the woman went into labor.

3. The patient in room 341 window has pancreatitis. His blood count is low as a result.

The patient in room 341 window has pancreatitis, which is the cause of his blood count.

4. The patient is a 3-year-old boy. He was jumping on the bed. There was a pencil on the bed. The boy fell. The pencil went into his eye.

The patient, a 3-year-old boy, was jumping on the bed when he fell and lodged a pencil into his eye.

5. Dr. Gutman referred Ted Brimes to our office. Dr. Gutman diagnosed Mr. Brimes with rotator cuff tendonitis.

Dr. Gutman referred Ted Brimes to our office and diagnosed him with rotator cuff tendonitis.

6. The nurse's aide transported the patient from the emergency room to the intensive care unit. The patient, Mr. White, began to arrest in atrial fibrillation. The nurse's aide began CPR in the middle of the hallway.

While the nurse's aide transported the patient from the emergency room to the intensive care unit, the patient, Mr. White, beginning to arrest in atrial fibrillation, forced the nurse's aid to begin CPR in the middle of the hallway.

7. The radiologist detected an abnormality on the patient's mammogram. The ultrasound exam of the patient's breast revealed a mass. The physician performed a biopsy.

As the radiologist detected an abnormality on the patient's mammogram, the ultrasound exam of the patient's breast revealed a mass, which encouraged the physician to perform a biopsy.

8. Samantha Green complained of sharp pain in her lower right quadrant. Her physician believed she had appendicitis. Ultrasound examination identified her problem as ovarian cysts.

As Samantha Green complained of sharp pain in her lower right quadrant, her physician believed she had appendicitis until the ultrasound examination identified her problem as ovarian cysts.

9. The patient arrived in the emergency room at 6:30 A.M. complaining of a migraine. By 6:40 A.M., the patient developed a temperature of 103° Fahrenheit. He began to have seizures at 6:45 A.M. His condition worsened rapidly.

   The patient arrived in the emergency room at 6:30 A.M. complaining of a migraine, developed a temperature of 103° Fahrenheit by 6:40 A.M., and began to have seizures at 6:45 A.M., when his condition worsened rapidly.

10. Margaret Levett had a stroke 6 months ago. She visits the speech therapist, physical therapist, and occupational therapist daily. Her functional skills are recovering quickly with the therapy.

    Suffering a stroke 6 months ago, Margaret Levett visits the speech therapist, physical therapist, and occupational therapist daily through which her functional skills are recovering quickly with the therapy.

PAGE 97
IDENTIFYING THE FOUR TYPES OF SENTENCES

Directions: Identify the following sentences as simple (**S**), compound (**CP**), complex (**CX**), or compound-complex (**CP-CX**).

1. Although the emergency room was full, the unit maintained strict schedule and tended to patients quickly. **CX**

2. The physical therapist recommends 6 weeks of therapy three times a week. **S**

3. When a patient visits the office complaining of chest pain, the nurses automatically record an ECG on the patient, and, if the doctor finds any problems, an ambulance rapidly transports the patient to the emergency room. **CP-CX**

4. Being a pediatric neurosurgeon requires immense dexterity, and it also demands extreme patience. **CP**

5. The patient prepared with physical therapy for 3 weeks prior to the surgery. **S**

6. The physician explained the traditional treatment for the patient's disease, but the patient decided to seek an unconventional intervention. **CP**

PAGE 97
COMBINING SIMPLE SENTENCES

Directions: Combine the following groups of simple sentences to form a compound, complex, or compound-complex sentence.

1. Dr. Hoffmann practices ophthalmology. He specializes in macular degeneration.
   Dr. Hoffmann practices ophthalmology, and he specializes in macular degeneration.

2. The doctor diagnosed Mr. Whitman with dermatitis. He referred the patient to a local dermatologist.
   Although the doctor diagnosed Mr. Whitman with dermatitis, he referred the patient to a local dermatologist.

3. All blood tests done on the patient returned normal. He was discharged in good health.
   Since all blood tests done on the patient returned normal, he was discharged in good health.

4. The emergency medical technician administered the Ambu bag. The victim suffered from heat exhaustion and collapsed.
   The emergency medical technician administered the Ambu bag because the victim suffered from heat exhaustion and collapsed.

PAGE 97
EXERCISES: PHRASES
IDENTIFYING TYPES OF PHRASES

Directions: In the following examples, identify the italicized phrases as participial, gerund, prepositional, or infinitive phrases.

1. *Reading the mammogram* proved more difficult than the radiologist expected. *(Gerund)*

2. *To begin the day*, the nurse recorded the vital signs of his 30 patients. *(Infinitive)*

3. The doctor informed the patient, *Mrs. Grouse, about the diagnosis, Raynaud's phenomenon, and the possible course of treatment. (Appositive, participial including an appositive)*

4. *Under the supervision of a faculty physician*, the resident correctly diagnosed over one

hundred cases *throughout the year*. *(Prepositional, prepositional)*

5. *Distracted by the activity in the emergency room*, the patient answered the doctor's questions incorrectly. *(Participial)*

6. The patient and the doctor jointly decided *to continue the chemotherapy treatment*. *(Infinitive)*

7. *Talking* remains the most effective therapy *for the families of the ill*. *(Gerund, prepositional)*

8. *Through extended discourse with other physicians*, Dr. Link determined the patient's diagnosis: gastric cancer. *(Prepositional, appositive)*

PAGE 98
USING PHRASES TO COMBINE SENTENCES

Directions: Combine the following sentences to create a participial, gerund, prepositional, appositive, or infinitive phrase.

1. The hospital specializes in trauma cases. It receives hundreds of trauma cases a week.

   Specializing in trauma, the hospital receives hundreds of trauma cases a week. *(Participial)*

2. The patient is a 45-year-old woman. She complains of abdominal pain and back pain.

   The patient, a 45-year-old woman, complains of abdominal pain and back pain. *(Appositive)*

3. The physician was not sure about the diagnosis. He discussed the case with other physicians.

   In order to be sure about the diagnosis, he discussed the case with other physicians. *(Prepositional)*

4. The patient underwent total knee replacement yesterday. She began physical therapy today. The therapist visited the patient in her room.

   Undergoing total knee replacement yesterday and beginning physical therapy today caused the therapist to visit the patient in her room. *(Gerund)*

5. The patient visited the lab to have blood drawn. He must have blood tests done weekly. His physician requires the tests to monitor his blood coagulation.

   To monitor his blood coagulation, the physician required that he have blood drawn weekly, and the patient visited the lab to have blood drawn. *(Infinitive)*

6. Tanya Brass has diabetes. The nurse checks her blood sugar every 2 hours. The patient required further testing to confirm a diagnosis. The podiatrist requested another appointment.

   Requiring further testing to confirm a diagnosis of diabetes, the podiatrist requested another appointment and ordered the nurse to check blood sugar of the patient, Tanya Brass. *(Participial, appositive)*

PAGE 100
EXERCISES: SENTENCE VARIETY IN THE ESSAY
CREATING SENTENCE VARIETY

Directions: Change the sentence structure in the following passage to create continuity and flow and to eliminate choppiness and/or wordiness.

Revisions will vary. Target areas involving diction and wording problems are in **bold** *type. Sentence monotony problems are in* **italics**. *All subject-verb combinations are underscored.*

The new manager of Buffalo Allied Health has submitted a report in which she has outlined several problems that she feels **are** responsible for the low production that has been plaguing her facility. *(Sentence drags on because of phrases and clauses attached to the end of the independent clause.)* The first problem that she identifies is that employees and therapists **are** working with equipment that they have not **been specifically** trained to use. *(Sentence is weakened with dependence on "to be" verbs.)* **There are** often significant differences that she has identified between the preparation workers have and the actual tasks that they are expected to perform. She feels that **this** is the primary reason for poor productivity. Her report also indicates that absenteeism in the Therapy Clinic is 15% higher than that which is experienced by the surrounding clinics and hospital facilities. **It is** also noted in her report that she can find no reason for the higher absenteeism. She is willing to speculate that **there is** a relationship between poor training and low morale. **This** can cause employees to be absent from work. The third problem in the clinic noted in her report is **that because** the Clinic operates some of the company's oldest equipment, down time and a lack of spare parts leave many workers idle for what she calls "extended periods." *(Was the second problem clearly identified?)* The manager speculates that these three problems could be the causes for low productivity. She adds that until the Clinic has newer equipment and better training for its personnel, productivity will continue to be a problem.

PAGE 101
SAMPLE STUDENT ESSAY: IDENTIFYING AND CORRECTING SENTENCE VARIATION PROBLEMS

Directions: Examine the following sample student essay and identify the problems in sentence variation. All sentences begin with the same format: S-V-O. Look for ways to combine sentences, coordinate, subordinate, or use the phrases and sentence types to make this work a readable piece.

Revisions will vary according to what writers consider is important enough to be included in independent clauses and what information can be subordinated into dependent clauses or phrases. All diction and wording problems that lead to sentence monotony or to confusion are in **bold** *type. All subject-verb combinations are underscored.*

MTV is a popular television station among teenagers. The videos MTV plays expose young people to **unnecessary** material. The material teens view in the videos is **highly** influential. Teens begin to duplicate the actions they see. Many people consider the material in music videos obscene. Something obscene is offensive to a group or person, includes indecent gestures, and contains degrading or immoral material *(parallel structure problem?)*.

In some music videos, artists make offensive references to different groups of people. The groups **most referred to** are gays and minorities. Videos offend the gay community by portraying gay relationships as being inappropriate. Teens viewing videos of this nature receive the impression that same-sex relationships are disgusting. The most offensive videos toward minorities are rap videos. Rap videos depict gang activity between groups. **This offends** minority groups because the videos give the impression that the groups portrayed are uncivilized. MTV makes no attempt to censor its material. It does blur some activities. These activities, however, are no secret. Young people will conclude that the images being hidden are exciting. They will want to replicate them even more.

The music videos played on MTV are obscene. They are obscene to many people for different reasons. The videos offend gays and minorities by portraying their lifestyles as wrong. The material in videos gives teenagers **the wrong impression**, teaches disrespect, and influences teens to follow in the same obscene behavior.

CHAPTER 5

Changes to sentences are provided in parentheses. In some cases, the italicized words are identified as targets for which various word choice or diction replacements could substitute.

PAGE 145
EXERCISES: EDITING, REVISING, AND PROOFREADING
EDITING

Directions: Revise the following passage by demonstrating your knowledge of professional/academic writing skills. You may consider reorganizing and rewriting the entire passage to make it a coherent whole.

The new director of physical therapy has submitted a report *(add comma)* which he has outlined several problems that he feels *is (are)* responsible for the department's failure to *receive* compensation for treatments. The first problem he identifies *is when (predication prob-*

lem) therapists are not *clear (what does this mean?)* in stating their rationale for treatment, *(comma splice. Change to semicolon)* additionally, he cites poor writing skills as the main reason for the following: *There are (diction)* often significant differences between therapists writing *(insert comma)* but he says that most students cannot organize his/her thoughts clear. *(This sentence does not use coordination effectively. Additionally, all sentences to this point begin with subject-verb monotony and can be more fluid with the addition of sentence variety strategies.)* Which is a major problem *(sentence fragment)*. Although many students are *taking* writing classes *(sentence fragment)*. After *taking* such writing classes, the documents *are often plagued (passive voice construction)* with other problems such as: *(colon is misused here because it does not end an independent clause)* sentence fragments, run on sentences and the therapists constantly write comma splices. *Another problem is not describing* the medical necessity of procedures. But *("But" should be used as a coordinating conjunction and not a sentence opener)* this *(unclear)* is *getting (weak verb)* better because students are being taught to define medical necessity in their documentation. Documentation should *say* the appropriateness of treatment too; *(semicolon is incorrect because it does not separate two independent clauses)* as this demonstrates that the Therapists *(capitalization and possession)* work is of the quality of meeting general medical standards. *It is* also found that documentation is needed to educate payors and patients as well. All therapists must be able to educate others *(other practitioners?)* or the profession will suffer. *And this brings us to statement five, (comma splice)* we need to *get* reimbursed for *your (pronoun agreement)* services which *(that)* are rendered. *It is* also a problem that writers/therapists' *(incorrect identification of possession)* don't know how to use commas, *(eliminate unnecessary comma)* or other marks of punctuation accurately. Writers/therapists also don't use *good* sentence variety. They have several short sentences that are choppy. They should have sentences that show the four types of sentences and the five types of

phrases. They use verbs that are weak and passive too. *(These are all short and choppy sentences, identified by the redundant starting word "They." Employ sentence variety strategies here.)* Sentence combination skills are required by many educated people to provide *this*. Because subordination and coordination of an idea is good for readers *(sentence fragment)*. Proofreading and editing skills are needed *(insert comma)* and therapists should always remember *what is needed* for documentation that is effective.

PAGE 145
REVISION

Directions: Employing the strategies of writing/revising that you have learned, rewrite the following essay.

The new manager of Buffalo Allied Health has submitted a report in which she has outlined several problems that she feels are responsible for the low production that has been plaguing her facility *(overuse of "that" clauses)*. The *first (does this word intend an order?)* problem that she identifies is that employees and therapists are working with equipment *that they have not been specifically trained to use (wordiness)*. *There are (diction)* often significant differences that she has identified between the preparation workers *have (weak verb)* and the actual tasks that they are expected to perform. She feels that *this (unclear)* is the primary reason for poor productivity. Her report also indicates that absenteeism in the Therapy Clinic is 15% higher than that which is experienced by the surrounding clinics and hospital facilities. *(Writer abandons order established by the previous use of "first." Also, sentence variety problem can be identified here because of the consistent form of each sentence: S-V-O.)* It is also noted in her report that she can find no reason for *the* higher absenteeism. She is willing to speculate that *there is* a relationship between poor training and low morale. This can cause employees to be absent from work. *(Again, choppiness and monotony can be changed with sentence variety strategies.)* The *third* problem in the clinic noted in her report *is that because* the Clinic operates some of the company's oldest equipment, down time and a lack of spare parts leave many workers idle for what she calls "extended periods." *(Identify what this quote means.)* The manager speculates that these three problems could be the causes for low productivity. She adds that until the Clinic has newer equipment and better training for its personnel, productivity will continue to be a *problem.*

PAGE 146
EDITING AND PROOFREADING AN EVALUATION

Directions: Find and fix all the problems with this evaluation.

Upon treating Jane Smith for the past four months, *she ("She" should be changed to "I," which would reinvent the entire sentence. This problem results from dangling modifier)* has gained movement, sensation, and balance *back* on her left side after *having* a stroke *last March (Give specific dates)*. Mrs. Smith is able to perform *some (vague)* of her daily functional activities. She has been discharged two weeks ago. *I would appreciate (Choose specific language to request reimbursement)* a reimbursement for the services rendered. *(short and choppy sentences)*

Dr. Thomas referred Jane to physical therapy. *(Coherence break between these two sentences)* She *desires* to ambulate a normal distance in order to *do* her daily activities. Jane, a 55-year-old female that *(who)* lives with her husband in an apartment *(This is a sentence fragment)*. She was a healthy person with *no* medical history prior to the stroke. She has been working as a library clerk for 20 years. Jane's goal is to *go back* to work after physical therapy. *(Coherence break)* She suffered a mild stroke. The most important exercises for Mrs. Smith at this time is maintaining her balance and coordination. Mrs. Smith did not *have* any physical therapy prior to her visit to the clinic. Upon evaluation, the patient has shown capability to stand and ambulate with one physical therapist assisting her. Transferring from chair to bed also *needs to be worked on.* The patient's left arm and leg requires strengthening exercises *(vague)*. To test

the patient's strength and ability, I *went through* some active and passive ROM. I wanted to evaluate how severely the stroke *effected (affected)* her. *(Language in this description is unprofessional and the thought processes are jumbled. The document requires reorganization.)*

PAGE 146
EDITING AND PROOFREADING A REIMBURSEMENT NARRATIVE

Directions: Find and fix the errors in all facets of the writing process.

Mr. James *recently (meaningless time reference)* arrived in the hospital emergency room with a *very* serious heart condition. James *happens* to be covered under *your* insurance policy for up to $500 for an emergency room visit. *In closely evaluating this policy, with reference to Mr. James' specific case, I (Why is the practitioner evaluating the policy?)* am fully aware that reimbursement for services rendered will only be satisfied when the *payor (confusing between second person and third person)* deems the patient's treatment "medically necessary." Therefore, I intend to validate the options of treatment that I administered to James and prove their crucial necessity.

Mr. James, referred to us by Dr. Carlton, *possesses* a history of ventricular fibrillation *(insert comma or change "which" to "that.")* which previously resulted in two cardiac arrests. In addition, he *suffered from a double by-pass surgery whereby he emerged with the presence of* a minimal functional strength deficit in both his lower extremities. A systematic evaluation of his electrocardiogram records over the past five years, beginning with his first cardiac arrest, illustrates a gradual *increase in the severity* of his ventricular fibrillation. Before his recent visit to the emergency room *(insert comma)* the fibrillation discomfort and general strength deficit have persisted as his only complaints.

James arrived by ambulance in full cardiac arrest. *Responding to the seriousness of the situation, he (dangling modifier)* underwent resuscitation. With no response, I immediately *defibrillated him to initiate* a steady heart rhythm.

PAGE 146

EDITING AND PROOFREADING:
SENTENCES AND PASSAGES

Directions: Find all the errors in the sentences and passages below and correct.

The therapists in this department are *going to work* with the patient to *get* his ROM and strength *back to where it needs to be* to function properly.

It is important to have early motion because it *decreases effusion, pain, and inhibits fear (parallel structure problem:* decreases effusion and pain, and it inhibits fear*)*. Weights should also be used early, but in *small* amounts and *little by little*.

It is essential for her to attend physical therapy to repair her ROM of the petellofemoral joint and *strength (parallel structure:* to strengthen*)* of the quadriceps and hamstring muscles.

She was able to *handle (lift)* 25 lbs. of weights.

The *onset began (redundancy)* when she fell.

The left biceps and triceps *had (measured)* 5 out of 5.

The patient *received* treatment for her right shoulder. The treatment *consists (verb-tense shift from past in "received" to present in "consists.")* of electrical stimulation, ultrasound, joint mobilization, and exercises from active-assisted and active-free ROM to active-resisted. The exercises included using pulleys, *(delete unnecessary comma)* and *pendulum*. The exercises *were used (passive)* to strengthen the patients' strength, *(delete unnecessary comma)* and ROM.

Patient's ability to perform daily activities should *show a little improvement*.

She has *problems going from* wheelchair to shower. The use of crutches *is a must*.

On the other hand, she will receive treatment.

No specific action was recalled by the patient. *(passive voice construction)*

The patient was requested *(passive voice construction)* to participate in exercises and *attending (parallel structure:* attend*)* therapy.

Edna fractured her right radius on 3/3/00. She injured her radius by slipping on ice. *(Try sentence combining strategies to provide flow to these short and choppy sentences.)*

The patient is not allowed *to put weight on* leg, *(Comma splice. Change comma to semicolon or add information to provide continuity between action and measurement.)* no coordination can be measured.

The pain can be *intense* at time, *(Comma splice. Change comma to semicolon)* on a scale of 1–10, she *says it can vary*.

The stairs will be *slow going, (insert semicolon to avoid comma splice)* however *(insert comma)* she will *have* a ramp to help these *things*.

She may lean to *(too)* far and *end up* hurting herself.

Patient should have been able to increase movement *back* to it's *(stands for "it is," which is not correct.)* original status. *Although the therapy proved unsuccessful because the patient still experiences problems. (sentence fragment)*

In evaluating the information obtained during the exam, they (dangling modifier) can be organized and interpreted in the following way.

Patient demonstrates normal ROM, and *this (unclear) is where (predication)* we will concentrate our efforts.

He will be encouraged to continue those exercises when he is not in the clinic *(insert comma)* and he will also be *given* additional exercises for home.

Good posture is essential for him because it will *help with* his aerobic capacity for sports, and it will benefit treatment because posture affects joint integrity *(insert comma)* which is *what we are trying to get the most out of*.

Dr. Meyers diagnosed the patient on 9/8/00 *(insert comma)* and on 9/15/00 *(insert comma using option to rule)* reconstructive surgery *was performed (passive)*.

The treatment that Mr. Smith *receives* on a *regular basis* would improve his ROM, *(delete unnecessary comma)* and strengthen his muscles *gradually (can he strengthen muscles in any other way?)*.

The patient *(insert comma)* being an avid basketball star *(insert comma to complete nonessential element)* has experienced many problems.

The patient will attend *5 ("5" should be written as a word)* sessions three or four times per week.

Some of the injuries are listed below, *(replace comma with colon)*
1. Torn ACL
2. Dislocated knee
3. Sprain to knee

(Use of numbers here is not necessary because the list does not indicate a specific order)

The patient engages in strenuous exercises such as; *(eliminate any mark of punctuation here as the list completes the sentence)* running, jumping, and swimming.

CHAPTER 8

PAGE 209
EXERCISE: BUILDING THE REFERENCES SECTION

Directions: Reinvent the following list of references according to an acceptable style manual format. Identify what type of source is listed; then apply the appropriate format. Be sure to identify and change problems in mechanics (capitalization, underlining) as well as simple formatting.

1. Lanshire, Phillip. "Why We Need Direct Access" Home page: http://www.chass.com
2. Snyder, Peter and Diane Olsen. "A Pore Segment: DEG in Channels." Journal of Biological Sciences, 1999, 24, p. 74. Chem Abstracts database, May 24, 2000, www.Chemabstracts.com/pore/
3. Bowling, A. (1997). Research Methods in Health: an Investigation of the Brain. Buckingham, Open Univ. Press.
4. Measuring Disease. Handbook of qualitative research. 2000. pp. 47–59.
5. Publication Manual of the American Psychological Association. (your edition)
6. Lewitus, A.J., R.V. Jesien, T.W. Kana, E. May, M. Herzog, J.H. Hawkins, and R.S. Cone.

1990. Species distribution of Ulcerative Lesions of Pimlico Sound Fish. Journal of Aquatic Research, 22, 1304.

Revision

American Psychiatric Association. (2001). *Publication manual of the American Psychological Association* (5th ed.). Washington, DC: Author.

Bowling, A. (1997). *Research methods in health: An investigation of the brain*. Buckingham: Open University Press.

Lanshire, P. (n.d.). *Why we need direct access*. Retrieved July 9, 2003 from http://www.chass.com.

Lewitus, A. J., Jesien, R. V., Kana, T. W., May, E., Herzog, M., Hawkins, J. H., et al. (1990). Species distribution of ulcerative lesions of Pimlico Sound fish. *Journal of Aquatic Research, 22,* 1304.

Measuring disease. (2000). *Handbook of qualitative research* (pp. 47–59).

Snyder, Peter, & Olsen, D. (1999). A pore segment: DEG in channels. *Journal of Biological Sciences, 24,* 74. Retrieved May 24, 2000, from Chem Abstracts database.

PAGE 213
EXERCISE: PARAPHRASING

Directions: Read the following passages and then write acceptable paraphrases of each.

1. The University of Michigan time-analysis data confer that traditional college-aged students spent the bulk of their lives in structured, adult-oriented activities. They are the most honed and supervised generation in human history. If they are group-oriented, deferential to authority, and achievement-obsessed, it is because we achievement-besotted adults have trained them to be. We have devoted our prodigious energies to imposing a sort of order and responsibility on our kids' lives that we never experienced ourselves. [from Brooks, D. (April 2001). The organizational kid. The Atlantic, 287(4): 40–54.]

2. Opiate poisoning is easily treated and reversed with naloxone. Large doses of naloxone may be needed to treat massive

opiate overdoses because it has a short half-life of only 15–20 minutes. Treating opiate overdose in chronic opiate user can precipitate acute withdrawal. Classic symptoms of acute withdrawal include vomiting, cramping, and yawning, and sweating. [from Salyer, S. W., & Battista, R. (2001). Managing the acutely poisoned patient. <u>Physician Assistant, 25</u>(6): 41–49.]

3. Following the fall salmon run, steelhead trout enter the Niagara River, feeding greedily on the millions of eggs deposited by the spawning salmon. Steelhead are a silvery lake-run version of rainbow trout, and the best time to fish for these hard fighters is December through March. Fishing is done with small "kwikfish" lures or by drifting egg skeins near the river bottom. [from Raykovicz, M. (2001). Niagara: River of opportunity. <u>New York State Conservationist, 55</u>(6): 19–21.]

Paraphrasing Examples

1. According to Brooks (2001), parents today have molded and shaped their teenage children into the responsible, ambitious, and respectful young adults that they were not.

2. Because of its fast decaying time, the drug naloxone is used to "treat and reverse" (p. 41) the effects of "opiate poisoning" (Salyer & Battista, 2001, p. 42). According to Salyer and Battista (2001), in some opiate addicts, use of naloxone causes severe "withdrawal symptoms" (p. 42) including nausea, regurgitation, and increased perspiration.

3. According to Raykovicz (2001), the optimal time to catch steelhead trout is during the winter months, owing to the abundance of other fish eggs remaining from the "fall salmon run" (p. 20) for the trout to feed upon. Anglers use smaller sized "lures" (p. 20) or real fish eggs to attract the feasting trout (Raykovicz, 2001).

PAGE 218
EXERCISE: REVISING THE RESEARCH PAPER

Directions: Revise and rewrite the following proposal to make it an acceptable document for standard, academic writing by employing any and all strategies that we have addressed thus far in this text. You must address writing issues on several levels: essay, paragraph, sentence, and word. You should also add or delete information when appropriate or reorganize the essay as needed to meet demands of logic and proportion. Additionally, the "References" section does not meet the standards represented by the APA style manual or any other style manual. Make the appropriate changes and also change the inaccurate information in the in-text citations.

Title: Media Effects on Body Image in College-Aged Women

Today, according to mass mediums, a thin fat-free body is seen as the ideal body in our culture. In a body image survey conducted by Psychology today, it was revealed that 15% of woman say they would sacrifice more than five years of their lives to be at their desired weight. (Spitzer et al 1999) Anything from soap operas to film to popular magazines are influencing women to set for what the most part is unrealistic and unattainable goals for how they want to see themselves. Which is called the Cinderella Syndrome. The ideal body weight portrayed by the media is one that is 13–19% below what is considered healthy (Schell 1998) yet it is one that woman use as a standard for comparing themselves. (Wilcox and Laird 2000) Body dissatisfaction and a desire to loose weight has become a norm for collage age woman which begins a lifetime of that thinking and feeling. Advertising, their friends, magazines, their mother, movies and their romantic partner are rated by Collage woman as more influential of their ideas about attractiveness then did men in a study done by Reed in 1998. Overall adolescent and collage-age woman are at the highest risk as their body fat and weight concern competes with biological reality. (Owen & Laurel-Seller 2000) Even with these alarming statistics role models in the media follows the trends of the Miss America Pageant winners, since the 1950's these woman's body sizes have decreased significantly as well as Playboy centerfolds; of whom one-third meet the Body Mass Index criterion for anorexia nervousa. In my study I plan on trying to find out if there is any relationship between brief media exposure and a decreased body satisfaction, drive for thinness and perfectionism. I also plan on comparing their Eating Disorder Inventory results with the participant's actual weight to see if there any that are overweight and if that has any affect on their perceptions. I plan to use clips from this years Miss America Pageant; to see if watching these woman on TV has an affect on their body image and satisfaction which I made up. There is also a control that I use half will watch a clip from the popular TV show The Price is Right. I am hoping to find that even brief exposure to these "skinny" woman can have affects on one's thoughts and feelings about their own body. I will use a measure of eating disorders, the Eating Disorder Inventory (EDI) before the participant watches the video clip and then I will question the participants after the video clip regarding drive for thinness and body satisfaction. I think I will find a relationship between woman who have a low score on body satisfaction, and also have some characteristics of having a eating disorder. I have enclosed the Eating Disorder Inventory. Members of Daemen College faculty have used this in the past, and find it a reputable measure.

Works Cited

Spitzer, D. and Jones, Michael, and Slade, Samuel. (1999). The Cinderella Syndrome. Psychology Today. Vol. 25. Number 6. Pages: 25–35

Reed, Marian (1998). Women and Men in College. Bantam, NY, pp. 215, 217, 299, and 306.

Schell, David. (1998). Media Measures and The Ideal Body. Journal of Adolescent Psychology, 2.6 (February): pages 6–12.

Wilcox, F. & Laird, Sandra. (2000). The Eating Disorder Inventory: theory and application. Eating Disorders Quarterly. Vol 6. Num. 1. Pages: 117–119.

Owen, William and Laurel, Seller. (2000). Eating Disorders and the Adolescent. Prentice Hall. 2000. New York and Tokyo. Pages 200–209.

Revision: Sample Student Response

Media Effects on Body Image in College-Age Women

Since the 1950s, women in the media, many of whom are role models to young women, appear more slender; thus, according to mass media, a majority of American women view the ideal body as thin and "fat-free" (Owen & Laurel, 2000; Reed, 1998). Women influenced by the media to set unrealistic and unattainable goals for their body image are identified as having the Cinderella syndrome. According to Schell (1998), the ideal body weight for women, as portrayed by the media, is 13–19% below the healthy weight. Although one-third of the women in the media are classified as having anorexia nervosa, college-age women continue to compare themselves to the ideal body weight (Wilcox et al., 2000). As a result, body dissatisfaction and a desire to lose weight have become a norm for college-age women. According to a body image survey conducted by Spitzer, Jones, and Slade (1999), 15% of women would sacrifice more than 5 years of their lives to attain their desired weight. In my study, I will identify the effects of brief media exposure on college-age women's perspective on their body image.

In order to correlate a relationship between mass media and body image of the participants, I will use various film and television clips showing slender young women, including the Miss America Pageant. Before the television clips, each of the participants will be weighed and then questioned about her body image perspective and satisfaction. The Eating Disorder Inventory (EDI) will be used to categorize each of the participant's weight into one of the following categories: healthy weight, overweight, or eating disorder. After the television clips, the participants will be questioned again about their body image perspective and satisfaction in order to legitimize the negative effects of brief media exposure on body image in college-age women.

References

Owen, W., & Laurel, S. (2000). *Eating disorders and the adolescent*. New York: Prentice Hall.

Reed, M. (1998). *Women and men in college*. New York: Bantam.

Schell, D. (1998, February). Media measures and the ideal body. *Journal of Adolescent Psychology*, *2*(6), 6–12.

Spitzer, D., Jones, M., & Slade, S. (1999). The Cinderella syndrome. *Psychology Today*, *25*(6), 25–35.

Wilcox, F., & Laird, S. (2000). The Eating Disorder Inventory: Theory and application. *Eating Disorders Quarterly*, *6*(1), 117–119.

CHAPTER 11

PAGE 273
EXERCISE: EDITING FOR CONTINUITY AND FLOW

Directions: Examine the following paper, submitted by a student as a rough draft, and consider the italicized text, which indicates problems, and correct. Then look at the paragraphs throughout the paper and find the ones that read like lists. Consider how you might draw transitions between these paragraphs to build continuity and coherence.

Additional corrections in style and mechanics have been made.

Christopher Adams, a 17-year-old high school student, started attending physical therapy on September 29, 2000. Dr. Matthew Myers referred Christopher to therapy after he underwent reconstructive surgery on his left patellofemoral joint (knee). Christopher entered physical therapy with pain and stiffness in his knee, which he was unable to flex or extend with ease. Since he first attended physical therapy a *(1?)* month ago, he has made significant progress and will be able to finish therapy at an earlier date than originally anticipated, if *there are* no complications. He will need to continue therapy for at least 3 more months for supervised exercising and strengthening to ensure that he does not further injure his knee. Chris has been attending therapy regularly three times a week for the past month *and* has only missed one visit due to lack of transportation.

When Chris started physical therapy, he was confined *(is this the right word? I don't think HE himself was confined to the brace.)* to a knee brace that limited his movement. He no longer needs the brace and has *progressed nicely (vague)* without it. Chris has made *excellent (vague)* progress on both active and passive range of motion for his patellofemoral joint. With active range of motion, he has increased in extension from 140° to 165° and in flexion from 90° to 100°. With passive range of motion, he has increased in extension from 160° to 175° and in flexion from 95° to 110°. This is an above *(hyphenate)* average increase considering he has been attending therapy for only 1 month.

Christopher also showed improvement in the manual muscle test for strength. For extension, he *progresses (past tense?)* from a two out of five to a four out of five. For flexion, he *progressed* from a three out of five to a four and a half out of five. *(Since you are using a numerical scoring method, you can use numbers here. Example: 4½.)*

Chris (appropriate?) reports decreased pain in his leg using the same scale of 1 to 10, with 10 being the worst pain. With walking, his pain has decreased from a 7 out of 10 to a 4 out of 10. During excessive movement, he now experiences a 5 out of 10 instead of a 9 out of 10, which is still his worst pain. He now sleeps much better since his pain has diminished from a 5½ out of 10 to a 2 out of 10. *(Relevance? Was sleep an issue?)*

Christopher's ability to perform his exercises has *enhanced (word choice)* to a level close to his previous capability of performance. He has now moved beyond simple stretching to more intense stretching along with leg presses and squat exercises on the Total Gym. While warming up, he continues to alternate between the bicycle and the treadmill. He also performs exercises at home two to three times a day. Even though he is progressing smoothly and effectively, his mother has reported that he is not performing the exercises on a regular schedule. I have talked with Christopher about *doing (word choice)* his exercises at home and explained to him the importance of them. *(Transition)* He will not receive therapy for an extended period of time and needs to continue his exercises in order to keep up his strength and mobility. The exercises are also important for him to reduce scar tissue, which can *immensely slow down (awkward and vague—find a single word as a substitute for these.)* his recovery process.

(Transition) Chris has progressed on the platform system for balancing. He now has the capability to bear full unilateral weight on his left leg and balance on his leg without the assistance of a therapist or a wall. A therapist does, however, stand by in case he loses his balance.

(Transition) Chris has electrical stimulation with cold packs applied to his left leg by a therapist to provide increased input to the quadriceps and hamstrings. This technique will alleviate pain and stiffness to the patellofemoral joint, making it easier for Chris to perform his exercises.

Physical therapy may not be required for the full 6 months, but *it is* in Christopher's best interest to continue therapy three times a week for at least 2 more months, after which he will be reevaluated on his progress. Chris needs to continue attending physical therapy for supervision while performing his rehabilitation program to alleviate any possibility of reinjury to his knee.

My short-term goals for Christopher's rehabilitation include a continuation of better range of motion of his patellofemoral joint and increase *(increased?)* strength of his lower extremity muscles. I would like to increase his range of motion 2–3° for both flexion and extension within the next week. The pain in Chris's knee should be alleviated within the next month.

Christopher desires to play football again along with other sports, *so* over the long term, I would like to return Chris's range of motion and strength to normal *so* he is capable of playing sports again. In relation to Chris's right knee, his left knee should possess full range of motion and full strength by the time therapy *is completed (passive)*.

PAGE 274
EXERCISE: EDITING FOR WORD CHOICE AND DICTION

Directions: Examine the following paper, which a student submitted as a rough draft, and consider the words and phrases highlighted in italics. Review each mark and determine why these comments are made.

Preliminary Assessment

Christopher Adams tore the anterior cruciate ligament (ACL) of his left knee at a high school football game, which required reconstructive surgery. *It is* essential for Chris to attend physical therapy to repair his range of motion of the patellofemoral joint (knee) and *to strengthen his* . . . strength of the quadriceps and hamstring muscles.

REFERRAL

An orthopedic surgeon, Dr. Matthew Myers, referred Chris to the Physical Therapy Department at St. Joseph's Hospital in order to advance with the recovery process following a weekend of rest.

Data Accompanying Referral

Dr. Myers diagnosed Chris on September 8, 2000 *(comma)* with a torn ACL *(comma)* and on September 15, reconstructive surgery was performed *(who performed? = passive voice. Dr. Myers performed . . .)* on Chris's knee. Dr. Myers prescribed ibuprofen for any pain and/or inflammation accompanying the surgery. Crutches and a functional knee brace will also be needed after surgery. For the first 2 to 3 weeks after surgery, the brace needs to be set with limitations of the final 20° extension and flexion to 90° or greater. Following those initial weeks after surgery, the brace is adjusted so *there is* unlimited flexion with some limitations on extension that progressively decrease until full extension is possible.

Patient History

- Name: Christopher Adams
- Date of birth: June 30, 1983
- Age: 17
- Gender: Male
- Start of care: September 29, 2000
- Primary complaint: stiffness and soreness in the knee and weakness in the muscles of the left leg

Referral Diagnosis

Christopher tore his ACL in a football game when he was tackled on a play. He was sent to the hospital for x-ray and MRI examinations to diagnose the injury. *These tests showed how serious the tear was (awkward)* and what type of treatment would be necessary.

Prior Therapy History

Chris has not undergone physical therapy prior to our first session.

EVALUATION

While the evaluation and tests were performed, the following data were collected about the patient's injury.

Baseline Evaluation Data

Christopher is *very (omit)* cooperative and follows direction well. He is anxious to get his rehabilitation program started so he can get back to his everyday activities, including football.

Posture

Chris's posture is excellent, which will *greatly (omit)* benefit his progress with rehabilitation. Good posture is essential for him because it will help with his aerobic capacity for sports, and it will benefit treatment because posture affects joint integrity and mobility *(comma)* which *is what we are trying to get the most out of (awkward and wordy)*.

AROM/PROM

Chris *demonstrates* normal range of motion for his injury, with his active range of motion (AROM) at 140° for extension, and for flexion, he *demonstrated (verb tense problem—is he currently demonstrating this or did he demonstrate in his tests at a previous date/time? [maintain consistency with verb tense throughout each section])* his AROM to be 90°. When testing passive range of motion (PROM), he demonstrated 160° for extension and 79° for flexion.

Before his injury of his left knee *and with his right knee (omit)*, Chris had full range of motion *(add: in both knees)*, which included 180° for extension and 70° for flexion.

Strength

During the manual muscle test for strength, Chris showed that his muscle strength of extension is a 2/5 and for flexion his strength is a 3/5. Normally, Chris shows full strength of 5/5 for both extension and flexion.

Pain

When asked about pain, Chris stated that he notices pain in his knee when walking or with excessive movement *(comma)* and when he is sleeping, it wakes him up when he rolls onto his left side. Based on a scale from 1 to 10, with 10 being the worst amount of pain, he describes his pain when walking to be a 7/10 *(comma)* and with excessive movement, *his pain is the worst being at a (awkward)* 9/10. When Chris sleeps, his pain is not unbearable, but it *is enough to* wake him up, being at about a 5.5/10.

Activity Tolerance

Chris performs the exercises well and has a high *tolerance to the activities (what does this mean?)*. He complains of pain and discomfort when his knee is stretched beyond his ability, making us aware of what he can handle and how fast we can progress his rehabilitation. He is able to walk upstairs and perform daily activities with a small level of difficulty and few complaints.

Wound Description

Chris does not possess *and* open wounds and shows good progress in the appearance of his scars. The scars do not show any signs of discoloration. The main scar is about 3 inches long and 2 centimeters wide. The smaller scar is a 1-centimeter-diameter circle *(relevance?)*.

Requirements to Return to Home, School, and/or Job

Christopher needs to be taken out of gym class and school and also needs to limit the number of stairs he climbs. At home, he needs to rest as much as possible and also *perform his exercises he is given to do by himself (wordy)*.

DIAGNOSIS

In evaluating the information obtained during the examination (this phrase must modify the next word: "it"?), it can be organized and interpreted in the following way.

Treatment Diagnosis

The patient has undergone reconstructive surgery of his ACL, which has caused some movement and strength limitations. Through the process of physical therapy, Chris will be able to increase his movement and strength ability back to *it's* original status.

Reason for Skilled Care

It is necessary for Chris to attend physical therapy because he needs to be watched and guided carefully. *It is* essential for Chris's rehabilitation to be gradual because if the process occurs too fast, his injury could regress. If he is not monitored closely during his program, he could develop effusion, laxity, and joint surface irritation.

PLAN OF CARE

It is important to have early motion because it decreases effusion, pain, and inhibition. Weights should also be used early, but in small amounts *and little by little*. Isometric, concentric, and eccentric techniques are needed where the patient is most deficient in the range of motion. In the early stages, flexion-adduction and flexion-abduction diagonal patterns are used so the knee can maintain flexion from 30° or greater. Extension-adduction and external rotation with knee extension are also needed in order to decrease the stress placed on the ACL.

When Chris gets his ROM at a better standing, he will progress to strength and endurance exercises. Using the leg press and squat exercises on the Total Gym offers a wide range of help to the patient with various degrees of incline and the ability to add weight resistance. Stationary bicycling will also be used when Chris has adequate ROM.

Balancing on the injured leg can be assisted through training on a platform system. He will begin with partial body weight on his injured leg and slowly progress to full unilateral weight bearing.

Electrical stimulation will be used to provide increased input to the quadriceps and hamstrings.

As Chris's strength increases, more exercises, including toe raises, squats, step-ups, resisted gait, reciprocal lower extremity extension, treadmill walking/running, and stair climbing, will be added to his program.

Frequency/Duration

Christopher needs to attend physical therapy two or three times a week for approximately 6 months. He will be reevaluated in 6 months to see how well he has progressed *(comma)* and if he has not progressed to the right standards *(comma)* then therapy will continue.

Patient Instruction

The patient will be instructed on how to perform all the exercises assigned to him in each of his sessions. He will be encouraged to continue those exercises when he is not in the clinic *(comma)* and he will also be given some additional exercises that can be done strictly at home and do not need a therapist's supervision to perform.

Short-Term Goals

The therapists in this department are going to work with Christopher to get his ROM and strength back to *where it needs to be* to function properly in everyday activities.

Long-Term Goals

Christopher would like to be able to play football and other spots again, so as therapists, we will perform to the best of our abilities to get Chris's ROM and strength *where it needs to be* in order for him to play sports again.

Rehabilitation Potential

The patient has a high potential for a full recovery from his injury. He is anxious to get started and willing to cooperate and work to return his knee to where it started.

Glossary

Abstract A short description of the ensuing article

Active voice Creating a WHO-DID-WHAT focus of sentences; allowing the subject to act as subject

Appendices Sections of text, outside of the standard chapters, that hold large bodies of information that cannot fit logically into the flow of text; often in the forms of charts, graphs, and tables

Appositive phrase A group of words renaming the noun before it

Argument Objectively stating claims, defending positions, and refuting opposition

Asynchronous Not occurring at the same time

Audience As a group, the intended or expected readers, which controls the type of language used

Authoritative Work that represents good science and can be verified

Authoritative source material Generally accepted by the profession and published in referenced publications

Bidirectional A cause-and-effect organizational pattern in which either an event may be explained by its causes or the effects of that event on the future may be explained

Block quote Direct quotes of more than 40 words, requiring format change

Body paragraphs The paragraphs that provide support for the thesis

Bullets Typographical symbols used to indicate elements for which a specific order is not necessary

Categorical approach In comparing/contrasting, analysis of both subjects through a predetermined set of categories

Categorical argument Attempts to prove that an entity (a term, object, person, and so on) fits into the parameters of an established design or mechanism

Causal argument Reasoning based on a chain of events that explain the problem or issue in reasonable and rational terms

Circular reasoning Evidence used to support the claim is essentially the claim itself

Classical argument structure A logical sequence to argument; strategy for outlining

Classification Organizes large bodies of information into categories

Coherence Maintaining a consistent line of thinking throughout the essay to create a logical flow of ideas

Comma splice Two independent clauses incorrectly joined by punctuation

Complex sentence One or more dependent clauses added to an independent clause

Compound sentence Two or more independent clauses

Compound-complex sentence One or more dependent clauses added to two or more independent clauses

Conclusion The paragraph or paragraphs at the end of the essay that reinforce that you have proved your stated thesis

Conversational language The type of language people use when speaking, which is not appropriate for writing

Coordination Making elements of equal importance equivalent in grammatical structure

Cover letter Business letter introducing a longer, more descriptive document

Critical analysis Reading and thinking about a subject to discover errors in reasoning or presentation; also called critical reasoning

Curriculum vitae A lengthy description of qualifications usually emphasizing educational experiences relevant to job

"Cut and paste job" Relying on the words of others to produce the flow of ideas in the text

Dangling modifier An introductory phrase that fails to modify its intended antecedent

Deduction The principle has categories; if an object fits a category, it fits the principle

Definitional argument Reasoning based on an expanded definition

Delimitations Considerations in determining the merits of the results and the application of the results to other avenues of research or practice

Dependent clause A group of words that contain a subject and a verb but does not make a complete thought

Descriptive review A summary of studies or research; most often used in literature reviews

Diction Choosing the words appropriate to audience

Direct patient education literature Specific instructions written for a specific patient

Direct quote Information taken directly from a source and indicated with quotation marks

Directional process analysis Explains how to accomplish a goal, for example, a recipe of giving directions to someone who is lost

Discharge report Documentation chronicling the patient's progress to recovery or discharge from care

Discussion The meaning of the results

Division Classifies the parts of the whole

Documentation The strategies that practitioners use to chronicle their work

Drafting Reinventing the document-in-progress according to a plan or formula of the recursive writing process, as needed to restructure the thesis, reorganize the support paragraphs, and reinforce conclusions to build unity and coherence

Drafting Reinventing the text according to a plan or formula addressing specific issues of the writing process

Editing Retooling sentences to address the formalities of language and grammar for precise communication

Editorial An informed opinion solicited by a publication

Electronic communication Writing in asynchronous environments using computer technology

Essential elements Elements that a sentence requires to maintain its meaning

Evaluative review A separate publication that evaluates the science of published information

Executive summary A description of a proposed business program—the introduction

Expanded definition Redefining terms or concepts through logic

Expository writing Writing that provides information, using patterns of organization to create well-reasoned text

First person Using "I" in the subjective case and "me" in the objective

Functional grammar Grammar learned for the sake of writing, not for the sake of knowing rules

General patient population literature Documents prepared that anticipate patients' concerns and frequently asked questions

Gerund phrase A group of words beginning with a word that ends in *ing* and acting as a noun in the sentence

Grant proposal A document seeking funding for support of research

Hasty generalization   A claim made with insufficient evidence

Heading   A signpost indicating to the reader that information is compartmentalized for convenience

Implicit argument   Writing that defends a position although the language and support is objective

Independent clause   A group of words that contains a subject and a verb and makes a complete thought (a sentence)

Induction   If several show the same principle, the principle applies to all

Infinitive phrase   A group of words beginning with a root form (to + verb construction) and acting as a modifier

Informational process analysis   Explains how a process works

Informative writing   States facts through synthesizing existing information; also called expository writing

Informed consent   A method of protecting the subjects' rights by providing subjects with clear instructions and options for participation or withdrawal

Initial evaluation   The report form that outlines a practitioner's first clinical experience with a patient

Introduction   The first paragraph or paragraphs of the essay that introduce the subject matter and that house the thesis statement

Investment potential   The type of investment offered and rates of return

Journals   Publications in specific fields that are governed by editorial boards and committees that referee submissions

Limitations   Outside forces that have been placed on the study and influenced results

Literature review   Summary of researchable material that directly influences the writer's research and/or experimentation

Market   The product or service in terms of the competition

Mechanics   Marks on the text that standardize text according to manuals or rules of usage (capitalization, italics, apostrophe, hyphen)

Methods   Principles used to gather data or conduct research

Mission statement   Language stating the overall direction of the organization; also called vision statement

Narration   Chronological sequencing of events; telling the story

Narrative   The description of the events that take place between patient and practitioner; story form

Negation   Defining an object or a concept by what it is not

Nonessential elements   Elements that a sentence does not require and therefore can be set off with commas

Notes   Brief sketches of procedures completed and conversations with patients, using a shorthand form of writing employing abbreviations and basic information

Noun-based language   Focus of sentence action is on noun instead of verb; often called nominalization

Numbers   Used to indicate order

Objective description   Clear statement of facts as they occur

One-to-one correspondence   Relationship between cause and effect in which only one factor is the cause of an event or a condition, with other factors discounted as causes

Organizing   Planning the presentation of ideas through outlining

Overhead   The facilities needed to be operational and the personnel associated with operations

Parallelism   Like elements in similar grammatical constructions are coordinated in form

Paraphrase   Information used that is reinvented in the writer's own language; not a direct quote

Participial phrase A group of words beginning with a word ending in *ing*, *t*, *d*, *ed*, or *n* and acting as an adjective describing the subject of the sentence

Passive voice Allowing the object to serve as the subject of the sentence

Persuasive writing Attempts to influence the reader to choose one position over another; also called argumentative writing

Plagiarism Using the works, ideas, or words of others without providing appropriate reference or citation; allowing the reader to assume that borrowed knowledge belongs to the author

Prepositional phrase A group of words showing relationship (in, on, under, of, to, at, and so on)

Primary evidence Data, such as results of experiments, that can be verified

Primary research Gathering data and performing experiments to create conclusions

Progress report Documentation supporting patient assessments

Projected revenues Estimated growth and development in relation to capital expenditures

Pronoun agreement The pronoun and its antecedent reflect each other grammatically

Proofreading Scouring the final draft for problems in mechanics and formalities

Punctuation Marks on the text that dictate separation of elements or help clarify meaning (comma, colon, semicolon, dash)

Purpose The thesis, which controls the information provided and the order of presentation

Recursive writing process A writing process that depends on revision for a successful and effective product

Red herring Misdirecting the reader to support other causes, not the original claim

References The list of bibliographic entries used as a basis for the research

Reimbursement Payment from a third party payer

Request for proposal (RFP) A document prepared by a company or grant-offering institution advertising for a project to be completed

Request for qualifications (RFQ) A document prepared by a supporting institution that ensures that the right organization has been targeted for a project

Results The evidence that allows the author to make a claim

Resume A brief description of qualifications usually emphasizing employment experience

Review A component of the scholarly dialogue that assesses the value of published information

Revising Reading, rethinking, and making appropriate wholesale changes to the draft

Run-on sentence Two independent clauses incorrectly joined without punctuation

Scholarly dialogue The "conversation" that exists between professionals to debate pertinent issues

Scholarly research Seeks to use information to launch original thinking

Second person Using "you" in subjective and objective case

Secondary evidence Data from studies conducted by others that are used by a writer

Secondary research Using the published works of others to support claims

Sentence fragment An incomplete thought posing as a complete thought

Simple definition The dictionary definition of a word, term, or concept

Simple sentence A single independent clause

SOAP note The accepted form for note taking, with four data categories: Subjective, Objective, Assessment, Plan

Style The attribute of writing that meets professional standards and accuracy while still maintaining the reader's interest by creating continuity and flow

Subject-verb disagreement Verbs do not match nouns in number or form

Subjective description Interpretation of the facts or events

Subordination Making information less important in a sentence by reducing it to a phrase or dependent clause

Summary A short description of a text's main points or message

Summary research Seeks only to gather information from a variety of sources and synthesize

Synthesis Summaries of texts combined into a paper

Third party payer An organization that pays health care providers for services rendered

Third person Telling the story using he, she, or they or using the passive voice

Tone The choice of words that dictates objectivity or subjectivity

Topical approach In comparing/contrasting, discussion of one subject first in its entirety and then another subject in its entirety

Transitions Sentences, phrases, or words that connect two related sentences or paragraphs to continue a line of thought

Unity Focusing all of the elements of the essay on a singular purpose, the thesis

Verb tense shift Unnecessarily changing verb tense within a sentence or paragraph

Verb-based language Focus of sentence action is on verb, not nouns

Word choice Choosing the exact word for precise meaning

Index